Cancer Chemotherapy
Pocket Guide

Cancer Chemotherapy Pocket Guide

Robert J. Ignoffo, Pharm.D.
Clinical Professor of Pharmacy and Oncology

Carol S. Viele, R.N.
Oncology Nurse Specialist
Associate Clinical Professor of Nursing

Lloyd E. Damon, M.D.
Associate Clinical Professor of Medicine

Alan Venook, M.D.
Associate Professor of Clinical Oncology
and Medicine

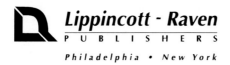

Lippincott - Raven
P U B L I S H E R S

Philadelphia • New York

Manufacturing Manager: Dennis Teston
Production Manager: Lawrence Bernstein
Production Editor: Lawrence Bernstein
Cover Designer: Karen K. Quigley
Indexer: Leon Kremzner
Compositor: Maryland Composition
Printer: Phoenix Offset

Printed and bound in China.

9 8 7 6 5 4 3 2 1

Library of Congress Cataloging-in-Publication Data

Cancer chemotherapy pocket guide / Robert J. Ignoffo . . . [et al.].
     p.   cm.
   Includes index.
   ISBN 0-397-51521-9
   1. Antineoplastic agents—Handbooks, manuals, etc.   2. Cancer–
Chemotherapy—Handbooks, manuals, etc.   I. Ignoffo, Robert J.,
1944–   .
   [DNLM: 1. Neoplasms—drug therapy—handbooks.   2. Antineoplastic
Agents—therapeutic use—handbooks.   QZ 39 C2149 1997]
RC271.C5C322192   1997
616.99′4061—dc21
DNLM/DLC
for Library of Congress

Every effort has been made to ensure the accuracy of the chemotherapy indications, drug doses and schedules, and combination drug regimens contained in this book. The editors recommend that the reader refer to the package insert information published by the manufacturer for specific drug information, and also refer to the listed literature references for details about combination chemotherapy protocols.

The authors, editors, and publisher have exerted every effort to ensure that drug selection and dosage set forth in this text are in accordance with current recommendations and practice at the time of publication. However, in view of ongoing research, changes in government regulations, and the constant flow of information relating to drug therapy and drug reactions, the reader is urged to check the package insert for each drug for any change in indications and dosage and for added warnings and precautions. This is particularly important when the recommended agent is a new or infrequently employed drug.

Some drugs and medical devices presented in this publication have Food and Drug Administration (FDA) clearance for limited use in restricted research settings. It is the responsibility of the health care provider to ascertain the FDA status of each drug or device planned for use in their clinical practice.

CONTENTS

IV. Chemotherapy Regimens in Pediatric Tumors

Bruce Shiramizu and Ken DeSantes

Pediatric Malignancies

Ewing's Sarcoma and Primitive Neuroectodermal Tumor (PNET)

CONTRIBUTORS

Betsy Althaus, Pharm.D.
Assistant Clinical Professor
Department of Clinical Pharmacy
University of California, San Francisco
521 Parnassus Avenue
San Francisco, CA 94143

Lloyd E. Damon, M.D.
Associate Professor of Medicine
Division of Oncology
University of California, San Francisco
521 Parnassus Avenue
San Francisco, CA 94143

Ken DeSantes, M.D.
Assistant Professor of Pediatrics
Pediatric Bone Marrow Transplantation Department
University of California, San Francisco
505 Parnassus Avenue, Room R679
San Francisco, CA 94143

Elaine Harney, Pharm.D.
At the time of preparation
Assistant Clinical Professor
Department of Clinical Pharmacy
University of California, San Francisco
521 Parnassus Avenue
San Francisco, CA 94143

Robert J. Ignoffo, Pharm.D.
Clinical Professor of Pharmacy and Oncology
Department of Clinical Pharmacy
University of California, San Francisco
521 Parnassus Avenue
San Francisco, CA 94143

Reginald S. King, Pharm.D.
Clinical Specialist, Oncology/BMT
Department of Pharmacy
Allegheny University Hospital/Hahnemann
MS 451, Broad and Vine Streets
Philadelphia, PA 19102

Donald W. Northfelt, M.D., F.A.C.P.
Assistant Clinical Professor
Department of Medicine
University of California, San Diego
Pacific Oaks Medical Group
1401 North Palm Canyon, Suite 100
Palm Springs, CA, 92262

Robert L. Robles, M.D.
Clinical Instructor
Department of Medicine
San Francisco General Hospital
Ward 84, 1001 Potrero Avenue
San Francisco, CA 94110

Hope S. Rugo, M.D.
Assistant Clinical Professor of Medicine
Division of Oncology
University of California, San Francisco
521 Parnassus Avenue
San Francisco, CA 94143

Bruce Shiramizu, M.D.
Associate Professor of Pediatrics
Department of Pediatrics
University of California, San Francisco
521 Parnassus Avenue
San Francisco, CA 94143

Alan Venook, M.D.
Associate Professor of Medicine
Division of Oncology
University of California, San Francisco
521 Parnassus Avenue
San Francisco, CA 94143

Carol S. Viele, R.N., M.S.
Assistant Clinical Professor
Department of Physiological Nursing
Clinical Nurse Specialist
Hematology/Oncology, Bone Marrow Transplant
University of California, San Francisco
School of Nursing
521 Parnassus Avenue
San Francisco, CA 94143

BODY-SURFACE AREA OF CHILDREN

NOMOGRAM FOR DETERMINATION OF BODY-SURFACE AREA FROM HEIGHT AND WEIGHT

Height	Body surface area	Weight

Height
cm 120 — 47 in
115 — 46
— 45
110 — 44
— 43
105 — 42
— 41
100 — 40
— 39
95 — 38
— 37
90 — 36
— 35
85 — 34
— 33
80 — 32
— 31
75 — 30
— 29
70 — 28
— 27
65 — 26
— 25
60 — 24
— 23
55 — 22
— 21
50 — 20
— 19
45 — 18
— 17
40 — 16
— 15
35 — 14
— 13
30 — 12
— 11
cm 25 — 10 in

Body surface area
1.10 m²
1.05
1.00
0.95
0.90
0.85
0.80
0.75
0.70
0.65
0.60
0.55
0.50
0.45
0.40
0.35
0.30
0.25
0.20
0.19
0.18
0.17
0.16
0.15
0.14
0.13
0.12
0.11
0.10
0.09
0.08
0.074 m²

Weight
kg 40.0 — 90 lb
— 85
35.0 — 80
— 75
30.0 — 70
— 65
— 60
25.0 — 55
— 50
20.0 — 45
— 40
15.0 — 35
— 30
10.0 — 25
9.0 — 20
8.0
7.0 — 15
6.0
5.0
4.5 — 10
4.0 — 9
3.5 — 8
3.0 — 7
— 6
2.5 — 5
2.0 — 4
1.5 — 3
kg 1.0 — 2.2 lb

From the formula of Du Bors and Du Bors, *Arch. intern. Med.*, 17, 863 (1916): $S = W^{0.425} \times H^{0.725} \times 71.84$, or $\log S = \log W \times 0.425 + \log H \times 0.725 + 1.8564$ (S = body surface in cm², W = weight in kg, H = height in cm). Reprinted from *Scientific Tables*, 7th edition, Ciba Geigy, 1971, pg. 537. Used with permission.

PREFACE

This pocket guide was developed by a multidisciplinary team of editors and is intended for all practitioners involved in the care of the cancer patient, including oncologists, nurses, pharmacists, fellows, and students. It is designed as a quick source of information on chemotherapeutic agents, commonly used or standard chemotherapy regimens, management of commonly encountered chemotherapy toxicities, and other information (i.e. formulas and conversions). Although it is not meant to be a comprehensive reference, it may be used as an aid in therapeutic decision-making for both adult and pediatric patients.

The authors and contributors have presented the material in a concise manner and have tabulated much of the information for easy access by the user. This publication covers all of the commercially available anticancer drugs, along with ancillary agents used in the treatment of cancer patients. In addition, some investigational agents are included that the authors believe to be important new therapies or which are soon expected to be approved for commercial use. The information for each drug monograph was generated from the primary literature as well as from several authoritative sources, such as *AHFS Drug Information* 1994 and 1995, American Society of Health-systems Pharmacists; *Facts and Comparisons,* Wolters and Kluwer 1995; *Cancer: Principles and Practice of Oncology, 4th edition,* Lippincott 1993 (DeVita, Hellman, and Rosenberg); *Cancer Chemotherapy Handbook, 2nd edition,* Elsevier 1993 (Dorr and Von Hoff), *The Cancer Chemotherapy Handbook, 4th edition,* Mosby 1993 (Fischer, Knopf, and Durivage), and *Handbook on Injectable Drugs, 8th edition,* American Society of Health-System Pharmacists, 1995.

Selected chemotherapy regimens were chosen on the basis of what is considered the standard of practice and from information published in the oncology literature. We have also included preparative regimens for bone marrow transplantation, and high-dose chemotherapy regimens requiring hematopoietic stem-cell rescue. For many cancers, there may be more than one chemotherapy regimen that is considered "standard." In such instances, the editors have chosen commonly used regimens and have provided commentary about the

application of these regimens. Older regimens that have been sup-
planted by newer, more effective regimens have not been included.

Robert J. Ignoffo, Pharm.D.
Carol S. Viele, R.N.
Lloyd E. Damon, M.D.
Alan Venook, M.D.

ACKNOWLEDGMENTS

We wish to thank several of our colleagues who have given advice and support for the development of this book. We also would like to thank Lippincott-Raven for giving us the opportunity to publish this work. The efforts of our editorial department, especially Amy Barach and Wendy Miller, are greatly appreciated. We appreciate the assistance of Eileen Jackson in the development of the graphics used in this book.

BODY-SURFACE AREA OF ADULTS

NOMOGRAM FOR DETERMINATION OF BODY-SURFACE AREA FROM HEIGHT AND WEIGHT

Height	Body surface area	Weight

From the formula of Du Bors and Du Bors, *Arch. intern. Med.*, 17, 863 (1916): $S = W^{0.425} \times H^{0.725} \times 71.84$, or $\log S = \log W \times 0.425 + \log H \times 0.725 + 1.8564$ (S = body surface in cm^2, W = weight in kg, H = height in cm). Reprinted from *Scientific Tables*, 7th edition, Ciba Geigy, pg. 538. Used with permission.

CHAPTER I

Cancer Chemotherapy Drugs and Guidelines for Prescribing of Cytotoxic Drugs

Robert J. Ignoffo

Carol S. Viele

Recent drug misadventures have resulted in efforts to assure the safe administration of cytotoxic drugs. The following guidelines have been adopted by our institution and are based on recent literature and those from other institutions.

All orders should contain the following information or be written as follows:

1. The patient's name, height, weight, and BSA (if applicable), so that the nurse or pharmacist can double-check the dosage calculation.

2. While common abbreviations are well known for many of the drugs, it is recommended that complete names be used when writing orders for chemotherapy drugs.

3. The total daily dose, written as "X mg/kg or mg/m^2 = Y mg on day 1" for single-day regimens. Indicate the duration of infusion if an IV infusion (i.e., 1 hour, 4 hours, etc.). Multi-day regimens should be written as "X mg/kg or mg/m^2 = Y mg daily for Z days."

4. Do not write a zero after a whole number (e.g., 2.0 mg). Leave off the decimal and zero (e.g., 2 mg). Decimal points are easily obliterated by the lines on order sheets, which can lead to serious errors in dosage.

5. Continuous infusions of vesicant drugs should only be given via a central line.

6. A co-signature by an attending physician is required for all transplant protocol orders.

7. A co-signature by the oncologist will be required within 24 hours if orders are faxed. Faxed orders **must** be written on an accepted institutional order form.

8. Write the method of drug administration as either "IV push" or "IV infusion".

9. The solution and volume may be specified for IV infusions of chemotherapeutic drugs. If not specified, the solution and volume will be determined by the pharmacist, based on the appropriate guideline.

10. Whenever possible, order practical doses of chemotherapeutic drugs. Pharmacy will confer with you on the rounding of certain drugs to their most practical doses as long as these do not vary by more than 5% of the original dose. The exceptions are vincristine, for which exact dosing is required, and vinblastine, mitoxantrone, and idarubicin, which should be rounded to the nearest **mg.**

11. Leave a space between the number and its unit value, e.g., 100 mg, not 100mg.

12. Changes in chemotherapy must be written by the fellow or attending physician (verbal orders to nurses or housestaff are not acceptable).

13. Orders should not contain Latin abbreviations. Specifically, do not use "qd," "bid" or, "qid." Use the term "daily" instead of "qd", q12h instead of "bid," etc.

14. Order antiemetics, hydration, and other supportive care on the same order form as used for chemotherapeutic drugs.

ANTICANCER DRUG MONOGRAPHS

Each drug monograph contains information on the *indications, mechanism of action, pharmacology/pharmacokinetics, drug interactions, dose, dosage forms, administration, compatibilities/incompatibilities, adverse reactions, practitioner interventions, and selected references.* This information was obtained from the primary literature and authoritative references including *AHFS Drug Information* 1996 and 1997, *Facts and Comparisons* 1997, *Cancer: Principles and Practice of Oncology 4th and 5th editions*, Lippincott 1993 and 1997 (DeVita, Hellman, and Rosenberg), *Cancer Chemotherapy Handbook 2nd edition* Elsevier, 1993 (RT Dorr and D Von Hoff), *The Cancer Chemo-*

therapy Handbook, 4th edition, Mosby 1993 (Fischer, Knopf, and Durivage), and *Handbook on Injectable Drugs, 9th edition,* American Society of Health-system Pharmacists, 1996.

Common abbreviations that will be used in the following monographs will include:

Abbreviation	Meaning
$/m^2$	Per meter squared (body surface area)
BSA	Body surface area
CNS	Central nervous system
D5W	5% dextrose and water
IM	Intramuscular
IP	Intraperitoneal
Ipl	Intrapleural
IT	Intrathecal
IU	International units
IV	Intravenous
LR	Lactated Ringer's (solution)
mg/kg	Milligram per kilogram
NS	Normal saline or 0.9% NaCl
PO	Oral
SC	Subcutaneous
Vd	Volume of distribution
$T_{1/2}\alpha$	Initial distribution half-life
$T_{1/2}\beta$	Second or terminal-phase half-life
$T_{1/2}\delta$	Terminal-phase half-life
Vd_{ss}	Volume of distribution at steady state

In the adverse drug reaction section, we have put each reaction in order of its dose-limiting toxicity or severity.

ALDESLEUKIN

Other Names:
Proleukin®, Interleukin-2, IL-2, T-cell growth factor.

Uses:
Aldesleukin is FDA-approved for use in renal-cell cancer. It also has minor activity in malignant melanoma.

Mechanism of Antitumor Action:

Interleukin-2 is an endogenous glycoprotein that is formed and released during helper T-cell activation. It mediates and is able to generate lymphokine activated killer (LAK) cells and tumor-infiltrating lymphocytes (TILs), which have antitumor properties.

Pharmacokinetics:

Absorption: Interleukin-2 is given only parenterally. After intramuscular administration, only 30% of IL-2 activity is evident systemically. After subcutaneous administration, peak levels are achieved in about 5 hours.

Distribution: The volume of distribution ranges from 7.5 to 13.3 L.

Protein Binding: Not bound to plasma proteins.

Metabolism: IL-2 is not metabolized to any significant extent by the liver. The drug is catabolized by the renal tubule to unknown breakdown products.

Half-life: Biphasic elimination occurs. The $T_{1/2}\alpha$ is rapid, ranging from 5 to 12 minutes, while the $T_{1/2}\beta$ ranges from 45 to 85 minutes.

Elimination: The drug is renally cleared, involving catabolism in the renal tubules.

Drug Interactions:

Glucocorticoids block IL-2 antitumor efficacy.

Nonsteroidal anti-inflammatory drugs lessen the clinical toxicity of IL-2, but may also worsen renal function. Indomethacin may enhance capillary leak syndrome.

Anthracyclines-treated arrhythmias may be exacerbated by IL-2.

Interferon-alfa combined with IL-2 may produce an enhanced antitumor response.

Dosage:

Renal-cell carcinoma: 600,000 IU/kg per dose as a 15 minute IV infusion every 8 hours, for 14 doses.

Dose Forms:
Proleukin® is available in a single use vial of lyophylized powder containing 22 million IU. When reconstituted with 1.2 mL of sterile water for injection, each mL contains 18 million IU (1.1 mg).

Administration:
The current FDA-approved form of IL-2 is for IV use only, but many clinicians deliver this drug both subcutaneously and intramuscularly.

Compatibilities: In simulated 1:1 mixtures, Y-site injection of IL-2 (Roche; 4,800 IU/mL in D5W) is compatible with amikacin sulfate, fat emulsions, gentamicin sulfate, morphine sulfate, piperacillin sodium, ticarcillin, tobramycin sulfate, and TPN solutions in a concentration of 4,800 IU/mL.

Drug delivery of aldesleukin in polyvinyl chloride (PVC; plastic) containers is more consistent and complete than in glass containers.

The preferred diluent for IV infusions of aldesleukin is D5W. NS or bacteriostatic water increases the aggregation of IL-2 and should not be used.

Incompatibilities: Aldesleukin should not be frozen or agitated excessively. In-line filters should not be used during the administration of aldesleukin.

Adverse Reactions:

 Capillary Leak: Hypotension during infusion, interstitial pulmonary edema, decreased peripheral vascular resistance, and weight gain.

 ***Pulmonary:*** Dyspnea, respiratory distress, pulmonary edema, and pleural effusion may occur (7 to 25% of patients) 2 days after starting IL-2.

 Renal: All patients develop an elevated serum creatinine level, which may reach as high as 8 mg/dL and oliguria beginning 48 hours after starting IL-2. This effect is completely reversible within 3 to 5 days after discontinuing IL-2. Dialysis is rarely required.

 Cardiac: Atrial arrhythmias and reflex tachycardia (common).

Dermatologic: Purpuric skin rashes, urticaria, facial swelling, and distal erythema may occur within 3 days after starting treatment.

 Hepatic: Hyperbilirubinemia is common but returns to baseline in about 5 days after stopping IL-2.

 CNS: Somnolence, delirium, and confusion are especially troublesome in elderly patients.

 Hematologic: IL-2 may cause bone-marrow suppression manifested by anemia, thrombocytopenia (13%), and neutropenia <500/mL (~5%).

Practitioner Interventions:

1. If delivering FDA-approved dose (600,000 IU/kg), the patient's vital signs must be monitored closely.
2. Premedicate patient prior to each dose with diphenhydramine, acetaminophen, and indomethacin. Avoid corticosteroids.
3. Give antiemetics 30 minutes before each dose.
4. Monitor stool output and perform guaiac test on all stools. Administer antidiarrheal agents as necessary.
5. Monitor O_2 saturation to keep above 90%.
6. Vital signs before each dose and every 30 minutes for 2 hours after an IV dose.
7. Strict input and output; weigh patient twice daily.
8. Monitor for ectopy or arrhythmias.
9. Laboratory work as ordered, monitor patient's complete blood cell count (CBC), platelet count, electrolytes, BUN, creatinine.
10. Monitor patient for restlessness, nightmares, somnolence.
11. Discontinue therapy for grade IV cardiovascular, renal, hepatic, gastrointestinal, or psychologic toxicity.

References:

1. Konrad MW, Hemstreet G, Hersh EM, et al. Pharmacokinetics of recombinant interleukin-2 in humans. Cancer Res 1990;50:2009–2017.
2. Kozeny GA, Nicolas JD, Creekmore S, et al. Effects of IL-2 immunotherapy on renal function. J Clin Oncol 1988;6:1170–1176.
3. Margolin KA, Raynor AA, Hawkins MJ, et al. Interleukin-2 and lymphocyte-activated killer cell therapy of solid tumors: Analysis of toxicity and management guidelines. J Clin Oncol 1989;7:486–498.

4. Parkinson DR. Interleukin-2 in cancer therapy. Semin Oncol 1988;15 (Suppl 6):10–26.
5. Thompson JA, Lee DV, Cox WW, et al. Recombinant interleukin-2 toxicity, pharmacokinetics, and immunomodulatory effects in a phase I trial. Cancer Res 1987;47:4202–4207.

ALTRETAMINE

Other Names:
Hexalen®, hexamethylmelamine, HMM.

Uses:
Ovarian carcinoma, lymphoma, lung cancer.

Mechanism of Antitumor Action:
Its exact mechanism is unknown, but altretamine probably acts like a DNA alkylating agent.

Pharmacokinetics:

Absorption: Oral absorption of altretamine is highly variable and peaks from 1 to 4 hours after dosing.

Distribution: Altretamine has a large Vd, indicating extensive intracellular binding.

Protein Binding: More than 90% bound to plasma protein.

Metabolism: Extensive first-pass metabolism in liver by hepatic microsomal enzyme system, yielding eight or more metabolites.

Half-life: Terminal $T_{1/2}$ = 4 to 10 hours (average 6.9 hours).

Elimination: About 60% of a dose is excreted in urine as demethylated metabolites.

Drug Interactions:

Cimetidine may increase the half-life and toxicity of altretamine.

Ranitidine does not affect altretamine catabolism.

Phenobarbital may decrease half-life and toxicity of altretamine. Monoamine oxidase inhibitors plus concurrent altretramine may cause severe hypotension.

Dosage:
The usual dose of altretamine is 260 mg/m^2/day given in four divided doses after meals and at bedtime for 14 to 21 days in a 28 day cycle.

Dose Forms:
Hexalin® is available in 50 mg capsules.

Administration:
Hexalen® is given orally in four divided doses daily, after meals and at bedtime, usually for 21 days. This cycle is repeated every 6 weeks.

Adverse Reactions:

Hematologic: Myelosuppression—neutropenia, thrombocytopenia, with minimum counts at 21 days. Recovery occurs by day 28.

Nausea and vomiting: Common, and may be severe at doses > 12 mg/kg/day.

Neurologic: Manifested as somnolence, lethargy, mood changes, paresthesias, and ataxia after prolonged therapy. This effect is reversible on discontinuation of treatment.

Gastrointestinal: Anorexia, abdominal cramps, and diarrhea occur occasionally.

Practitioner Interventions:
1. Use gloves to protect against handling altretamine.
2. Give altretamine 2 hours after meals and at bedtime.
3. Monitor nausea and vomiting, and give mild antiemetic if needed.
4. Assess patient for signs of neurologic toxicity.
5. Vitamin B$_6$ may be administered concurrently to decrease neurologic complications.

References:
1. Hahn DA. Hexamethylmelamine and pentamethylmelamine: An update. Drug Intell Clin Pharm 1983;17:418–424.

2. Hande K, Combs G, Swingle R, et al. Effect of cimetidine and ranitidine on the metabolism and toxicity of hexamethylmelamine. Cancer Treat Rep 1986;70:1443.

AMIFOSTINE

Other Names:
Ethyol®, WR2721.

Uses:
Ethyol® is indicated to reduce the cumulative renal toxicity associated with repeated administration of cisplatin in patients with advanced ovarian cancer. It may also protect against cisplatin myelosuppression and neurologic toxicity, and against other cytotoxic chemotherapy.

Mechanism of Antitumor Action:
Amifostine is a prodrug, which after dephosphorylation by membrane alkaline phosphatase to an active metabolite (WR1065), protects normal cells from the effects of free radicals produced by alkylating agents or radiation therapy, and also binds directly to alkylating metabolites. It is preferentially taken up by normal cells because of a higher pH as well as a higher concentration of alkaline phosphatase as compared with tumor cells, resulting in a higher free thiol content within the cell. A higher concentration of free thiol will bind, and therefore detoxify, reactive metabolites and act as a scavenger of free radicals.

Pharmacokinetics:

Absorption: Amifostine is not active orally. It is given by the intravenous route.

Distribution: Unmetabolized amifostine has a small Vd (about 7 to 8 L), indicating that the drug is largely confined to the intravascular space. The distribution phase of amifostine is very rapid (0.88 minute), and is consistent with its rapid conversion in plasma. Less than 10% of the drug is present in plasma 6 minutes after administration. Maximum concentration of WR1065 is achieved about 15 minutes after administration. The drug distributes into a variety of tissues including kidney, liver, salivary gland, intestinal mucosa, lung, and other tissues, but very little distributes into brain or skeletal muscle.

Protein Binding: Low.

Metabolism: At doses of 740 to 910 mg/m^2 plasma amifostine is rapidly metabolized to its active metabolic WR1065.

Half-life: More than 90% of amifostine is cleared from the plasma in 10 minutes.

Elimination: Membrane alkaline phosphatase rapidly converts amifostine to active and inactive metabolites. Only 1 to 2% of the parent drug is eliminated by the kidneys. Similarly, 1 to 4% of amifostine metabolites are excreted in the urine.

Drug Interactions:
Amifostine decreases the renal clearance of **carboplatin** and increases the area-under-the-curve of total platinum, carboplatinum, and ultrafilterable platinum by 20 to 25%. This results in an increase of 64% in the carboplatin half-life.

Dosage:
The FDA approved dose is 910 mg/m^2 IV once daily over a period of 15 minutes, 30 minutes prior to chemotherapy. However, a dose of 740 mg/m^2 once daily is equally effective and better tolerated.

Dose Forms:
Ethyol® is available in 10 mL vials of 500 mg of amifostine plus 500 mg of mannitol.

Administration:
Amifostine is administered in 50 mL of NS by slow IV infusion over a period of 10 to 15 minutes with monitoring of blood pressure. Patients should be adequately hydrated prior to administration. If diastolic pressure falls significantly, the infusion should be discontinued until the blood pressure returns to baseline, and should then be completed by 15 minutes. Do not extend the infusion beyond 15 minutes rate.

Compatibilities: Ethyol® is stable in PVC bags for 5 hours at room temperature, and for 24 hours when refrigerated at 2 to 8°C.

Incompatibilities: The compatibility of Ethyol® in solutions other than NS is unknown at this time.

Adverse Reactions:

 Nausea and vomiting: Common. Antiemetics should be given prior to amifostine.

 Hypotension: occurs in about one-fourth of patients treated with usual doses of amifostine, but is usually asymptomatic.

 Somnolence: dose related and occurs more frequently in women than in men.

 Sneezing and hypersensitivity-like symptoms: reported during infusions of amifostine. Other, less common adverse effects of amifostine include a metallic taste, flushing, fever, rash, chills, hypocalcemia, and hiccups.

Practitioner Interventions:

1. Adequate prehydration with 500–1000 mL of NS prior to amifostine.
2. Amifostine is a moderate to severe emetogen. The antiemetics prescribed for emetogenic chemotherapy should be given prior to amifostine. Recommended antiemetics include a serotonin antagonist, diphenhydramine, H_2 antagonist, and dexamethasone.
3. Infuse amifostine in NS over a period of 15 minutes.
4. Monitor systolic and diastolic blood pressure every 5 minutes during infusion and 10 minutes after infusion.

Guideline for Interrupting Amifostine (Ethyol®) Infusion

Baseline systolic blood pressure (mmHg)	<100	100-119	120–139	140–179	≥180
Reduction in systolic blood pressure during infusion (mmHg)	20	25	30	40	50

References:

1. Ethyol® Package Product Information. Alza Pharmaceuticals, March 1996.
2. Kemp G, Rose P, Lurain J, et al. Amifostine pretreatment for protection against cyclophosphamide and cisplatin-induced toxicities: Results of a randomized controlled trial in patients with advanced ovarian cancer. J Clin Oncol 1996;14:2101–2110.

3. Ignoffo, RJ. Chemoprotectants in Oncology. Cancer Pract 1994;2:157–159.
4. Schucter LM, Glick JH. The current status of WR 2721 (amifostine): A chemotherapy and radiation therapy protector. Biologic therapy of Cancer Updates vol 3. 1–10.
5. Spencer CM, Goa KL. Amifostine: A review of its pharmacodynamic and pharmacokinetic properties, and therapeutic potential as radioprotector and cytotoxic chemoprotector. Drugs 1995;50:1001–1031.

AMINOGLUTETHIMIDE

Other Names:
Cytadren®.

Uses:
Breast cancer.

Mechanism of Antitumor Action:
Aminoglutethimide is a nonsteroidal inhibitor of corticosteroid biosynthesis. It produces a chemical adrenalectomy, thereby decreasing the formation of endogenous estrogen, androgen, and cortisol.

Pharmacokinetics:

Absorption: Aminoglutethimide is well absorbed when given orally. Peak plasma concentrations occur within 0.7 to 1.5 hours.

Distribution: Aminoglutethimide is concentrated about 1.4 to 1.7 times more in cells than in plasma.

Protein Binding: 20 to 25%.

Metabolism: Aminoglutethimide is metabolized by the liver to N-acetyl aminoglutethimide (NAG). The parent drug induces its own metabolism.

Half-life: The initial half-life of aminoglutethimide is 13.3 hours, but decreases to 7 to 9 hours after chronic dosing. NAG has a half-life of 7 to 10 hours.

Elimination: Dose-dependent renal elimination, with about 50% of a 500-mg dose excreted after administration, compared to 40% for a 250-mg dose.

Drug Interactions:
Aminoglutethimide interferes with levels and enhances clearance of ***warfarin, antipyrine, theophylline***, and ***digitoxin***. Aminoglutethimide also enhances the metabolism of ***dexamethasone***, but not of hydrocortisone.

Dosage:
The usual dose of aminoglutethimide is 250 mg PO given twice daily × 2 weeks, followed by 250 mg PO four times daily. Concurrent oral hydrocortisone is given at a dose of 20 mg in the morning, 20 mg at 2 pm, and 60 mg at bedtime for 2 weeks, followed by 40 mg in three divided doses (10 mg in the morning, 10 mg at 2 pm, and 20 mg at bedtime).

Dose Forms:
Cytadren® is available in 250 mg tablets.

Administration:
The daily dose of aminoglutethimide is given in two to three divided doses.

Adverse Reactions:
About 50% of patients experience side effects of aminoglutethimide.

Dermatologic: A maculopapular rash is frequently seen during the first 2 weeks of therapy. It is usually self-limiting and abates in about a week. If the rash persists after 1 week, the drug should be discontinued. Increasing the dose of hydrocortisone to 50 mg twice daily may help control acute dermatologic reactions.

Neurologic: Another common adverse effect of aminoglutethimide is lethargy, which often occurs in the first week of therapy. This problem can be very severe in some patients, and necessitates discontinuing the drug. Lethargy may take about a month to resolve. Dizziness, nystagmus, and ataxia are less common.

Endocrine: Hypothyroidism has been reported after several weeks of therapy. Thyroid function should be monitored periodically.

Hematologic: Pancytopenia, leukopenia, and thrombocytopenia have been reported in less than 1% of patients, but have resulted in mortality. The mechanism of this reaction is unknown.

Other: Nausea, vomiting, and anorexia are uncommon and mild. Adrenal insufficiency is uncommon but is manifested by postural hypotension and hyponatremia. This problem is prevented with the use of concurrent hydrocortisone therapy.

Practitioner Interventions:

1. Monitor patient for any signs of hypothyroidism, i.e., postural hypotension and hyponatremia. Limit free water intake.
2. Observe patient for skin reactions—rash is usually observed in the first week of therapy and disappears after 5 to 8 days.
3. Observe patient for signs of somnolence, dizziness, blurring of vision, and fatigue.
4. Administer antiemetics as needed.

References:

1. Barton-Burke M, Wilkes G, Engeversen K. Chemotherapy Care Plans, Designs For Nursing Care. Jones & Bartlett, Boston, 1993, pp. 93–96.
2. Cocconi G, Basaghi G, Ceci G, et al. Low dose aminoglutethimide with and without hydrocortisone replacement as first-line endocrine treatment in advanced breast cancer: a prospective, randomized trial of the Italian Oncology Group for Clinical Research. J Clin Oncol 1992;10: 984–989.
3. Santen RJ, Worgul TJ, Samojlik E, et al. A randomized trial comparing surgical adrenalectomy plus hydrocortisone in women with advanced breast cancer. N Engl J Med 1981;305:545–551.

ANASTROZOLE

Other Names:
Arimidex®.

Uses:
Anastrozole is used for advanced breast cancer in postmenopausal women who have disease progression following tamoxifen therapy.

Mechanism of Antitumor Action:
Anastrozole is a potent and selective nonsteroidal aromatase inhibitor.

Pharmacokinetics:

Absorption: After oral administration of tablets or solutions, anastrozole is rapidly absorbed within 2 hours. Food does not affect its absorption.

Distribution: Anastrozole is widely distributed throughout the body.

Protein Binding: Unknown

Metabolism: Mostly hepatic (85%), to metabolites that are inactive. N-dealkylation breaks the two rings and results in free triazole. Hydroxylation also occurs, producing metabolites that are glucuronidated and excreted in the urine.

Half-life: The half-life of anastrozole in postmenopausal women is about 50 hours, and does not appear to change with age.

Elimination: Renal elimination of the parent compound accounts for about 11% of the dose. Most of the drug is eliminated as glucuronide metabolites in the urine.

Drug Interactions:

Anastrozole in very high doses inhibits cytochrome P450 1A2, 2C8/9, and 3A4. The drug does not affect cytochrome P450 2A6 or 2D6 *in vitro*. Thus, it is unlikely that 1 mg doses of anastrozole will result in clinically significant inhibition of cytochrome P450 enzyme activity or of the metabolism of drugs affected by this enzyme, such as **coumarin, warfarin, dextromethorphan, nifedipine, tolbutamide,** or **phenacetin.** Doses of cimetidine up to 1,200 mg daily do not affect the metabolism of anastrozole.

Dosage:

The usual initial oral dose of anastrozole in adults is 1 mg PO daily. In patients with moderate to severe liver dysfunction, plasma concentrations of anastrozole may increase by less than 30%, and this probably does not necessitate dose reduction, but patients should be monitored for increasing side effects. The metabolism and clearance of anastrozole have not been studied in patients with severe liver dysfunction.

In patients with renal failure, the dose of anastrozole need not be altered, because only 10% of the dose is cleared by the kidney.

Dose Forms:
Arimidex® is available in 1 mg tablets.

Administration:
Anastrozole may be given orally at any time during the day without regard to food intake.

Adverse Reactions:
Anastrozole is generally well tolerated.

Cardiovascular: Hot flushes occur in about 12% of patients receiving anastrozole. Edema occurs in about 7% of patients. Thromboembolic disease has been reported in about 3% of patients. Weight gain has occurred in about 1% of patients.

Dermatologic: A dry, scaling rash occurs in about 5% of patients.

Gastrointestinal: Nausea and vomiting are uncommon and mild. Mucositis and stomatitis are commonly seen with large doses. Anorexia may also occur.

Practitioner Interventions:

1. Monitor patient for any signs and symptoms of gastrointestinal effects.
2. Monitor patient's bilirubin/liver function tests every 3 months.
3. Instruct patient about the possibility of hot flushes.

References:

1. Arimidex® Product Information. Zeneca Pharmaceuticals, January 1996.
2. Jonat W, Howell A, Blomqvist C, et al. A randomized trial comparing two doses of the new selective aromatase inhibitor anastrozole (Arimidex®) with megestrol acetate in postmenopausal patients with advanced breast cancer. Eur J Cancer 1996;32A:404–412.
3. Plourde PV, Dyroff M, Dowsett M, et al. Arimidex: a new oral, once-a-day aromatase inhibitor. J Steroid Biochem Mol Biol 1995;53:175–179.
4. Budzar A, Jonat W, Howell A, et al. Anastrozole (Arimidex®), a potent and selective aromatase inhibitor, versus megestrol acetate in postmenopausal women with advanced breast cancer: results of an overview analysis of two phase III trials. J Clin Oncol 1996;2000–2011.

ASPARAGINASE

Other Names:
Elspar®, L-asparaginase.

Uses:
The FDA-approved indication for asparaginase is in the treatment of acute lymphocytic leukemia (ALL). It is usually used together with daunorubicin, vincristine, and prednisone.

Mechanism of Antitumor Action:
Asparaginase is an enzyme that acts indirectly to inhibit protein synthesis in tumor cells that are dependent on asparagine, which is a nonessential amino acid in humans.

Pharmacokinetics:

Absorption: After intravenous administration, asparaginase remains in the vascular compartment. After intramuscular injection, peak plasma concentrations are half of those achieved after IV administration.

Distribution: Very little asparaginase distributes outside of the vascular compartment.

Protein Binding: Unknown

Metabolism: Unclear. Asparaginase has minimal urinary and biliary excretion.

Half-life: The elimination half-life of asparaginase ranges from 8 to 30 hours.

Elimination: Asparaginase is slowly cleared from plasma. Only a small amount is cleared renally.

Drug Interactions:

Cytarabine when used concomitantly with asparaginase, has antitumor synergism.

Vincristine neurotoxicity may be enhanced when used with asparaginase.

Prednisone enhances hyperglycemia; asparaginase transiently inhibits insulin synthesis.

Dosage:

Test Dose: An initial 2 IU intradermal dose of asparaginase should be given prior to each cycle of asparaginase.

Pediatric ALL: In combination with vincristine and prednisone, asparaginase may be used in a dose of 1000 IU/kg/day for 10 days or 6000 IU/m^2 every 3 days starting on day 4 and going through day 28.

Adult ALL: A commonly used regimen is 6,000 to 10,000 IU given IM in 12 injections. The injections are given every 1 to 3 days starting on day 17. Another regimen is 20,000 IU/m^2 IM/SC three times weekly.

Dose Forms
Elspar® is provided as 10,000 IU in lyophilized powder in 10 mL vials.

Administration:
The recommended route of administration of asparaginase is intravenous or intramuscular, but several institutions have also given the drug subcutaneously. An intravenous solution in 50 to 100 mL of NS or D5W may be given over a period of 15 to 30 minutes. Avoid vigorous agitation during preparation and administration.

Compatibilities: D5W and NS.

Incompatibilities: None known, but because asparaginase is a protein and easily degradable, it is recommended that other drugs not be admixed with it or given via Y-site administration.

Adverse Reactions:
Allergic: Hypersensitivity can occur in 20 to 35% of patients treated with asparaginase. Reactions may be life threatening or mild, with an urticarial rash noted. Anaphylaxis may also occur. Patients experiencing severe allergic reactions from *Escherichia-coli*-derived asparaginase may be treated with pegasparaginase or *Erwinea*-derived L-asparaginase.

Hepatic: Increased bilirubin, alkaline phosphatase, and SGOT occur frequently, sometimes leading to fatal liver failure.

Coagulation: Antithrombin III levels are depressed. Bleeding or clotting may occur. Fibrinogen is usually decreased. There is also a risk of disseminated intravascular coagulation (DIC).

 Gastrointestinal: About 40 to 50% of patients treated with asparaginase complain of anorexia, mild nausea, and vomiting.

Pancreatitis: Has been reported in about 5% of patients.

 Neurologic: CNS symptoms are noted in about 20 to 30% of adults, most frequently as lethargy and somnolence.

Practitioner Interventions:

1. Monitor patient for signs of allergic reactions. Keep Ambu bag at bedside, along with diphenhydramine, hydrocortisone, and epinephrine.
2. Monitor patient for 30 minutes after IV dose and 60 minutes after IM dose.
3. Monitor laboratory data weekly, including liver function tests, complete blood count with differential, platelets, antithrombin III levels, and amylase.
4. Evaluate patient for CNS toxicity and pancreatic symptoms.
5. Instruct patient and family to contact physician if pain occurs in right upper quadrant or increasing fatigue is noted.

References:

1. Barton-Burke M, Wilkes G, Ingevesen K. Chemotherapy Care Plans. Jones & Bartlett, Boston, 1993, pp. 219–225.
2. Kucuk O, Kwaan HC, Gannar W, et al. Thromboembolic complications associated with L-asparaginase therapy. Cancer 1985;55:702–706.
3. Oettgen HF, Stephenson PA, Schwartz MK, et al. Toxicity of *E. coli* L-asparaginase in man. Cancer, 1970;25:253–278.

AZACITIDINE

Other Names:
AZA-CR, 5-Azacytidine.

Uses:
Azacitidine is a group C investigational drug that is used for refractory acute myelogenous leukemia, (AML) and myelodysplastic syndrome.

Mechanism of Antitumor Action:
Azacitidine is an antimetabolite that acts by interfering with nucleic acid metabolism, being incorporated into RNA and DNA, and eventually decreasing protein synthesis.

Pharmacokinetics:

Absorption: Rapid and efficient after SC administration; peak plasma levels are seen in about 30 minutes and are equal to levels seen after IV dosing.

Distribution: The Vd is slightly less than the total body water content.

Protein Binding: Binding to albumin is minimal.

Metabolism: Metabolism occurs in the liver, yielding 5-azauridine and other inactive metabolites.

Half-life: The plasma half-life of azacitidine ranges from 3.5 to 4.2 hours.

Elimination: More than 90% of azacitidine is excreted in urine; 20% is unchanged drug.

Drug Interactions:
No reported drug interactions.

Dosage:

Intravenous: In AML - doses of 100 to 250 mg/m^2 biweekly, 150 to 400 mg/m^2/d $\times$ 5 days IV, or continuous dosing of 150 to 400 mg/m^2/day $\times$ 5 or 10 days. In myelodysplasia - 75 mg/m^2/day SC or continuous IV $\times$ 7 days.

Subcutaneous: 250 to 850 mg/m^2 (total) given over 10 days, or 35 to 90 mg/m^2/week.

Dose Forms:
Azacitidine is supplied as a powder in 30 ml vials, containing 100 mg of drug and 100 mg of mannitol.

Administration:
Azacitidine may be given by rapid, continuous, IV infusion or SC injection. When given by rapid IV infusion, the drug should be prepared in 250 to 500 mL of lactated Ringer's solution and given over a period of 2 to 3 hours. Continuous infusions should not last more than 3 hours. 5-Azacytidine is very unstable in solution, having a shelf-life of about 4.5 hours in aqueous solution. The drug is most stable at a pH between 6.2 and 6.5 (in lactated Ringer's solution).

Compatibilities: Lactated ringer's solution.

Incompatibilities: Acidic or basic solutions may accelerate drug degradation. The recommended diluent is lactated Ringer's solution.

Adverse Reactions:
 Hematologic: Leukopenia is the dose-limiting toxicity of azacitidine. Prolonged leukopenia may occur in leukemia patients. The nadir occurs at about day 25. Thrombocytopenia is also dose dependent.

 Gastrointestinal: Nausea and vomiting may be severe and occur frequently. Diarrhea has also been reported. Continuous infusions are less toxic than rapid infusion.

 Hepatic: Liver failure has occurred in elderly patients or those with significant liver metastases. Azacitidine should be avoided in patients with significant liver dysfunction.

 Neurologic: General muscle pain, weakness, and lethargy have been reported in early studies.

Other: Fever may occur at up to 24 hours after dosing.

Practitioner Interventions:
1. Administer antiemetics 30 minutes prior to each dose and for 24 hours after dosing.
2. Monitor patient's laboratory data for neutropenia, thrombocytopenia.

3. Monitor patient for any elevation in liver function test results.
4. Evaluate neurologic status during drug infusion and for 24 hours after infusion is complete.
5. Evaluate vital signs on a regular basis.

References:
1. Bellett RE, Mastrangelo M, Engstrom PF, Custer RP. Hepatotoxicity of 5-azacytidine. Neoplasma 1973;20:303–309.
2. Gaynon PS, Baus EM. Continuous infusion of 5-azacytidine as induction for acute nonlymphocytic leukemia in patients with previous exposure to 5-azacytidine. Oncology 1983;40:92–94.
3. Glover AB, Leyland-Jones BR, Chun HG, et al. Azacytidine: 10 years later. Cancer Treat Rep 1987;71:737–746.
4. Goldberg J, Gryn J, Raza A, Bennett J, et al. Mitoxantrone and 5-azacytidine for refractory/relapsed ANLL or CML in blast crisis: a leukemia intergroup study. Am J Hematol 1993;43:286–290.
5. Israili ZH, Vogler WR, Mingioli ES, Pirkle JC, et al. The disposition and pharmacokinetics in humans of 5-azacytidine administered intravenously as a bolus or by continuous infusion. Cancer Res 1976;36:1453–1461.
6. Pinto A, Zagonel V. 5-Aza-2′-deoxycitidine and 5-azacytidine in the treatment of acute myeloid leukemias and myelodysplastic syndromes: past, present, and future trends. Leukemia 1993;1(Suppl 7):51–60.

BLEOMYCIN SULFATE

Other Names:
Blenoxane®, BLEO.

Uses:
Testis cancer; lymphoma; Hodgkin's disease; head and neck cancer; squamous cell cancer of the skin, penis, cervix and vulva; malignant pleural effusions.

Mechanism of Antitumor Action:
Bleomycin binds to the guanosine and cytosine portions of DNA through intercalation mechanisms. The drug may also produce oxygen free radicals that cause scission of both single- and double-stranded DNA, which inhibits DNA synthesis.

Pharmacokinetics:

Absorption: Bleomycin is not absorbed when given orally. After IM administration, peak levels are obtained in about 30 to 60 minutes, but are only one-third of the level obtained after an intravenous dose. After intrapleural and intraperitoneal administration, about 50% of the drug is absorbed systemically.

Distribution: Bleomycin distributes into intra- and extracellular fluid, having a Vd of 20 to 30 L.

Protein Binding: Less than 10% of bleomycin is bound to plasma proteins.

Metabolism: Significant cellular metabolism. Tissue enzymatic metabolism is rapid, especially in the liver and kidney. There is a notable lack of drug inactivation in skin and lung tissue.

Half-life: After an IV bolus dose, there is an initial rapid distribution half-life of 10 to 20 minutes and a terminal half-life of 2 to 4 hours. $T_{1/2}$ may be prolonged for up to 21 hours in patients with renal dysfunction or those previously treated with cisplatin.

Elimination: About 50% of the dose of bleomycin is recovered in urine, 20 to 40% as active drug.

Drug Interactions:

Phenothiazines may enhance the cytotoxicity of bleomycin. ***Cisplatin*** decreases bleomycin elimination and may enhance toxicity. Concurrent hyperoxia and radiation may increase the pulmonary toxicity of bleomycin.

Bleomycin is inactivated *in vitro* by ***hydrogen peroxide*** and ***ascorbic acid***.

Dosage:

Test dose in lymphoma patients optional: 1–2 U IM/IV prior to full dose.

Standard: 10 to 20 U/m² IV bolus or IM injection once or twice weekly.

In combination with chemotherapy: 3 to 4 U/m² IV bolus or IM injection.

Continuous infusion: 15 U/m^2 IV over 4 days. (5.75 mg/m^2/day)

Intrapleural: The most commonly used dosages are 60 to 90 U/m^2 via intrapleural tube.

Intraperitoneal: The usual dose is 60 to 150 U/m^2 in 1000 mL of NS (or in 1 to 2 L NS or dialysate) instilled into ascites fluid.

Dose Modification:
In patients with renal dysfunction:

CrCl (mL/min)	% of normal Dose
>35	100%
20–30	50%
<20	40%

Dose Forms:
15 U vial (1 U = 1 mg).

Administration:

Test dose: Give 1–2 U IV in 50 mL over a period of 15 minutes and observe patient for 1 hour.

Intravenous: IV bolus over 10 minutes or rapid infusion diluted in 25 mL of D5W or NS and given over 15 minutes. Continuous infusions are diluted in 500 to 1000 mL of NS (preferred) and delivered from a glass container only, over a period of 24 hours.

Intramuscular: IM injection of 2 mL or less is recommended.

Intraperitoneal: Dose is dissolved in 1 to 2 L of NS, or dialysate is instilled via a peritoneal catheter. The catheter is clamped for 8 to 24 hours.

Intrapleural: The dose is dissolved in 50 mL of NS and instilled into the pleural space. Tubing should be flushed with an additional 25 mL of NS.

Compatibilities: In Y-site infusion, bleomycin sulfate is compatible with: allopurinol sodium, cefepime HCl, cisplatin, cyclophosphamide, dexamethasone sodium phosphate, diphenhydramine HCl, doxorubicin HCl, droperidol, filgrastim, fludarabine phosphate, fluorouracil, gentamicin sulfate, heparin sodium, hydrocortisone sodium phosphate, leucovorin calcium, melphalan HCl, methotrexate sodium, metoclopramide HCl, mitomycin, ondansetron HCl, phenytoin sodium, sargramostim, sodium chloride 0.9%, tobramycin sulfate, vinblastine sulfate, vincristine sulfate, vinorelbine tartrate.

Incompatibilities: Amino acids, ascorbic acid, cefazolin, diazepam, furosemide, hydrocortisone sodium succinate, methotrexate sodium (in admixtures), mitomycin (in admixture), nafcillin sodium, penicillin G sodium, terbutaline sulfate.

Adverse Reactions:

 Hypersensitivity: Anaphylactoid reactions to bleomycin are rare, but most common in lymphoma patients (1 to 8% incidence). Fever and hypotension may also occur. In lymphoma patients, give a test dose of 2 U prior to the first two treatments. If no reactions occur, full dosage may then be given. Fever with or without chills is common.

 Dermatologic: Skin hyperpigmentation, edema, and erythema, and thickening of nail beds are common. Alopecia is a common occurrence, and may or may not be total.

 **Pulmonary:** Alveolar damage is uncommon but dose-related. It is manifested as a dry cough, dyspnea, rales, and a nodular infiltrate on chest x-ray. The lung toxicity can progress to pulmonary fibrosis and can occasionally be fatal. Patients receiving high-dose oxygen (as in general anesthesia) are at increased risk for bleomycin pulmonary toxicity. Carbon monoxide diffusing capacity (DLco) is the most sensitive monitoring tool for risk of toxicity. Toxicity is dose- and age-related, occurring most frequently in patients over 70 years of age and in those who have received more than 400 mg of bleomycin. Younger patients have developed toxicity with total doses of less than 200 mg.

 Cardiovascular: Rare cases of myocardial infarction, stroke, or Raynaud's phenomena have been reported in patients given bleomycin.

 Hematologic: Myelosuppression is mild if it occurs at all.

Practitioner Interventions:

1. Before the first two treatments with bleomycin, a test dose of 2 U should be given. Bleomycin may be prepared in 2 to 50 mL of D5W or NS and given over a period of 15 minutes. Follow the patient's blood pressure, and monitor for chills, or fever.
2. Have at bedside an anaphylaxis kit that includes diphenhydramine, epinephrine, hydrocortisone, and an Ambu bag.
3. Instruct patients that fever and chills can occur for up to 6 hours after administration of bleomycin. Fever may be prevented with acetaminophen and diphenhydramine.
4. Inform patient about local pain from both SC and IM injections.
5. Premedicate patient with acetaminophen 30 minutes prior to dosing and every 6 hours for 24 hours if fever is noted.
6. Monitor for signs of pulmonary dysfunction such as shortness of breath, dyspnea, and low O_2 saturation. Pulmonary function tests, especially DLco, should be monitored and evaluated at baseline and every 3 months while patient is receiving bleomycin.
7. After IP administration, peritoneal drainage should decrease to <100 mL/24 hours before the instillation tube is removed.

References:

1. Alberts DS, Chen HSG, Liv R, et al. Bleomycin pharmacokinetics in man. Cancer Chemother Pharmacol 1978;1:1–5.
2. Barton-Burke M, Wilkes G, Ingwersen K. Chemotherapy Care Plans. Jones & Bartlett, Boston, 1993, pp. 107–114.
3. Bitran JD, Gbrown C, Desser RK, et al. Intracavitary bleomycin for the control of malignant effusions. J Surg Oncol 1981;16:273–277.
4. Dorr RT. Bleomycin pharmacology: mechanism of action and resistance, and clinical pharmacokinetics. Semin Oncology 1992;2(Suppl 5):3–8.
5. Trissel LA. Handbook of Injectable Drugs, 9th Ed., American Society of Hospital Pharmacists, Bethesda, 1996.
6. Van Barneveld PWC, Sleijfer DT, Van Der Mark TW, et al. Natural course of bleomycin-induced pneumonitis. Am Rev Respir Dis 1987;135:48–51.

BUSULFAN

Other Names:
Myleran®, BU.

Uses:
Chronic myelogenous leukemia (CML). High doses are useful as a preparative regimen for bone marrow transplantation in refractory leukemias, lymphomas, and advanced pediatric solid tumors.

Mechanism of Antitumor Action:
Busulfan is an alkylating agent, it produces a small amount of DNA (interstrand) crosslinking and a large amount of DNA–protein crosslinking.

Pharmacokinetics:

Absorption: Low doses of busulfan are well absorbed orally, with peak levels achieved within 2 to 4 hours after administration.

Distribution: Busulfan distributes rapidly in plasma and crosses the blood–brain barrier. The drug distributes readily into saliva.

Protein Binding: Binding to plasma protein is low, at about 7%.

Metabolism: Via the liver; sulfoxane, 3-hydroxysulfoxane, and other metabolites are formed and excreted in the urine.

Half-life: 2.5 hours after both high and low doses.

Elimination: The metabolites of busulfan are excreted renally. Only 1% of busulfan is excreted unchanged in the urine.

Drug Interactions:
None known.

Dosage:
Initially 4 to 12 mg/day for several weeks. The maintenance dose is 1 to 3 mg/day. The dose for bone marrow transplantation is 4 mg/kg/day for 4 days, to a total dose of 16 mg/kg.

Dose Forms:
Myleran® is available in 2 mg scored tablets.

Administration:
Busulfan is administered orally and may be taken any time during the day. Low doses of busulfan are generally very well tolerated. How-

ever, in bone marrow transplantation regimens, moderate to severe nausea and vomiting are common.

Adverse Reactions:

Hematologic: Leukopenia is the major toxicity at standard doses. Neutropenia nadirs range from 11 to 30 days; recovery occurs in 24 to 54 days after treatment is stopped. Anemia also occurs, especially with high doses (bone marrow transplantation).

Pulmonary: Occurs after long-term therapy. Symptoms include anorexia, cough, dyspnea, and fever.

Endocrine: Hormonal effects with occasional gynecomastia, and addisonian symptoms.

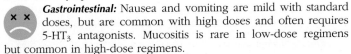

Gastrointestinal: Nausea and vomiting are mild with standard doses, but are common with high doses and often requires 5-HT$_3$ antagonists. Mucositis is rare in low-dose regimens but common in high-dose regimens.

Dermatologic: Hyperpigmentation is a result of increased melanin synthesis and/or dispersion in the skin. It is noted at skin creases, particularly in the hands and nail beds.

Neurologic: Generalized seizures have been reported to occur on day 3 or 4 of daily high-dose therapy with busulfan. Phenytoin (300 mg PO daily) or clonazepam infusion (0.1 mg/kg/day IV) prior to busulfan is effective in preventing seizures.

Practitioner Interventions:

1. Monitor patient's complete blood cell count (CBC) on a weekly basis.
2. Monitor patient's respiratory status on a monthly basis.
3. Instruct patient to notify provider if any swelling occurs in the breast, or any signs of Addison's disease.
4. Administer antiemetics before use of busulfan in bone marrow transplantation.
5. Instruct patient on possible skin changes, such as hyperpigmentation and nail-bed changes.
6. Warn patient about hypersensitivity to sun.
7. Instruct patients on high dose to shower twice daily during drug administration.

References:
1. Ehrsson H, Hassan M, Ehrnebo M, Beeran M. Busulfan kinetics. Clin Pharmacol Ther 1983;34:86–89.
2. Grigg AP, Shepherd JD, Phillips GL. Busulphan and phenytoin. Ann Intern Med 1989;111:1049–1050.
3. Hassan M, Oberg G, Ehrsoon H, et al. Pharmacokinetics and metabolic studies of high-dose busulphan in adults. Eur J Clin Pharmacol 1986;36: 525–530.
4. Louis J, Limarzi LR, Best W. Treatment of chronic granulocytic leukemia with Myleran. Arch Intern Med 1956;97:299–308.
5. Marcus RE, Goldman M. Convulsions due to high-dose busulfan. Lancet 1984;2:1463.

CARBOPLATIN

Other Names:
Paraplatin®, CBDCA.

Uses:
Ovarian cancer, head and neck cancer, lung cancer, testis cancer, bladder cancer, endometrial cancer.

Mechanism of Antitumor Action:
The exact mechanism of antitumor action of carboplatin is unknown. It binds to DNA, producing DNA–DNA crosslinks and DNA–protein crosslinks.

Pharmacokinetics:

Absorption: Not orally absorbed.

Distribution: Carboplatin distributes into body fluids, including cerebrospinal fluid. It can penetrate into malignant pleural effusions and ascites.

Protein Binding: About 30% bound to plasma protein.

Metabolism: Carboplatin is not metabolized to any great extent. Most of the drug is excreted unchanged by the kidneys.

Half-life: $T_{1/2}\alpha$ = 1.5 hours (free drug and free platinum), and $T_{1/2}\beta$ = 6-9 hours (free drug).

Elimination: In patients with CrCl > 60 mL/min, 65% of carboplatin is excreted in 24 hours. Hemodialysis clears the drug at 25% of the renal clearance rate. Peritoneal dialysis is ineffective for removing carboplatin from the body.

Drug Interactions:
Aluminum needles can react with carboplatin and produce an inactive complex.

Dosage:
The usual dose of carboplatin ranges from 300 to 400 mg/m^2 as an IV bolus.

High doses used for bone marrow transplantation are 800 to 2000 mg/m^2 IV.

The dosage should be modified for patients with renal dysfunction, using the Calvert formula given below:

Dose (mg/m^2) = 4 to 6 (GFR + 25), previously treated patient
Dose (mg/m^2) = 7 to 9 (GFR + 25), previously untreated patient
GFR = glomerular filtration rate or estimated creatinine clearance (ECC).
Estimated creatinine clearance may be determined by the Cockcroft and Gault formula:

$$ ECC = \frac{(140 - age)}{(serum\ cr\ in\ mg/dL)} \times \frac{(wt\ in\ kg)\ (0.85\ if\ female)}{(72)} $$

Dose Forms:
Carboplatin is available in 50 mg, 150 mg and 450 mg vials.

Administration:
Doses ≤ 500 mg may be given as a bolus over a period of 30 to 60 minutes, or as a continuous infusion.

Doses > 500 mg should be given over a period of 1 to 2 hours or as a continuous infusion.

Compatibilities: In simulated Y-site infusion, carboplatin is compatible with allopurinol sodium, cefepime HCl, etoposide, filgrastim, fludarabine phosphate, ifosfamide, melphalan HCl, ondansetron HCl, paclitaxel, piperacillin sodium-tazobactam sodium, sargramostim, and vinorelbine tartrate.

Incompatibilities: Fluorouracil, mesna, and sodium bicarbonate solutions.

Adverse Reactions:

Hematologic: Bone marrow suppression and especially thrombocytopenia, is the dose-limiting toxic effect of carboplatin. The nadir occurs 3 weeks after chemotherapy, with recovery by 4 weeks after the end of therapy.

Gastrointestinal: Nausea and vomiting are much less severe than with cisplatin, and are usually controlled with phenothiazine or low-dose 5-HT$_3$ antagonists with or without dexamethasone.

Kidney: Nephrotoxicity and ototoxicity are rare, but loss of serum electrolytes, especially magnesium, is common.

Neurologic: Peripheral neuropathy occurs in a small percentage of patients.

Practitioner Interventions:

1. Check patient's complete blood cell count and platelet count prior to the initiation of carboplatin.
2. Check serum creatinine and estimate creatinine clearance, and adjust dosage if necessary.
3. Give antiemetics 30 minutes prior to carboplatin.
4. No pre- or post-treatment hydration is necessary.

References:

1. Baltzer L, Berkery R. Oncology Pocket Guide to Chemotherapy. CV Mosby, St. Louis, 1994, pp. 32–35.
2. Calvert AH, Newell DR, Gumbull LA, et al. Carboplatin dosage: Prospective evaluation of a simple formula based on renal function. J Clin Oncol 1989;7:1748–1756.

3. Woloschuk DM, Pruemer JM, Cluxton RJ. Carboplatin: A new cisplatin analog. Drug Intell Clin Pharm 1988;22:843–849.

CARMUSTINE

Other Names:
BiCNU®, Bischloronitrosourea, BCNU.

Uses:
Brain tumors—especially glioblastoma; multiple myeloma; refractory Hodgkin's disease; and non-Hodgkin's lymphoma

Mechanism of Antitumor Action:
Carmustine acts primarily as an alkylating agent through chloroethyl metabolites. It inhibits a number of key enzymatic reactions involved with DNA synthesis through DNA–protein and/or DNA–DNA crosslinks.

Pharmacokinetics:

Absorption: Carmustine is not absorbed orally.

Distribution: Carmustine is a very lipid-soluble drug that distributes into fat. It achieves prolonged plasma levels and crosses the blood–brain barrier.

Protein Binding: About 67% bound to plasma protein after high-dose regimens.

Metabolism: Partial activation by hepatic microsomal enzymes.

Half-life: Carmustine has a very short biologic half-life due to rapid metabolism. After rapid infusion, it has a $T_{1/2}\alpha$ of 6.1 minutes and a $T_{1/2}\beta$ of 21.5 minutes. After high-dose carmustine (300 to 750 mg/m²), the half–life is 22 minutes, which is similar to that with conventional doses.

Elimination: Sixty to 70% of a dose of carmustine is excreted in urine after 4 days, as metabolites. Ten percent is excreted in respiratory CO_2.

Drug Interactions:

Cimetidine potentiates the toxicity of carmustine in humans.

Phenytoin and corticosteroids do not inhibit carmustine toxicity.

Dosage:

Intravenous:

1. 75 to 100 mg/m^2 IV × 2 days every 6 weeks.
2. 200 mg/m^2 IV × 1 dose for brain cancers every 6 weeks.
3. 450 to 600 mg/m^2 IV × 1 dose for bone marrow transplantation.

Dose Forms and Storage:

BiCNU® is available as a 100 mg powder in a 30 ml amber vial, with a separate 3 mL vial of absolute alcohol diluent.

Administration:

Intravenous: Administer over a period of 1 to 2 hours in 100 to 250 mL D5W or NS.

Compatibilities: In simulated Y-site infusion of 100 mg/L of carmustine, the drug is compatible with cefepime HCl, filgrastim, fludarabine phosphate, melphalan HCl, ondansetron HCl, piperacillin sodium–tazobactam sodium, sargramostim, and vinorelbine tartrate.

Incompatibilities: Sodium bicarbonate solutions rapidly degrade carmustine.

Adverse Reactions:

 Hematologic: Delayed hematopoietic toxicity is the dose-limiting toxic effect of carmustine. Leukopenia and thrombocytopenia peak at 3 to 5 weeks after administration, and may persist for 1 to 3 weeks.

 Gastrointestinal: Nausea and vomiting are severe and begin 2 hours after dosing, lasting for 4 to 6 hours.

 Neurologic: Encephalopathy—neurologic deterioration and seizures have been reported.

Hepatic: Transient elevations in liver enzymes to twice normal values occur in about 90% of patients within a week after treatment is begun. Venoocclusive disease has been reported after high doses of carmustine in bone marrow transplantation protocols. This may be a fatal complication in 5 to 20% of patients.

 Pulmonary: Severe interstitial pneumonitis and frequent opportunistic infections have been reported in about 20% of patients after high-dose therapy with carmustine.

 Vascular: Facial flushing may occur during IV administration. Local burning at the injection site and along the vein may be evident. Slowing the infusion rate or use of a more dilute solution may decrease local burning.

Practitioner Interventions:

1. Initiate a new peripheral IV site prior to carmustine administration.
2. Make sure that infusions run for at least 1 hour when infusing peripherally.
3. Monitor peripheral infusion site for pain, erythema, or burning. If noted, decrease rate and increase keep open D5W or NS solution.
4. Administer antiemetics 30 minutes prior to initiating infusions of carmustine, and continue to evaluate emesis for 12 hours following infusion.
5. In bone marrow transplantation patients:
   a. Monitor patient's neurologic status and liver function tests at least twice weekly.
   b. Instruct patient to monitor his or her own respiratory status following discharge. If any shortness of breath or increase in respiratory rate occurs, patient should notify the physician immediately.

References:
1. Holoye PY, Jenkins DE, Greenberg SD. Pulmonary toxicity in long-term administration of BCNU, Cancer Treat Rep 1976;60:1691–1693.
2. Lokich JJ, Drum DW, Kaplan W. Hepatic toxicity of nitrosurea analogues. Clin Pharmacol Ther 1974;16:363–367.

3. Peters WP, Shpall EJ, Jones RB, et al. High-dose combination alkylating agents with bone marrow support as initial treatment for metastatic breast cancer. J Clin Oncol 1988;6:1368–1376.

CHLORAMBUCIL

Other Names:
Leukeran®.

Uses:
The most common uses of chlorambucil are in chronic lymphocytic leukemia (CLL) and Hodgkin's and non-Hodgkin's lymphoma. Chlorambucil has also been used in choriocarcinoma, ovarian and breast carcinoma, and Waldenstrom's macroglobulinemia.

Mechanism of Antitumor Action:
Chlorambucil is a classic alkylator, a cell-cycle-nonspecific agent that binds to DNA.

Pharmacokinetics:

Absorption: The oral bioavailability of chlorambucil when taken with meals is about 75%.

Distribution: The distribution of chlorambucil in humans has not been studied. In animals, chlorambucil is widely distributed in all tissues, especially fatty tissues.

Protein Binding: Over 90% of the drug is bound to albumin and other gamma globulins.

Metabolism: Extensive metabolic degradation of chlorambucil occurs, with 60% of drug metabolites eliminated within 24 hours.

Half-life: The terminal half-life ranges from 2 to 8 hours.

Elimination: Chlorambucil is eliminated via the renal and hepatic systems. A significant amount of the drug is metabolized and excreted in the urine; only about 1% of the drug is excreted unchanged in the urine.

Drug Interactions:
Chlorambucil has increased toxicity when given to patients previously treated with ***barbiturates***.

Dosage:
Chronic lymphocytic leukemia—0.1 to 0.2 mg/kg PO daily for 3 to 6 weeks, followed by 2 to 4 mg PO daily for maintenance.

Dose Forms and Storage:
Leukeran® is available as a 2-mg sugar-coated tablet.

Administration:
Give tablets of chlorambucil all at one time and with food.

Adverse Reactions:

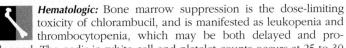
Hematologic: Bone marrow suppression is the dose-limiting toxicity of chlorambucil, and is manifested as leukopenia and thrombocytopenia, which may be both delayed and prolonged. The nadir in white cell and platelet counts occurs at 25 to 30 days; recovery occurs within 40 to 45 days. Lymphocytopenia may also occur with prolonged use of chlorambucil, and irreversible bone marrow damage has been reported.

Gastrointestinal: Dyspepsia may occur, but is usually mild.

Pulmonary: Lung fibrosis, alveolar damage, and pneumonitis are rare, but can be life-threatening and are dose related.

Neurologic: Seizures and coma have been described when large cumulative doses are ingested.

Dermatologic: Rashes, urticaria, plaque, and urticarial lesions on the face and scalp occasionally occur. Alopecia is uncommon.

Carcinogenic: Second malignancies have occurred in patients taking chlorambucil for a prolonged period. Patients with breast cancer have developed acute leukemia.

Reproductive: Chlorambucil is known to induce amenorrhea/azoospermia, and is a teratogen. It should be avoided during pregnancy.

Practitioner Interventions:

1. Instruct patient to take chlorambucil as a whole dose with meals.
2. Monitor complete blood cell count (CBC), including platelets, on a weekly basis.
3. If patient experiences nausea, premedicate with an oral antiemetic agent (e.g., prochlorperazine) at 30 minutes before chlorambucil dose.
4. Monitor patient for skin toxicity (i.e., rash, urticaria).
5. Instruct patient to take only the prescribed dose. Warn family, significant others of seizure potential in cases of overdose.
6. Counsel patients on possible second malignancy if drug is taken over a prolonged period.
7. Counsel patients about appropriate precautions to prevent pregnancy.

References:
1. Berk PD, Goldberg JD, Silverstein MN, et al. Increased incidence of acute leukemia in polycythemia vera associated with chlorambucil therapy. N Engl J Med 1981;304:441–447.
2. Byrne TN, Moseley TA, Finer MA. Myoclonic seizures following chlorambucil overdose. Ann Neurol 1981;9:191–194.
3. Peterman A, Braunstein B. Cutaneous reaction to chlorambucil therapy. Arch Dermatol 1986;122:1358–1360.
4. Sawitsky A, Rai KR, Colidewell O, et al. Comparison of daily versus intermittent chlorambucil and prednisone therapy in the treatment of patients with chronic lymphocytic leukemia. Blood 1977;50:1049–1059.

CISPLATIN

Other Names:
Cis-platinum, cis-diamminedichloroplatinum (II), CDDP, DDP, Platinol®, Platinol-AQ®.

Uses:
Testis cancer, ovarian cancer, head and neck cancer, bladder cancer, lung cancer, esophagus cancer, lymphoma.

Mechanism of antitumor action:
Cisplatin is activated to an aquated form, which then binds to DNA, resulting in inter- and intrastrand crosslinking. The drug acts like a bifunctional alkylating agent.

Pharmacokinetics

Absorption: Cisplatin is not absorbed by the oral route. After IP administration, systemic absorption is rapid and complete. Peak concentrations are greater after IP administration, which results in a 15 to 30% increase in intraperitoneal exposure as compared with IV administration.

Distribution: Cisplatin is widely distributed into all cells, but the highest concentrations are observed in renal, prostate, and liver tissues. The drug distributes readily into pleural effusions and ascites, but CNS penetration is variable, ranging from 5 to 100% of concurrent plasma levels. The Vd ranges from 20 to 80 L.

Protein Binding: After aquation or hydroxylation in plasma, cisplatin is highly bound (over 90%) to plasma proteins. This binding is slowly reversible to active alkylating forms.

Metabolism: Cisplatin is rapidly activated through an aquation reaction with plasma and cellular water. It is also hydroxylated to several reactive species.

Half-Life: Depending on the dose and schedule of IV administration, plasma elimination of cisplatin may be monophasic or biphasic. The $T_{1/2}\alpha$ and $T_{1/2}\beta$ of unbound platinum are 20 minutes and 70 minutes, respectively. The terminal phase half-life of the bound drug ranges from 12 to 24 hours.

Elimination: Between 15 and 35% of the dose is excreted in the urine within 48 hours. About 50% of a cisplatin dose is slowly eliminated by the kidneys over a 96-hour period, while another 40% of the dose is excreted even more slowly over the next several days. Less than 10% of the drug is eliminated by biliary excretion. Patients with moderate or poor renal function should not receive cisplatin because of the increased risk for nephrotoxicity.

Drug Interactions:
Concurrently administered nephrotoxins, such as ***aminoglycosides*** and ***amphotericin B***, may increase the risk of cisplatin nephrotoxicity.

Cisplatin may decrease the renal excretion and increase the accumulation of other drugs cleared by renal mechanisms, such as ***bleomycin***, ***cytarabine***, ***methotrexate***, and ***ifosfamide***, leading to enhanced toxicities.

In patients previously treated with cisplatin, the peripheral neurotoxicity of ***paclitaxel*** may be increased.

Cisplatin may enhance the cytotoxicity of ***etoposide***. In contrast, ***dipyridamole*** increases the cytotoxicity of cisplatin by enhancing cellular uptake of the drug.

Sodium thiosulfate and ***mesna*** directly inactivate cisplatin when given concurrently.

In animal models, ***probenecid*** may decrease the renal tubular secretion of cisplatin and enhance its nephrotoxicity. ***Cimetidine*** enhances cisplatin cytotoxicity *in vitro*.

Dosage:
Intravenous: Several dosage regimens for cisplatin have been used, including:

1. 50 to 120 mg/m^2 IV over 2 to 24 hours every 3 to 4 weeks.
2. 20 mg/m^2 IV daily over 2 to 24 hours for 5 days every 3-4 weeks.

Intraperitoneal: 100 mg/m^2 in 1500 to 2000 mL of dialysate monthly.

Dose Modification:

Creatinine Clearance	Dose
>60 mL/min	100%
<60 mL/min	Avoid

Dose Form
Platinol® is available in vials of 10 and 50 mg of powder. Platinol-AQ® is an aqueous solution of cisplatin and is available as 50 or 100 mg vials.

Administration:

Intravenous: Several methods of cisplatin administration have been used. Cisplatin should be administered in a slow infusion in order to minimize its nephrotoxic potential. Assuring good urine output (> 150 ml/hr) will decrease nephrotoxicity. Thus, prehydration with 1 to 2 L of NS is often recommended. In addition, cisplatin may admixed with 12.5 to 50 g of mannitol to ensure diuresis of the drug. Avoid the use of aluminum needles when administering cisplatin, since a precipitate will form.

Doses of ≥ 50 mg/m^2 should be diluted in NS in a concentration of 1 mg/mL, and given no faster than 1 mg/min. Doses of ≥ 20 mg/m^2 should also be diluted to a concentration of 0.4 mg/mL in NS and given over a period of 60 minutes.

Intraperitoneal: Administration is accomplished through a Tenckhoff catheter or an implanted port device. A volume of 1,500 to 2,000 mL is required to adequately bathe the peritoneal surface with the chemotherapeutic agent. The solution is instilled over a period of 30 of 90 minutes into the peritoneal cavity, depending on patient tolerance. The dwell time is variable.

Compatibilities: In Y-site simulation of 1 mg/mL, cisplatin is compatible with bleomycin sulfate, chlorpromazine HCl, cimetidine HCl, cyclophosphamide, diphenhydramine HCl, doxorubicin HCl, droperidol, etoposide, famotidine, floxuridine, fludarabine phosphate, fluorouracil, furosemide, ganciclovir, granisetron, heparin sodium, ifosfamide, leucovorin calcium, melphalan HCl, methylprednisolone sodium succinate, methotrexate sodium, magnesium sulfate, metoclopramide HCl, morphine sulfate, mitomycin, ondansetron HCl, paclitaxel, prochlorperazine edisylate, promethazine HCl, sargramostim, vinblastine sulfate, vincristine sulfate, and vinorelbine tartrate.

Incompatibilities: Cefepime HCl, mesna, sodium thiosulfate, thiotepa.

Adverse Reactions:

 Hematologic: Bone marrow suppression after single agent therapy is common but is mild with cisplatin in its usual doses. In contrast, higher doses may produce severe myelosuppression.

Leukopenia and thrombocytopenia are maximum at 7 days, and recovery occurs by day 21.

 Neurologic: The major dose-limiting toxicity of cisplatin is neurologic. Neurologic toxicity is manifested as peripheral neuropathy (paresthesias, numbness), which may slowly reverse or not reverse at all. The neuropathy worsens with higher cumulative doses of the drug. It presents in a typical stocking–glove distribution in the hands and feet. Numbness and sensory loss may also occur. Focal encephalopathy has been reported but is rare.

Nausea and Vomiting: Cisplatin produces severe emesis, depending on the dose given. The emesis is common with high-dose therapy. $5HT_3$ antagonists and corticosteroids are recommended for prophylaxis.

Nephrotoxicity: Cisplatin may cause acute or chronic renal insufficiency in about one-third of patients treated. Oliguria and elevated serum creatinine of acute onset have been observed within 48 hours of administration. Cisplatin also produces renal magnesium wasting, resulting in clinical hypomagnesemia. These effects are reversible in 7 to 14 days, but magnesium levels usually do not return completely to baseline. Chronic renal insufficiency is manifested primarily as a slow increase in the serum creatinine to two to three times baseline values over a period of 4 to 6 weeks. Hyperhydration with saline solutions prior to and during cisplatin therapy usually prevents acute renal insufficiency.

 Mucositis: Mouth sores are rare.

 Ototoxicity: Cisplatin frequently causes hearing loss in the high-frequency range, especially when given in high doses. Slower infusions may decrease the incidence of ototoxicity.

 Hypersensitivity: Acute anaphylactic reactions have occurred, and are manifested by facial edema, bronchospasm, and hypotension. Corticosteroids, antihistamines, and epinephrine should be used to treat such reactions.

 Vascular: Cellulitis and fibrosis have rarely occurred after cisplatin extravasation.

Practitioner Interventions:

1. Give antiemetics 30 minutes prior to cisplatin. Use post-chemotherapy antiemetics for 3 to 5 days to prevent delayed emesis.
2. IV fluids should be given as 100 to 150 mL/hr of NS prior to, during, and for 12 to 24 hours following cisplatin administration.
3. Avoid concurrent nephrotoxins during cisplatin administration.
4. Periodically assess the patient's neurologic status. Grade 4 neuropathy usually requires discontinuation of the drug.
5. Monitor renal function during each day of cisplatin therapy and with each clinic visit. Discontinue cisplatin if creatinine clearance is less than 60 mL/min.
6. Hypomagnesemia may be treated with oral magnesium salts, such as magnesium oxide 400 mg PO twice daily.

References:

1. Andrews PA, Howell SB. Cellular pharmacology of cisplatin perspectives on mechanisms of acquired resistance. Cancer Cells 1990;2:35–43.
2. Brock J, Alberts DS. Safe, rapid administration of cisplatin in the outpatient clinic. Cancer Treatment Rep 1986;70:1409–1414.
3. Dentine M, Luft FC, Yrem MN, et al. Long term effect of cis-diamminedichloride platin (CDD) on renal function and structure in man. Cancer 1978;41:1274–1281.
4. Frick GA, Ballentine R, Driever CW, Kramer WG. Renal excretion kinetics of high dose cis-dichloroammineplatin (II) administered with hydration and mannitor diuresis. Cancer Treat Rep 1979;63:13–16.
5. Gormley PE, Bull JM, LeRoy AF, Cysyk R. Kinetics of cisdichlorodiammineplatinum. Clin Pharmacol Ther 1979;25:351–357.
6. Gregg RW, Molepo JM, Monpetit VJ, et al. Cisplatin neurotoxicity: The relationship between dosage, time, and platinum concentration in neurologic tissues, and morphologic evidence of toxicity. J Clin Oncol 1992;10:795–803.
7. Himmelstein KT, Patton TE, Belt RJ, et al. Clinical kinetics of intact cisplatin and some related species. Clin Pharmacol Ther 1981;29:658–664.
8. Howell SR, Pfeifle CE, Wung WE, et al. Intraperitoneal cisplatin with systemic thiosulfate protection. Ann Intern Med 1982;97:845–851.
9. Hutchinson FS, Perez EA, Gandara DR, et al. Renal salt wasting in patients treated with cisplatin. Ann Intern Med 1988;108:21–25.
10. Khan A, Hill JM, Grater W, et al. Atopic hypersensitivity to cisdichlorodiammineplatinum (II) and other platinum complexes. Cancer Res 1975;35:2766–2770.
11. Loehrer PJ, Einhorn LH. Cisplatin. Ann Intern Med 1984;100:704–713.

12. Patterson WP, Reams JP. Renal toxicities of chemotherapy. Semin Oncol 1992;19:521–528.
13. Schilsky RL, Anderson T. Hypomagnesemia and renal magnesium wasting in patients receiving cisplatin. Ann Intern Med 1979;90:929–931.

CLADRIBINE

Other Names:
Leustatin®, 2-CdA, 2-chlorodeoxyadenosine.

Uses:
Hairy cell leukemia, non-Hodgkin's lymphoma (low grade), chronic myelogenous leukemia (CML).

Mechanism of Antitumor Action:
Cladribine is activated intracellularly to the triphosphate, which is incorporated into DNA and inhibits several enzymes, including DNA polymerase and ligase, and ribonucleotide reductase, resulting in DNA strand breakage. The drug also decreases nicotine adenine dinucleotide (NAD) concentration, causing ATP depletion.

Pharmacokinetics:

Absorption: About 50% of cladribine was bioavailable after administration of an investigational oral solution. After subcutaneous injection, about 97% is bioavailable.

Distribution: The Vd (steady state) is about 9L/kg.

Protein Binding: About 20% of cladribine is bound to plasma proteins.

Metabolism: Very little is known about its metabolism.

Half-life: $T_{1/2}\alpha = 35$ min; $T_{1/2}\beta = 6.7$ hours.

Elimination: After discontinuation of a 7 day infusion, cladribine is completely cleared from the plasma by renal excretion.

Drug Interactions:

Mechlorethamine: In vitro studies demonstrate cross-resistance with cladribine.

Dosage:
Leustatin® is available as a 10 mL (1 mg/mL) vial.

Administration:
One milligram or less of cladribine is diluted in 500 to 1,000 mL of NS and given over 24 hours. The drug is stable in polyvinyl chloride (PVC) plastic containers. It is stable for 7 days in the Pharmacia Deltec® cassette system.

Compatibilities: Not studied.

Incompatibilities: D5W is not recommended as a diluent for cladribine.

Adverse Reactions:

 Hematologic: Myelosuppression is the dose-limiting toxicity of cladribine. The neutrophil nadir occurs within 7 to 14 days and usually resolves within 4 weeks.

Immunosuppression: A decrease in CD4 and CD8 T-cells is evident in most patients and lasts about 6 months. Infections are common, owing to immunosuppression. Fungal infections occur in about one-fourth of patients.

 Hypersensitivity: About half of patients with hairy cell leukemia experience a maculopapular rash.

 Gastrointestinal: Nausea and vomiting are not usually problems with cladribine.

Practitioner Interventions:

1. If patient is seen on a daily basis, check for fever, which may be related to tumor lysis.
2. Instruct patients to monitor their temperature and other signs of infection, especially oral thrush.

References:

1. Carson DA, Wasson DB, Kaye J, et al. Deoxycytidine kinase-mediated toxicity of deoxyadenosine analogs toward malignant human lymphocytes *in vitro* and toward murine L-1210 leukemia *in vivo*. Proc Natl Acad Sci USA 1980;77:6865–6869.
2. Estey EH, Kurzrock R, Kantarjian HM, et al. Treatment of hairy cell leukemia with 2-chlorodeoxyadenosine (2-CdA). Blood 1992;79:882–887.
3. Lillemark J, Juliusson G. On the pharmacokinetics of 2-chloro-2′ deoxyadenosine in humans. Cancer Res 1991;51:5570–5572.

CYCLOPHOSPHAMIDE

Other Names:

Cytoxan®, Neosar®, CTX, CPM.

Uses:

Non-Hodgkin's lymphoma, adult acute leukemia, breast cancer, endometrial cancer, ovarian cancer, small-cell lung cancer, and multiple myeloma.

Mechanism of Antitumor Action:

Cyclophosphamide is a cell-cycle-nonspecific alkylating agent with major activity against rapidly proliferating cells.

Pharmacokinetics:

Absorption: Cyclophosphamide is well absorbed orally, with 90% bioavailability.

Distribution: Both cyclophosphamide and its metabolites are well distributed throughout the body, including brain and CSF. The drug also distributes into breast milk and saliva.

Protein Binding: Binding to plasma proteins is minimal. In contrast, the phosphoramide mustard metabolite of cyclophosphamide is about 60% bound to plasma protein.

Metabolism: A large fraction of cyclophosphamide is eliminated by hepatic enzyme metabolism. The majority of the drug is metabolized by microsomal enzymes in the liver to 4-hydroxycyclophosphamide (active), ketocyclophosphamide (inactive), and aldophosphamide, which may be enzymatically metabolized to carboxyphosphamide (inactive), phosphoramide mustard (active), and acrolein (active).

Half-life: The plasma $T_{1/2}$ of the parent compound after doses of 6 to 80 mg/kg ranges from 4 to 6.5 hours.

Elimination: Although a large amount of cyclophosphamide is metabolized by the liver, the kidney exclusively excretes both the drug and its metabolites. However, because of avid tubular reabsorption, only about 60% of cyclophosphamide and a larger amount of its metabolites appear in the urine. There may be significantly prolonged retention of the more polar metabolites in patients with severe renal dysfunction. However, there have been no reports of excessive myelosuppression in patients with severe renal failure.

Drug Interactions:

Allopurinol may increase the incidence of bone marrow suppression by prolonging the half-life of cyclophosphamide.

Barbiturates and other inducers of hepatic microsomal enzymes, such as *phenytoin* and *chloral hydrate*, may increase the rate of hepatic conversion of cyclophosphamide to its toxic metabolites.

Corticosteroids may inhibit microsomal enzyme metabolism and decrease the conversion of cyclophosphamide to its active metabolites, decreasing its activity.

Succinylcholine metabolism may be decreased during cyclophosphamide therapy.

Alfa interferon in doses exceeding 3 MU increases the myelosuppressive effect of cyclophosphamide.

Chloramphenicol metabolism is decreased by cyclophosphamide.

Halothane and *nitrous oxide* anesthesia in conjunction with cyclophosphamide has been associated with mortality.

Dosage:

Intravenous-continuous: The usual continuous IV dose of cyclophosphamide is 60 to 120 mg/m^2/day or 1 to 2.5 mg/kg/day, and is titrated to the myelosuppressive response.

Intravenous-bolus: Most IV regimens for cyclophosphamide use 500 to 1,500 mg/m^2 or 30 to 40 mg/kg per treatment course. A maximum bolus dose of 7 g/m^2 without bone marrow transplantation has been used.

Intravenous-high dose bone marrow transplant: The standard IV regimen of cyclophosphamide, used in combination with radiation therapy for allogeneic bone marrow transplantation, employs a dose of 60 mg/kg × 2 days.

Oral: The usual oral dose of cyclophosphamide in the treatment of breast cancer is 100 mg/m^2 daily for 14 days.

Dose Forms:

Cyclophosphamide is available in oral form as 25 and 50 mg tablets (Cytoxan®). Cyclophosphamide for IV infusion (Cytoxan®, Neosar®) is available in vials of 100, 200, 500, 1000 and 2000 mg.

Administration:

Oral tablets may be given as a single dose or in divided doses. A cyclophosphamide oral solution may be prepared by dissolving cyclophosphamide powder for injection in aromatic elixir in a concentration of 1 to 5 mg/mL. The manufacturers state that such solutions are stable for 14 days in glass containers under refrigeration.

Parenteral: cyclophosphamide may be given as a push over a period of 3 to 5 minutes, a bolus infusion over 15 to 30 min, or as a slow infusion over 1 to 24 hours.

Compatibilities: In simulated Y-site infusions at a concentration of 10 mg/mL in NS, cyclophosphamide is compatible with allopurinol sodium, melphalan HCl, sargramostim, and vinorelbine tartrate.

In simulated Y-site infusions of cyclophosphamide in concentrations of 10 mg/mL in D5W, cyclophosphamide is compatible with cefepime HCl, chlorpromazine HCl, cimetidine HCl, dexamethasone sodium phosphate, diphenhydramine HCl, droperidol, famotidine, filgrastim, fludarabine phosphate, furosemide, ganciclovir sodium, heparin sodium, hydromorphone HCl, lorazepam, melphalan HCl, methylprednisolone sodium succinate, metoclopramide HCl, morphine sulfate, ondansetron HCl, paclitaxel, piperacillin sodium–tazobactam sodium, prochlorperazine edisylate, promethazine HCl, ranitidine HCl, sargramostim, and vinorelbine tartrate.

In simulated Y-site infusions of cyclophosphamide in concentrations of 4 mg/mL in D5W, cyclophosphamide is compatible with idarubicin HCl.

In simulated Y-site infusions at a concentration of 20 mg/mL in D5W, cyclophosphamide is compatible with amikacin sulfate, bleomycin sulfate, cefamandole naftate, cefazolin sodium, cefoperazone sodium, cefotaxime sodium, cefoxitin sodium, cefuroxime sodium, cephalothin sodium, cephapirin sodium, chloramphenicol sodium succinate, cisplatin, clindamycin phosphate, doxorubicin HCl, doxycycline hyclate, droperidol, erythromycin lactobionate, fluorouracil, furosemide, gallium nitrate, gentamicin sulfate, heparin sodium, kanamycin sulfate, methotrexate sodium, metoclopramide HCl, metronidazole, mezlocillin sodium, minocycline HCl, mitomycin, moxalactam disodium, nafcillin sodium, ondansetron HCl, oxacillin sodium, penicillin G potassium, piperacillin sodium, ticarcillin disodium, ticarcillin disodium–clavulanate potassium, tobramycin sulfate, trimethoprim–sulfamethoxazole, vancomycin HCl, vinblastine sulfate, and vincristine sulfate.

Incompatibilities: None reported.

Adverse Reactions:

Hematologic: Leukopenia is the dose-limiting toxicity of cyclophosphamide. The leukocyte nadir occurs at 8 to 14 days, with recovery by day 18 to 25. Thrombocytopenia may also occur, especially with high-dose therapy.

Bladder: Sterile hemorrhagic cystitis may occur in patients treated with cyclophosphamide, and is associated with either large single doses or chronic low-dose therapy.

Gastrointestinal: Nausea, vomiting, and anorexia are common with high oral doses. Their incidence is 33% at doses below 400 mg/m^2 and 77% at doses above 400 mg/m^2.

Dermatologic: Alopecia is severe in at least 50% of all patients treated with cyclophosphamide. Sterile phlebitis has been reported after IV administration of the drug.

Pulmonary: Pneumonitis is rare and is similar to "busulfan lung." It may be lethal after high-dose therapy.

Cardiac: Cardiomyopathy may occur with high doses (120 to 279 mg/kg) of cyclophosphamide administered over periods of a few days. After 8 years from the beginning of therapy, about 3% of patients treated with high dose cyclophosphamide develop cardiomyopathy.

 Reproductive: Testicular atrophy, and sometimes reversible oligospermia and azoospermia can occur in patients treated with cyclophosphamide. Amenorrhea with ovarian failure may also be noted.

 Hypersensitivity: Anaphylaxis has occurred in rare instances.

Second malignancy: Urinary bladder cancers and skin cancers tend to predominate in patients receiving prolonged low-dose therapy with cyclophosphamide (12% of patients taking the drug for 12 years).

Endocrine: SIADH (syndrome of inappropriate antidiuretic hormone secretion) is noted at doses above 50 mg/kg and is a limitation and consequence of fluid loading.

Practitioner Interventions:

1. Give oral cyclophosphamide during the daytime to accomodate diuresis.
2. Ensure an adequate oral fluid intake of at least 2 to 3 L/day.
3. Avoid patient use of caffeine-containing products.
4. Encourage patients to empty bladder at least every 2 hours.
5. Give appropriate antiemetic therapy 30 minutes prior to dosing with cyclophosphamide.
6. Warn patients about impending alopecia.
7. Initiate a new IV site prior to infusion of cyclophosphamide.
8. Counsel patients on reproductive effects of cyclophosphamide. Prior to dosing in bone marrow transplantation, allow time for men to sperm bank and women to evaluate egg banking.
9. Counsel patients who will receive cyclophosphamide over a long term about risks of possible second malignancy.
10. Have appropriate equipment available for rare cases of anaphylaxis.

References:
1. American Hospital Formulary Service, Published by the American Society of Health System Pharmacists, 1996, pp. 581–85.
2. Bagley CM, Bosllick, FW DeVita VT. Clinical pharmacology of cyclophosphamide. Cancer Res 1973;33:226–233.
3. Braverman AC, Antin JH, Plappert MT, et al. Cyclophosphamide cardiotoxicity in bone marrow transplantation: A prospective evaluation of new dosing regimens. J Clin Oncol 1991;9:1215–1223.
4. DeVita VT, Hellman S, Rosenberg SA. Cancer Principles and Practice of Oncology, 5th Ed. Lippincott/Raven, Philadelphia, 1997.
5. Juma FD, Rogers HJ, Trounce JR. The pharmacokinetics of cyclophosphamide and alkylating activity in men after intravenous and oral administration. Br J Clin Pharmacol 1979;8:209–217.

CYTARABINE

Other Names:
Cytosar-U®, AraC, cytosine arabinoside.

Uses:
Acute myelogenous leukemia (AML), acute lymphoblastic leukemia (ALL), malignant lymphoma, CNS leukemia or lymphoma, myelodysplastic syndrome (MDS).

Mechanism of antitumor action:
Cytarabine is a pyrimidine antimetabolite and competitive inhibitor of DNA polymerase.

Pharmacokinetics:

Absorption: Oral absorption is poor (only 20%).

Distribution: Cytarabine distributes well into CSF fluid. After IV doses of 100 mg/m^2, CSF levels are about 40 to 50% of plasma levels. The Vd is the total body water. After high-dose regimens, cytarabine is present in high concentration in tears. After intrathecal administration, cytarabine is slowly cleared from the CSF.

Protein Binding: Unknown.

Metabolism: Within the cell, cytarabine is rapidly metabolized by deoxycytidine deaminase to the inactive metabolite ara-uridine (ara-

U). Intracellular cytarabine that avoids rapid metabolism by deaminase enzymes will be activated by dexoycytidine kinase to the phosphorylated metabolites ara-cytosine triphosphate (ara-CTP). After high doses of cytarabine, more drug is converted to active metabolites, which favors greater cytotoxicity.

Half-life: After IV administration, the initial half-life of cytarabine is 10 to 15 minutes, followed by a slower terminal phase of 2.5 to 3.0 hours. After intrathecal administration, the half-life of cytarabine ranges from 2 to 11 hours.

Elimination: The spleen and liver are major sites of metabolism and elimination of cytarabine.

Drug Interactions:

Cytarabine has been shown to decrease the cellular uptake of **methotrexate**, thereby inhibiting the latter drug's activity.

In vitro tumor models have demonstrated that cytarabine enhances the cytotoxicity of **asparaginase**.

Dipyrimadole may block cytarabine toxicity by inhibiting the uptake of cytarabine into cells.

Methotrexate may increase the intracellular activation of cytarabine and potentially enhance cell killing.

Sargramostim (GM-CSF) may increase the incorporation of cytarabine into myeloid leukemia cells.

Nephrotoxins (cisplatin, aminoglycosides, amphotericin B) may decrease renal clearance of cytarabine, increasing the risk of neurotoxicity.

Dosage:

Intravenous
AML

The conventional IV dose of cytarabine is 100 to 200 mg/m^2/day by continuous infusion for $\times$ 5 to 7 days.

The high dose IV infusion is 1-3 g/m^2 every 12 to 24 hours over a period of 1 to 2 hours $\times$ 6 to 12 doses

The low dose IV infusion is 5-30 mg/m^2 every 12 to 24 hours, given daily.
Lymphoma

Cytarabine is given in a dose of 2 g/m^2 IV every 12 hours $\times$ 2 doses every month.

Subcutaneous
AML
   Cytarabine is given in a dose of 5 to 30 mg/m² SC, administered daily.

Intrathecal
CNS leukemia or lymphoma:
   Cytarabine is given in a dose of 30 to 50 mg/m² intrathecally in non-preserved saline twice a week until the CSF is clear, followed by the same dose given weekly for maintenance.

Intraperitoneal
Ovarian Cancer
   The dose of cytarabine is 30 to 2,000 mg in 2 L of dialysate given monthly.

Dosage Modification:

Creatinine Clearance	Usual Dose 2 gm/m²	Dose Modification
> 60 mL/min	2 g/m²	n.a.
< 60 mL/min	n.a.	1 g/m²

Dose Forms:
Cytosar-U® is available in 100 mg, 500 mg, 1 g, and 2 g vials.

Administration:

Intravenous: Diluent with 0.9% benzyl alcohol—5 mL for 100 mg, 10 mL for 500 mg and 1 g; 20 mL for 2g. More concentrated solutions may be prepared for SC administration. Reconstituted solutions from 20 to 250 mg/mL are stable for 7 days at room temperature in D5W or NS.
   For 1-hour infusion: further dilution in 50 to 100 mL D5W or NS.
   For 24-hour infusion: further dilution in 500 to 1,000 mL D5W or NS.

Subcutaneous: 10 to 30 mg in 1 mL NS.

Intraperitoneal: Administration is accomplished through a Tenckhoff catheter or a Portacath® device. A volume of 1500 to 2000 mL is required to adequately bathe the peritoneal surface with the chemotherapeutic agent. The solution is instilled into the peritoneal cavity (dwell time) for at least 5 hours, and is drained prior to the next belly bath.

Compatibilities: Cytarbine is compatible with D5W, 5% dextrose in lactated Ringer's solution (D5LR), NS, 5% dextrose in normal saline (D5NS), and LR. *In simulated Y-site infusions of 50 mg/mL,* cytarabine is compatible with the following drugs:
Amsacrine, cefepime HCl, chlorpromazine HCl, cimetidine HCl, dexamethasone sodium phosphate, diphenhydramine HCl, droperidol, famotidine, filgrastim, fludarabine phosphate, furosemide, heparin sodium, hydromorphone HCl, Idarubicin HCl, lorazepam, melphalan HCl, methprednisolone sodium succinate, metoclopramide HCl, mitoxantron HCl, morphine sulfate, ondansetron HCl, paclitaxel, piperacillin sodium–tazobactam sodium, prochlorperazine edisylate, promethazine HCl, ranitidine HCl, sargramostim, teniposide, vincristine sulfate, and vinorelbine tartrate.

Incompatibilities: Allopurinol sodium, fluorouracil, regular insulin, nafcillin sodium, oxacillin sodium, penicillin G sodium, gallium nitrate, ganciclovir sodium.

Adverse Reactions:

 Myelosuppression: Leukopenia and thrombocytopenia, with a nadir in cell counts at 7 days and recovery by day 21.

 Neurologic: Manifested as ataxia, lethargy, and confusion, which may occur in about 10% of patients. Risk factors include age > 40 years and decreased renal (Cr_{Cl} < 60 mL/min)

 Mucositis: Mouth sores and diarrhea may occur concurrently or individually.

 Nausea and vomiting: Cytarabine is moderately to severely emetogenic, depending on the dose given.

 Pulmonary: Noncardiogenic pulmonary edema with diffuse infiltrates occurs in 13% of patients after high-dose therapy. This manifests several days after therapy, and is often fatal.

 Ocular Toxicity: Conjunctivitis is common and is due to drug distribution into tears. Conjunctivitis can be prevented by using a topical corticosteroid, such as dexamethsone 0.1%.

Practitioner Interventions:

1. Give antiemetics 30 minutes prior to cytarabine.
2. Give allopurinol 300 to 600 mg PO daily.

3. Give IV fluids at 100 to 150 mL/hr to enhance urate excretion.
4. Give concurrent corticosteroid eye drops (e.g., dexamethasone 0.1% thrice daily) with high dose therapy.
5. Avoid concurrent nephrotoxins during cytarabine administration.
6. Assess neurologic status daily during cytarabine therapy.
7. Use prophylactic mouth care.
8. Use chlorhexidine mouthwash during therapy.
9. Monitor patient daily for mucositis.
10. Monitor liver function two to three times weekly.
11. Monitor renal function daily during cytarabine administration, and modify dosage accordingly.
12. Discontinue cytarabine if neurologic toxicity is grade 3 or higher.

References:
1. Damon LE, Mass R, Linker CA. The association between high dose cytarabine neurotoxicity and renal insufficiency. J Clin Oncol 1989;7:1563–1568.
2. Graves T, Hooks MA. Drug induced toxicities associated with high dose cytosine arabinoside infusions. Pharmacotherapy 1989;9:23–28.
3. Lazarus HM, Herzig RH, Herzig GP, et. al. Central nervous system toxicity of high dose systemic cytosine arabinoside. Cancer 1981;48:2577–2582.

DACARBAZINE

Other Names:
DTIC-Dome®, DTIC.

Uses:
Malignant melanoma, soft-tissue sarcoma, Hodgkin's disease, neuroblastoma, malignant glucagonoma.

Mechanism of Antitumor Action:
Monoalkylation of DNA, RNA, and proteins. Dacarbazine also acts as an antimetabolite, inhibiting purine bases. Additionally, it binds to sulfhydryl groups on proteins.

Pharmacokinetics:

Absorption: Erratic and incomplete oral absorption.

Distribution: The Vd is 0.2 L/kg. Dacarbazine is not widely distributed. Less than 15% of the drug crosses the blood–brain barrier.

Protein Binding: Only 5% of dacarbazine is bound to plasma protein.

Metabolism: Rapid hepatic metabolism to the active metabolite, 5-aminoimidazole-4-carboxamide.

Half-life: After an IV bolus, $T_{1/2}\beta = 40$ min. The mean half-life of the primary metabolite is about 70 minutes.

Elimination: 40 to 50% of dacarbazine is excreted unchanged in the urine 6 hours after an IV bolus.

Drug Interactions:

Phenobarbital and *phenytoin* induce the metabolism of dacarbazine. *Interleukin-2* alters dacarbazine pharmacokinetics, specifically enhancing dacarbazine clearance. Dacarbazine inhibits *xanthine oxidase* and enhances the effects of *allopurinol* on azathioprine or mercaptopurine metabolism.

Dosage:

250 mg/m^2 IV daily $\times$ 5 days, or 850 mg/m^2 IV $\times$ 1 day. Cycles are repeated every 3 or 4 weeks. In severe renal dysfunction, doses should be reduced.

Dose Forms:

DTIC-Dome® is available in 100 mg and 200 mg vials.

Administration:

An IV push may be performed with 5 to 10 mL of D5W or NS, but short 15- to 30-minute infusion is recommended to minimize venous irritation. The solution should be protected from light.

Compatibilities: In simulated Y-site infusion of 4 mg/mL in NS, dacarbazine is compatible with melphalan HCl, sargramostim, and vinorelbine tartrate.

In simulated Y-site infusion of 4 mg/mL in D5W, dacarbazine is compatible with filgrastim, fludarabine phosphate, ondansetron HCl, and paclitaxel.

In simulated Y-site infusion of 10 mg/mL in NS, dacarbazine is compatible with heparin sodium (see incompatibilities below).

Incompatibilities: Allopurinol sodium, cefepime HCl, piperacillin sodium–tazobactam sodium.

In simulated Y-site infusion of 25 mg/mL in NS, dacarbazine is incompatible with heparin sodium.

Adverse Reactions:

 Myelosuppression is the dose-limiting toxicity of dacarbazine. Leukopenia and thrombocytopenia are equally severe, occuring at about 21 days after treatment is begun.

 Flu-like reaction: Uncommon, and consists of fever and/or malaise.

 Gastrointestinal: Nausea and vomiting are common and often severe. 5HT$_3$ antagonists should be given prophylactically.

 Hypotension: Occurs with high single-dose regimens. The infusion rate may be decreased to the patient's level of tolerance.

 Hepatic: Transaminase elevation is uncommon. Hepatic failure is rare.

 Hypersensitivity: Facial flushing and edema may occur. Photosensitivity can be severe.

Practitioner Interventions:

1. Give aggressive antiemetic prophylactic therapy before chemotherapy.
2. Give diluted dacarbazine over a period of 15 to 30 minutes in 250 to 500 mL D5W or NS. The solution should be protected from light.

3. Monitor the patient's blood pressure during the infusion.
4. Use acetaminophen to prevent flulike symptoms if this was a problem on prior cycles.
5. Assess patient's blood cell counts at 3 weeks after beginning of chemotherapy.

References:
1. Baltzer L, Bekery R. Oncology Pocket Guide to Chemotherapy, DTIC. CV Mosby, St. Louis, 1994, pp. 56–58.
2. Carter SK. Proceedings of the sixth new drug seminar: DTIC. Cancer Treat Rep 1976;60:123–214.
3. Ceci G, Bella M, Melissar M, et al. Fatal hepatic vascular toxicity of DTIC: is it really a rare event? Cancer, 1988;61:1988–1991.

DACTINOMYCIN

Other Names:
Cosmegen®, Actinomycin D.

Mechanism of Antitumor Action:
Intercalation between DNA base pairs; DNA-dependent ribosomal RNA and mRNA are selectively inhibited.

Uses:
Wilm's tumor, rhabdomyosarcoma, Ewing's sarcoma, nonseminomatous testicular cancer, gestational choriocarcinoma, Kaposi's sarcoma, melanoma.

Pharmacokinetics:

Absorption: Poor oral absorption.

Distribution: Dactinomycin distributes in high concentration into bone marrow and leukocytes.

Protein Binding: Specific data are unknown, but dactinomycin appears to be highly tissue bound.

Metabolism: Dactinomycin undergoes a minor amount of metabolism to an inactive monolactone metabolite.

Half-life: The plasma $T_{1/2}$ = 3-36 hours.

Elimination: Biliary excretion eliminates 50% of dactinomycin, while urinary excretion is about 10%.

Drug Interactions:
Enflurane and *halothane* hepatotoxicity may be enhanced.

Dosage:
Adult: 1.25 to 2 mg/m² IV every 3 to 4 weeks; or 0.5 mg daily × 5d q 3–5 wks

Pediatric sarcomas: 450 μg/m²/day (maximum: 600 mg/m²/d × 5 days) IV daily for 5 days.

Dose Forms:
Dactinomycin is available in a 500 μg vial.

Administration:
Constitute vial with 1.1 mL of non-preserved sterile water for injection. Dactinomycin is given only by IV injection as a slow intravenous push (10 to 15 minutes) in the side arm of a free-flowing IV line. Discard remaining drug. Do not give by intermittent or continuous infusion (because of adsorption to glass, plastic, and in-line filters).

Compatibilities: In Y-site infusion of 0.01 mg/mL, dactinomycin is compatible with allopurinol sodium, cefepime HCI, fludarabine phosphate, dacarbazine, mephalan HCI, ondansetron HCL, sargramostin, and vinorelbine tartrate.

Incompatibilities: Preserved diluents, filgrastim.

Adverse Reactions:

Hematologic: Bone-marrow suppression is common; neutrophils and platelets are equally affected. The onset is from 7 to 10 days after treatment is begun, with a nadir at 14 to 17 days. Recovery occurs by day 21 to 28.

Gastrointestinal: Emesis can be severe and may last up to 20 hours. It is usually well controlled with antiemetics. Mucositis, diarrhea, and proctitis can be severe. Cheilitis has also been infrequently reported.

Dermatologic: Alopecia is common but reversible. Skin changes may occur and include acne, erythema, hyperpigmentation, maculopapular rash, radiation recall reactions, and extravasation reactions.

Hepatic: Elevated transaminases, hepatitis, and hepatomegaly occur in 2 to 14% of patients, depending on the dose and schedule of dactinomycin. Daily schedules are associated with a higher incidence of severe hepatotoxicity.

Practitioner Interventions:

1. Check nadir of patient's complete blood cell count (CBC) and platelets count.
2. Give 5HT$_3$ antagonists prior to dactinomycin.
3. Establish a new, free-flowing IV line for dactinomycin infusion.
4. Administer dactinomycin in the side arm of a free flowing IV set-up over a period of 5 minutes.

References:

1. Baltzer L, Barkery R. Oncology Pocket Guide to Chemotherapy. CV Mosby, St. Louis, 1994, pp. 58–61.
2. Frei E III. The clinical use of actinomycin. Cancer Chemother Rep. 1974;58:49–54.
3. Green DM, Norkool P, Breslow NE, et al. Severe hepatic toxicity after treatment with vincristine and dactinomycin using single-dose or divided dose schedules: a report from the National Wilms' Tumor Study. J Clin Oncol 1990;8:1525–1530.

DAUNORUBICIN

Other Names:
Cerubidine®, DNR, Rubidomycin.

Uses:
Acute myelogenous leukemia (AML), acute lymphocytic leukemia (ALL) (children).

Mechanism of Antitumor Action:
Daunorubicin produces anthracycline intercalation between DNA base pairs, leading to inhibition of DNA synthesis. It inhibits DNA-dependent RNA and DNA polymerases. In addition, it interferes with

the enzyme topoisomerase II. Daunorubicin also generates oxygen free radicals, leading to cell-membrane damage.

Pharmacokinetics:

Absorption: Daunorubicin is a vesicant compound and must be given only by the IV route.

Distribution: Daunorubicin is widely distributed into tissues, with highest concentrations found in heart, liver, lung, kidneys, and spleen. The drug penetrates poorly into cerebrospinal fluid.

Protein Binding: Not well described, but daunorubicin has a large Vd, suggesting that it is highly protein bound.

Metabolism: The liver converts the parent compound to the 13-hydroxylated metabolite daunorubicinol, which has about 10% of the potency of daunorubicin.

Half-life: Daunorubicin has an elimination half-life of about 20 hours, while that of daunorubicinol is 28 to 40 hours.

Elimination: Both the parent compound and its metabolite daunorubicinol are excreted extensively into feces via the biliary system. Only 20% of the drug and its metabolites are excreted in the urine.

Drug Interactions:

Iron chelators such as ***dexrazoxane (ICRF-187)*** block the cardiotoxic effects of daunorubicin. Drugs that modulate the MDR efflux mechanism ***(amphotericin, verapamil)*** may enhance the effects of daunorubicin.

Dosage:

The usual dose for induction for adult AML ranges from 30 to 60 mg/m^2/day for 3 days. In pediatric acute lymphocytic leukemia, the dose ranges from 25 to 45 mg/m^2 IV. The frequency of dosing depends on the combination of chemotherapy employed. The dose should be modified for hepatic dysfunction as follows:

Dose Modification:

Serum bilirubin (mg/dL)	% Dose
<1.2	100
1.2–3.0	75
>3.0	50

Dose Forms:
Cerubidine® is available as a lyophilized powder in a 20 mg vial containing 100 mg mannitol.

Administration:
Daunorubicin is extremely irritating to tissues and should not be given IM or SC. Caution should be taken not to extravasate the drug. Only fresh intravenous lines should be used for IV administration of daunorubicin. Constitute with 4 mL of sterile water. Withdraw the desired dose into a syringe containing 10–15 mL of NS and infuse over a period of 2 to 5 minutes into the side arm of free-flowing IV infusion of D5W or NS, followed by 10 mL of D5W or NS to flush the line. Some practitioners prefer to dilute the drug in 50–100 mL of D5W or NS and administer the drug over a 15- to 30-minute period *(but this should be via a central line only).*

Compatibilities: In admixtures daunorubicin HCl is incompatible with dexamethasone sodium phosphate and heparin sodium. In simulated Y-site infusion of 1 mg/mL in NS, daunorubicin HCl is compatible with melphalan HCl, teniposide (0.1 mg/mL), and vinorelbine tartrate.

In simulated Y-site infusion of 12 mg/mL in D5W, daunorubicin HCl is compatible with ondansetron HCl.

Incompatibilities: Allopurinol sodium, cefepime HCl, fludarabine phosphate, piperacillin sodium-tazobactam sodium.

Adverse Reactions:

Hematologic: Myelosuppression occurs in all patients treated with daunorubicin and includes leukopenia, anemia, and thrombocytopenia. The nadir in cell counts occurs between days 10 and 14, and recovery between days 21 and 28.

Cardiac: Acute arrhythmias (within 48 hours) are common but usually asymptomatic, and include ST–T wave abnormalities, a low-voltage QRS complex and T-waves, sinus tachycardia, premature ventricular contractions, and heart block. These effects diminish over 2 to 3 days. A more significant cardiac toxicity is a dose-dependent cardiomyopathy, which is manifested by classic congestive heart failure. About 1 to 2% of patients treated with a cumulative dose of 550 mg/m^2 of daunorubicin may develop congestive heart failure, but the incidence increases with higher cumulative doses.

Gastrointestinal: Nausea and vomiting are common and moderately severe, lasting about 24 hours after administration of daunorubicin. Stomatitis can occur from 5 to 7 days after chemotherapy, and remits as myelosuppression remits.

  Dermatologic: Alopecia is common and includes hair loss on the scalp and in axillary and pubic areas. Hair growth resumes 4 to 6 weeks after daunorubicin is discontinued. Transverse hyperpigmentation of nail beds is common, and reverses as nails grow out. There have been rare cases of rashes, dermatitis, and urticaria. Recall dermatitis has been reported in skin areas exposed to local radiation.

 Skin Reactions: Local skin necrosis occurs after extravasation. Some patients develop severe necrosis requiring surgical debridement and grafting. Local antidotes should be used to treat extravasations (see practitioner intervention No. 8).

 Hepatic: Transient elevations of serum glutamic oxaloacetic transaminase (SGOT) and alkaline phosphatase.

 Urinary: Daunorubicin will turn urine orange or red for about 24 hours after administrations.

Practitioner Interventions:

1. Check bilirubin and adjust the dose of daunorubicin according to the guideline given above.
2. Give antiemetics 30 to 60 minutes prior to daunorubicin.
3. Start a new free-flowing IV line with NS.
4. Administer daunorubicin over a period of 2 to 5 minutes in the sidearm of the IV infusion set-up. Every 1 minute, check for signs of drug extravasation (local pain, flow-rate decrease). Flush line.
5. Remind patient about change in urine color over the next 1 to 2 days after infusion begins.
6. Keep a running tab on the cumulative dose of daunorubicin.
7. Have extravasation kit at bedside.
8. Extravasation Management.
   a. Stop infusion immediately and do not remove needle.
   b. Aspirate as much vesicant as possible.

c. Notify physician.

d. Instill antidote per institutional protocol.

References:

1. Cerubidine® Product Information. Bedford Laboratories, May, 1996.
2. Gottlieb AJ, Weinberg V, Ellison R, et al. Efficacy of daunorubicin in the therapy of adult acute lymphocytic leukemia: a prospective randomized trial by CALGB. Blood 1984;64:267–274.
3. Linker CA, Levitt LJ, O'Donnell M, et al. Treatment of adult acute lymphoblastic leukemia with intensive cyclical chemotherapy: a followup report. Blood 1991;78:2814–2822.
4. Von Hoff DD, Rozencweig M, Layard, et al. Daunomycin-induced cardiotoxicity in children and adults: A review of 110 cases. Am J Med 1977;62:200–208.

DAUNORUBICIN CITRATE, LIPOSOMAL

Other Names:
DaunoXome®

Uses:
HIV-associated Kaposi's Sarcoma

Mechanism of Antitumor Action:
While in the circulation, liposomal daunorubicin (DunoXome®) is protected from chemical and enzymatic degradation, protein binding, and distribution into normal cells. Once within the cell, daunorubicin is slowly released, enabling it to bind to DNA to inhibit nucleic acid synthesis.

Pharmacokinetics:

Absorption: Liposomal daunorubicin is administered only by the IV route.

Distribution: In contrast to the very large Vd of daunorubicin HCl (about 1000 L), liposomal doxorubicin has a small Vd (about 6 L), indicating that it remains primarily within the intravascular compartment.

Protein Binding: Minimal within the blood circulation.

Metabolism: Daunorubicinol is the primary metabolite of daunorubicin, but appears only in very small concentrations after DaunoXome® administration.

Half-life: After a dose of 40 mg/m^2, DaunoXome® has an elimination half-life of 4.4 hours.

Elimination: Plasma clearance of DaunoXome® (liposomal daunorubicin) is 17 mL/min, in contrast to 240 mL/min for daunorubicin HCl.

Drug Interactions:
Drug interactions between DaunoXome® and antiretroviral, antiviral and anti-infective agents have not been evaluated to date.

Dosage:
The standard starting dose of DaunoXome® is 40 mg/m^2 IV every 2 weeks. The dose should be adjusted in patients with liver dysfunction. Serum bilirubin measurement is recommended prior to chemotherapy. If the serum bilirubin is 1.2 to 3.0 mg/dL, the dose should be decreased by 25%; if the serum bilirubin is > 3.0 mg/dL, the dose should be decreased by 50%.

Dose Forms:
DaunoXome® is available in a 50 mg vial.

Administration:
DaunoXome® is given as an IV infusion in a concentration of 1 mg/mL in D5W over a period of 60 minutes. Diluted DaunoXome® should be refrigerated and given within 6 hours after preparation.

Compatibilities: DaunoXome® should not be mixed with other drugs or with the preservative benzyl alcohol.

Incompatibilities: Not determined to date.

Adverse Reactions:
Hematologic: Myelosuppression is the dose-limiting toxicity of DaunoXome®. Leukopenia is maximum at 10 to 14 days; recovery occurs by day 21. Thrombocytopenia is rarely severe ($<50,000$/mm^3). About 6% of patients develop a neutrophil nadir of less than 500/mL.

Dermatologic: While daunorubicin HCl is a vesicant, DaunoXome® has not been proven as a vesicant in animal studies. Until further experience is reported, caution should be taken not to extravasate DaunoXome®. Mild to moderate alopecia occurs in about 8% of patients and is reversible 3 months after discontinuation of DaunoXome®. Palmar–plantar erythrodysethesia is uncommon, occurring in about 1% of patients. This can be a very problematic manifestation of skin toxicity. Local therapy includes the use of topical steroids and moisturizing lotions.

 Cardiotoxicity: A triad of mild to moderate back pain, flushing, and chest tightness has been reported in about 14% of patients treated with DaunoXome® and in about 3% of treatment cycles, occuring during infusion of the drug. Cardiac events consisting of palpitations, syncope, and tachycardia have been reported in less than 5% of patients. Cardiomyopathy from DaunoXome® has not been fully elucidated. Special attention should be given to the potential cardiac toxicity of DaunoXome®. The left ventricular ejection fraction should be measured at total cumulative doses of 320 mg/m², 480 mg/m², and every 240 mg/m² thereafter.

 Gastrointestinal: Nausea and vomiting are common and moderately severe, occurring in about 50% of patients, and are often controlled with prophylactic antiemetics in addition to dexamethasone plus a 5-HT3 antagonist. Mucositis occurs in about 10% of patients.

 Urinary: Within 24 hours after administration of DaunoXome®, the urine may turn reddish-orange because of the urinary excretion of the parent compound, doxorubicin. This effect disappears by 24 hours after discontinuation of the drug.

Acute infusion-associated reactions: Reactions such as flushing, shortness of breath, facial swelling, headache, chills, back pain, and hypotension occur in about 7% of patients and may be infusion-rate-related. Slowing or discontinuing the infusion results in resolution of these reactions over the course of several hours to a day.

Practitioner Interventions

1. Monitor patient's complete blood cell count (CBC) and platelet count on a weekly basis.
2. Initiate new IV infusion prior to initiating therapy in order to prevent extravasation.

3. Evaluate electrocardiogram prior to initiating therapy.
4. Check ventricular ejection fraction prior to dosing with DaunoXome®.
5. Evaluate liver function; reduce dose in case of elevated bilirubin.
6. Premedicate patient with antiemetics, including dexamethasone plus a 5-HT3 receptor antagonist. Mucositis occurs in about 20% of patients.
7. Instruct patient about risk of total alopecia and orange-colored urine.
8. Keep an ongoing tabulation of total DaunoXome® dosage.
9. Extravasation management.
   - Stop infusion immediately and do not remove needle.
   - Aspirate as much extravant as possible.
   - Apply an ice pack for 15 minutes four times daily for 2 days.
10. The infusion should be given over a minimum of 60 minutes. If the patient experiences flushing, shortness of breath, or facial swelling, the infusion should be discontinued until the symptoms subside, and should be reinstituted at half the infusion rate.
11. Have an anaphylaxis kit consisting of hydrocortisone, diphenhydramine, epinephrine, and an Ambu bag at the bedside.

References:
1. DaunoXome® Product Information. NeXstar Pharmaceutical, Inc, April 1996.
2. Gill PS, Espina BM, Muggia F, et al. Phase I/II clinical and pharmacokinetic evaluation of liposomal daunorubicin. J Clin Oncol 1995;13:996–1003.
3. Money-Kyrle JF, Bates F, Ready J, et al. Liposomal duanorubicin in advanced Kaposi's sarcoma; a phase II study. Clinical Oncol 1993;5:367–371.

DEXRAZOXANE

Other Names:
Zinecard®, ADR-529, ICRF-187.

Uses:
Prevention of cardiac toxicity in advanced breast cancer patients who have received a cumulative dose of 300 mg/m^2 of doxorubicin

and who would benefit from continuing therapy. It is not recommended for use with initial doxorubicin therapy.

Mechanism of Action:
The exact mechanism of dexrazoxane is unknown. Dexrazoxane is rapidly hydrolyzed to ICRF-198, which is a potent intracellular chelator of heavy metals and binds to the hydrolysis product of doxorubicin-generated, iron-based oxygen-free radicals, thereby protecting myocardial cells from mitochondrial lipid peroxidation and thiol oxidation.

Pharmacokinetics:

Absorption: Dexrazoxane is administered only IV.

Distribution: Dexrazoxane is rapidly distributed to all body tissues.

Protein Binding: About 30% of dexrazoxane is bound to plasma proteins.

Metabolism: Dexrazoxane enters cells, where it is hydrolyzed to an ethylene diaminetetraacetic acid-like product.

Half-life: The elimination half-life of dexrazoxane is 2 to 3 hours.

Elimination: The kidney excretes 35 to 50% of dexrazoxane unchanged in the urine. A substantial amount of the drug is metabolized in the liver.

Dosage:
The recommended dose is a dexrazoxane: doxorubicin ratio of 10:1 given IV 30 minutes prior to doxorubicin.

Dose Forms:
Zinecard® is available in 250 and 500 mg lyophilized powder vials.

Administration:
Dexrazoxane is given by IV infusion in 50 to 100 mL of D5W or NS over a period of 15 to 30 minutes. Longer infusions (for up to 8 hours) have been given.

Compatibilities: Not studied.

Incompatibilities: Not studied. However, the manufacturer recommends that Zinecard® (dexrazoxane) not be mixed with other drugs.

Adverse Reactions:

 Leukopenia: Dexrazoxane may enhance the leukopenia caused by doxorubicin.

 Gastrointestinal: Mild nausea and vomiting.

 Cardiovascular: Deep venous thrombosis is uncommon.

 Liver: Elevated transaminase and bilirubin levels.

 Hair loss: Alopecia may be accentuated.

Practitioner Interventions:

1. Prepare dexrazoxane with supplied diluent (1/6 molar, preservative-free sodium lactate).
2. Administer dexrazoxane just prior to doxorubicin.

References:

1. Jakobsen P, Sorensen B, Bastholt L, Mirza MR, et al. The pharmacokinetics of high dose epirubicin and of the cardioprotector ADR-529 given together with cyclophosphamide, 5-fluorouracil, and tamoxifen in metastatic breast cancer patients. Cancer Chemother Pharmacol 1994;35: 45–52.
2. Malisza KL, Hasinoff BB. Doxorubicin reduces the iron (III) complexes of the hydrolysis products of the antioxidant cardioprotective agent dexrazoxane (ICRF-187) and produces hydroxyl radicals. Arch Biochem Biophys 1995;316:68–688.
3. Seifert CF, Nesser ME, Thompson DF. Dexrazoxane in the prevention of doxorubicin-induced cardiotoxicity. Ann Pharmacother 1994;28: 1063–1072.
4. Speyer J, Green MD, Zeleninch-Jacquotte A, et al. ICRF-187 permits longer treatment with doxorubicin in women with breast cancer. J Clin Oncol 1992;10:117–127.

DOCETAXEL

Other Names:
Taxotere®.

Uses:
Docetaxel is active in adenocarcinomas of the breast; in ovarian, non-small-cell lung and pancreatic cancer; and in soft-tissue sarcomas.

Mechanism of Antitumor Action:
Docetaxel stabilizes cell microtubule assembly by inhibiting the depolymerization of tubulin. This results in an inhibition of mitosis.

Pharmacokinetics:
Docetaxel has been studied in more than 500 patients receiving intravenous doses of 20 to 115 mg/m^2. The kinetics were not influenced by age, gender, ethnicity, or dexamethasone.

Absorption: Docetaxel is given intravenously.

Distribution: The mean Vd is 115 L after doses of 70 to 115 mg/m^2. Systemic and tumor exposure is proportional to the dose given.

Protein Binding: Docetaxel is highly bound (94%) to plasma and cellular proteins, and albumin. Dexamethasone does not influence the protein binding of docetaxel.

Metabolism: Hepatic metabolism by cytochrome P450 3A enzymes.

Half-life: The $T_{1/2}\alpha$ of docetaxel is 4 minutes; the $T_{1/2}\beta$ is 0.5 hour; the $T_{1/2}\gamma$ is 11 hours.

Elimination: The mean total body clearance in 21 L/m^2/hr. Fecal excretion is the primary route of elimination of docetaxel, accounting for about 75% of the dose given, 8% of which is active drug and the rest split among three other unknown metabolites. Renal excretion is approximately 6%. Plasma elimination is triexponential, with the half-lives given above.

Drug Interactions:
None known, but quinidine, cyclosporine, terfenadine, ketoconazole, erythromycin may induce or inhibit cytochrome P450 3A4. Since docetaxel is metabolized by the same isoenzyme, these drugs may

cause a significant drug interaction (potentiation of docetaxel by inhibitors and antagonism by inducers of cytochrome P450 3A4) and verapamil.

Dosage:

For locally advanced or metastatic breast carcinoma: 60 to 100 mg/m^2 IV over a period of 1 hour, given every 3 weeks. The usage of docetaxel in patients under the age of 16 years has not been established. All patients should be premedicated with oral dexamethasone 8 mg twice daily for 5 days starting one day prior to docetaxel.

In patients with hepatic or renal dysfunction, or the elderly: Patients with bilirubin levels elevated above the upper limit of normal should not receive docetaxel. Also, patients with elevated alkaline phosphatase or transaminase enzymes (AST or ALT) should not receive docetaxel. There is no dosage adjustment in elderly patients or those with renal impairment.

Dose Forms:
Taxotere® is available in 20 and 80 mg vials.

Administration:
The appropriate amount of diluent is added to a vial to produce a 10 mg/mL premix solution. Doses of up to 240 mg are further diluted with 250 mL of D5W or 0.9% sodium chloride. Doses greater than 240 mg require a larger volume, so that a concentration of 0.9 mg/mL Taxotere® is not exceeded. Unclear solutions should be discarded. Diluted solutions should be used as soon as possible. However, the diluted solutions are reported to be stable for 8 hours over a range of concentrations of 0.02 mg/mL to 0.9 mg/mL. Precipitation may occur at solution concentrations greater than 0.9 mg/mL.

Docetaxel should be given in polypropylene or polyolefin bags or glass bottles over a 1 or 24-hour time period. Due to plasticizer leaching, PVC containers and administration sets should not be used.

Compatibilities: none reported.

Incompatibilities: none reported.

Adverse Reactions:

Hematologic: The dose-limiting toxicity of docetaxel is neutropenia, with a nadir in the neutrophil count at 10 days and recovery by 15 days. Grade 4 neutropenia (<500 cells/mm^3) is frequent in patients given 60–75 mg/m^2 (75–80%). Thrombocytopenia is marked by a nadir at 10 days and recovery at 15 to 18 days.

Cardiovascular: Flushing, hypotension, urticaria, and diaphoresis are less frequent than with paclitaxel. Premedication with diphenhydramine and dexamethasone is not generally required unless reactions are evident. A fluid-accumulation syndrome has been noted, and might require diuretics.

Hypersensitivity: Anaphylaxis is rare but patients should be observed closely for reactions especially during the 1st and 2nd infusions. Severe hypersensitivity is characterized by rapid-onset shortness of breath or bronchospasm requiring epinephrine, hypotension requiring bolus fluid or pressor therapy, and generalized rash or erythema. Injectable hydrocortisone and diphenhydramine are used to treat anaphylactic reactions.

Dermatologic: Alopecia occurs in 80% of patients. A maculopapular rash and phlebitis occur in about 20% of patients.

Gastrointestinal: Nausea and vomiting are mild to moderate, and are controlled with antiemetics. Mucositis and diarrhea are uncommon.

Neurologic: In contrast to paclitaxel, peripheral neuropathy is rare with docetaxel.

Practitioner Interventions:

1. Premedicate the patient with 8 mg dexamethasone PO twice daily, starting one day prior to the injection of docetaxel and continue for 5 days. The patient should be given a reminder card or phone call to initiate dexamethasone in a timely fashion.
2. Monitor patient's complete blood cell count (CBC) with differential and platelet counts on a weekly basis.
3. Monitor fluid input, output, and weight weekly. Patients with edema may be treated with standard therapy (salt restriction, oral diuretics).

4. Instruct patient about risk of infection and when to contact the health-care provider.
5. Instruct patient about precautions for thrombocytopenia and to monitor for bleeding from gums, epistaxis, hematuria, hematemesis, and a change in stool color.
6. Have anaphylaxis kit at bedside, containing epinephrine, diphenhydramine, cimetidine/ranitidine, an Ambu bag, and hydrocortisone.
7. Counsel patients about probability of alopecia.
8. Make sure a new IV line is inserted peripherally prior to administration of docetaxel.
9. Instruct patient about signs and symptoms of phlebitis.

References:
1. Bissett D, Setanoians A, Cassidy J, et al. Phase I and pharmacokinetic study of taxotere administered as a 24-hour infusion. Cancer Res 1993;53:523–527.
2. Bruno R, Sanderink GJ. Pharmacokinetics and metabolism of taxotere (docetaxel). Cancer Surv 1993;17:305–313.
3. Fumoleau P, Chevallier B, Kerbrat P, et al. Current status of taxotere (docetaxel) as a new treatment in breast cancer. Breast Cancer Res Treat 1995;33:39–46.
4. Kaye SB. Docetaxel (Taxotere) in the treatment of solid tumors other than breast and lung cancer. Semin Oncol 1995;22(2 Suppl 4):30–33.
5. Pazdur R, Kudelka AP, Kavanagh JJ, et al. The taxoids: paclitaxel (Taxol®) and docetaxel (Taxotere®). Cancer Treat Rev 1993;19:351–386.
6. Piccart MJ, Gore M, Ten Bokkel Huiniuk, et al. Docetaxel: an active drug for the treatment of advanced epithelial ovarian. J Natl Canc Inst 1995;87:676–681.
7. Taxotere® Product Information. Rhone-Poulenc Rorer Pharmaceuticals, Inc., May 1996.

DOXORUBICIN HCl

Other Names:
Adriamycin®, Rubex®, hydroxydaunorubicin.

Uses:
Sarcoma, adenocarcinoma, melanoma, lymphoma, leukemia, non-Hodgkin's lymphoma, Hodgkin's disease, breast cancer, ovarian cancer, transitional cell bladder carcinoma, thyroid carcinoma, gastric carcinoma, and small-cell lung cancer. Doxorubicin may also be useful

in multiple myeloma, Kaposi's sarcoma, cervical cancer, pancreatic cancer, and testicular carcinoma.

Mechanism of Antitumor Action:
Doxorubicin intercalates between base pairs in the DNA double helix and inhibits DNA topoisomerase I and II.

Pharmacokinetics:

Absorption: After intraperitoneal administration of doxorubicin, systemic absorption is 10-fold lower than after a 60 mg IV dose.

Distribution: Doxorubicin is rapidly distributed in body tissues.

Protein Binding: Doxorubicin is 75% bound to plasma proteins, principally albumin.

Metabolism: Doxorubicin is metabolized extensively in the liver to glucuronide conjugates and the hydroxylated metabolite doxorubicinol.

Half-life: 30 to 40 hours.

Elimination: Only 5 to 10% of doxorubicin is excreted in the urine. The drug is primarily excreted in bile and feces, accounting for about 40% of the administered dose.

Drug Interactions:
Several potential drug interactions may occur with doxorubicin, but only a few are well documented in humans, including ***alfa interferon, cimetidine, ranitidine, streptozocin, dexrazoxane,*** and ***verapamil***. The disposition of doxorubicin is altered with concurrently administered ***alfa-interferon*** or ***streptozocin,*** resulting in increased toxicity. The ***H_2-antagonists*** decrease doxorubicin metabolism by inhibiting cytochrome P450, and may increase the toxicity of the drug. ***Verapamil*** increases the Vd and half-life of doxorubicin and decreases its clearance. ***Dexrazoxane*** inhibits doxorubicin–iron complexation as well as the formation of oxygen radicals, both of which may protect against myocardial toxicity.

Dosage:

Single agent: 60 to 90 mg/m^2 IV every 3 weeks.

Combination therapy: 45 to 60 mg/m^2 IV every 3 weeks.

Weekly IV injections: 20 mg/m^2.

Continuous infusion: 60 to 90 mg/m^2 IV given over a period of 96 hours.

Maximum lifetime cumulative dose is 550 mg/m^2: If radiation is involved, 450 mg/m^2 is the recommended lifetime dose.

Dose modification:

Bilirubin Level	% of Full Dose
<1.2 mg/dL	100
1.2–3 mg/dL	50
>3 mg/dL	25

Dose Forms:
Doxorubicin HCl is available in 10, 20, 50, 100 and 150 mg vials at various brands.

Administration:

Intravenous: Dilute in D5W and/or NS. Solutions that will not be used within 8 hours of reconstitution should be protected from light (these solutions are stable for several weeks). Push or bolus doses may be given over a 3- to 10-minute period in the side arm of a free-flowing IV line. Continuous infusions should be given only via a central line. Heparin locks are not recommended, since doxorubicin is incompatible with heparin.

Intraarterial: For regional perfusion

Topical bladder instillation: This has been used for superficial bladder cancer.

Compatibilities: In a concentration of 0.2 mg/mL in D5W, doxorubicin is compatible with chlorpromazine HCl, cimetidine HCl, dexamethasone sodium phosphate, diphenhydramine HCl, droperidol, famotidine, furosemide, heparin sodium, hydromorphone HCl, lorazepam, methylprednisolone sodium succinate, metoclopramide HCl, morphine sulfate, prochlorperazine edisylate, promethazine HCl, and ranitidine HCl.

In a concentration of 2 mg/ml, doxorubicin is compatible with bleomycin sulfate, cisplatin, cyclophosphamide, droperidol, filgrastim, fludarabine phosphate, fluorouracil, leucovorin calcium, melphalan HCl, methotrexate sodium, metoclopramide HCl, mitomycin, ondansetron HCl, paclitaxel, sargramostim, vinblastine sulfate, vincristine sulfate, and vinorelbine tartate.

Incompatibilities: In a concentration of 2 mg/mL, doxorubicin is incompatible with allopurinol sodium, cefepime HCl, furosemide, gallium nitrate, heparin sodium, and piperacillin sodium–tazobactam sodium.

In a concentration of 0.2 mg/mL, doxorubicin is incompatible with ganciclovir sodium.

Doxorubicin admixed with the following drugs in solution are incompatible: aminophylline, cephalothin sodium, dexamethasone sodium phosphate, diazepam, hydrocortisone sodium succinate, furosemide, heparin sodium, and fluorouracil.

Adverse Reactions:

 Hematologic: Myelosuppression is the dose limiting toxicity of doxorubicin. Leukopenia is maximum at 10 to 14 days, with recovery by day 21. Thrombocytopenia is rarely severe ($<50,000/mm^3$).

 Dermatologic: Local skin and deep tissue damage occurs with extravasations. Alopecia is common but reversible 3 months after discontinuation of doxorubicin.

 Cardiotoxicity: Acute electrocardiographic changes occur within 24 hours after the beginning of doxorubicin treatment. These are not dose related, and last about a day. Most of these arrhythmias are asymptomatic. Delayed cardiomyopathy is dose related and presents as a syndrome identical to classic congestive heart failure. It is usually irreversible, but its symptoms can be managed with standard medical therapy.

 Gastrointestinal: Nausea and vomiting are common but moderately severe, and can usually be controlled with prophylactic antiemetics. Mucositis may occur, especially with daily or continuous infusion regimens.

 Urinary: Within 24 hours of administration of doxorubicin, the urine may turn reddish-orange because of the urinary excretion of the drug. This effect disappears within 24 hours after discontinuation of the drug.

Practitioner Interventions:

1. Monitor patient's complete blood cell count (CBC) and platelet count on a weekly basis.
2. Initiate a new IV line prior to initiating therapy, in order to prevent extravasation.
3. Evaluate the patient's electrocardiogram prior to initiating therapy with doxorubicin.
4. Check patient's ejection fraction prior to dosing.
5. Evaluate liver function; reduce dose in cases of elevated bilirubin.
6. Instruct patient about risk of total alopecia.
7. Keep an ongoing tabulation of total doxorubicin dosage; do not exceed 550 mg/m^2 lifetime dose.
8. Extravasation management. (refer to Table 1.2, pg. 223–225)
   a. Stop infusion immediately and do not remove needle.
   b. Aspirate as much extravasant as possible.
   c. Notify physician.
   d. Instill antidote per institutional protocol.

References:

1. Benjamin RS, Riggs CE, Baschur NR. Plasma pharmacokinetics of adriamycin and its metabolites in human with normal hepatic and renal function. Cancer Res 1977;37:1416–1420.
2. Dorr RT. Antidotes to vesicant chemotherapy extravasations. Blood Rev 1990;4:41–60.
3. Garnick MB, Weiss GR, Stelle GD dr, et al. Clinical evaluation of long-term, continuous-infusion doxorubicin. Cancer Treat Rep 1983;67:133–142.

DOXORUBICIN HCL, LIPOSOMAL

Other Names:
Doxil®.

Uses:
Kaposi's sarcoma.

Mechanism of Antitumor Action:
Liposomal doxorubicin binds DNA to inhibit nucleic acid synthesis.

Pharmacokinetics:

Absorption: Liposomal doxorubicin is administered only by the IV route.

Distribution: In contrast to the very large Vd (volume of distribution) of doxorubicin HCl (20-30 L/kg), liposomal doxorubicin has a small Vd ($2L/m^2$), indicating that it is mainly confined to the vascular fluid compartment.

Protein Binding: Unknown, but the protein binding of doxorubicin is about 70%.

Metabolism: Doxorubicinol is the primary metabolite of doxorubicin, but it appeared only in very small concentrations after Doxil® administration.

Half-life: After doses of 10 to 20 mg/m^2, Doxil® has two distribution half-lives, of 5 and 55 hours, respectively.

Elimination: The plasma clearance of Doxil® is 0.041 $L/hr/m^2$, in contrast to that of doxorubicin, which is 24-35 $L/h/m^2$.

Drug Interactions:
Drug interactions between Doxil® and antiviral agents have not been evaluated.

Dosage:
The standard starting dose of Doxil® is 20 mg/m^2 IV every 3 weeks. The dose should be adjusted in patients with liver dysfunction. Serum bilirubin measurement is recommended prior to chemotherapy. If the serum bilirubin is 1.2 to 3.0 mg/dL, the dose of Doxil® should be decreased by 50%; if the serum bilirubin is >3.0 mg/dL, the dose should be decreased by 75%.

Dose Forms:
Doxil® is available in a 20 mg/10 mL vial.

Administration:
Doxil® is given as an IV infusion in 250 mL of D5W over a period of 30 minutes. Diluted Doxil® should be refrigerated and given within 24 hours after preparation. In-line filters should not be used because they may alter the characteristics of Doxil®.

Compatibilities: Doxil® should not be mixed with other drugs or with the preservative benzyl alcohol.

Incompatibilities: Not determined to date.

Adverse Reactions:

Hematologic: Myelosuppression is the dose-limiting toxicity of Doxil®. Leukopenia is most severe at 10 to 14 days, with recovery by day 21. Thrombocytopenia is rarely severe ($<$50,000/mm^3). About 6% of patients develop a nadir of less than 500 neutrophils/mL.

Dermatologic: Doxil® is an irritant in animal studies, but does cause as severe a local human skin reaction as doxorubicin solutions. Caution should be taken not to extravasate Doxil®. Only transient erythema, tenderness, and edema were noted about the infusion site in several cases of Doxil® extravasation. Alopecia is common but reversible 3 months after discontinuation of Doxil®. Palmar–plantar erythrodysethesia is uncommon, occurring in about 1% of patients. This can be a very problematic manifestation of skin toxicity from Doxil®. Local therapy includes the use of topical steroids and moisturizing lotions.

Cardiotoxicity: Long-term cardiac effects of Doxil® have not been adequately compared to those with conventional doxorubicin HCl therapy. Cardiac events definitely related to Doxil® have been reported in about 4% of treated patients. Only 1% were considered severe cardiac events. Acute electrocardiographic changes occur within 24 hours. These are not dose-related, and last about a day. Most of these arrhythmias are asymptomatic. Delayed cardiomyopathy is dose related and presents as a syndrome identical to classic congestive heart failure. The cardiomyopathy is usually irreversible, but symptoms can be managed with standard medical therapy.

Gastrointestinal: Nausea and vomiting are uncommon and mild, occurring in about 18% of patients. Conventional antiemetics are effective in preventing emesis from Doxil®. Mucositis occurs in about 7% of patients.

Urinary: Within 24 hours of administration of Doxil®, the urine may turn reddish-orange because of the urinary excretion of the parent compound, doxorubicin. This effect disappears within 24 hours after the administration of the drug.

Acute infusion-associated reactions: Reactions such as flushing, shortness of breath, facial swelling, headache, chills, back pain, and hypotension occur in about 7% of patients and may be infusion-rate-related. Slowing or discontinuing of the infusion results in resolution over the course of several hours to a day.

Practitioner Interventions:

1. Monitor patient's complete blood cell count (CBC) and platelet count on a weekly basis.
2. Initiate new IV infusion prior to initiating therapy with Doxil® in order to prevent extravasation.
3. Evaluate patient's electrocardiogram prior to initiating therapy.
4. Check patient's baseline cardiac ejection fraction prior to dosing with Doxil®.
5. Evaluate liver function; reduce dose in case of elevated bilirubin.
6. Instruct patient about risk of total alopecia and orange-colored urine.
7. Keep an ongoing tabulation of total doxorubicin dosage; do not exceed 550 mg/m² lifetime dose. The total lifetime anthracycline dose should take into account any previous or concomitant therapy with related drugs such as daunorubicin or epirubicin.
8. Instruct the patient about palmar–plantar erythema; use moisturizers initially, then progress to topical hydrocortisone as needed. Pain management may be needed for more severe cases.
9. Monitor for local extravasation. For extravasation:
   - Stop infusion immediately and do not remove needle.
   - Aspirate as much vesicant as possible.
   - Apply an ice pack for 15 minutes four times daily for 2 days.
10. Infusions of Doxil® should be given over a minimum of 30 minutes. If the patient experiences flushing, shortness of breath, or facial swelling, the infusion should be discontinued until the symptoms subside, and should be reinstituted at half the infusion rate.
11. Have an anaphylaxis kit at the bedside, consisting of hydrocortisone, diphenhydramine, epinephrine, and an Ambu bag.

References:
1. Doxil® Product Information. Sequus Pharmaceuticals, Inc., November 1995.
2. Harrison M, Tomlinson D, Stewart S. Liposomal-entrapped doxorubicin: an active agent in AIDS-related Kaposi sarcoma. J Clin Oncol 1995;13: 914–920.
3. Madhavan S, Northfelt DW. Lack of vesicant injury following extravasation of liposomal doxorubicin. J Natl Cancer Inst 1995;87:1556–1557.

ERYTHROPOIETIN

Other Names:
Procrit®, Epogen®, Epoetin alfa, EPO.

Uses:
Erythropoietin is an endogenous glycoprotein that stimulates red cell (erythrocyte) production. Synthetic recombinant erythropoietin is used in cancer patients receiving chemotherapy who develop anemia. It is also used to treat anemia in zidovudine-treated human immuno-deficiency virus (HIV)-infected patients.

Mechanism of Action:
Erythropoietin has no antitumor activity. Its major effect is to stimulate erythrocyte synthesis and proliferation.

Pharmacokinetics:

Absorption: Because erythropoietin is a protein, it is degraded rapidly in the gastrointestinal tract and poorly absorbed. Thus, it must be given parenterally, either by the IV or SC route. Systemic absorption is delayed and incomplete after SC injection, but produces low, sustained levels compared to IV injection. Absorption is greater following SC injection into the thigh than after SC administration into the arm or abdomen.

Distribution: Erythropoietin has an apparent Vd of about plasma volume. The drug may accumulate after multiple SC doses due to delayed, prolonged systemic absorption.

Protein Binding: None.

Metabolism: The metabolism of recombinant erythropoietin is unclear. Hepatic metabolism causes desialylation and removal of oligosaccharide side chains. Bone marrow may also catabolize erythropoietin.

Half-life: 4 to 13 hours.

Elimination: About 10% of erythropoietin is eliminated in the urine in unchanged form. Elimination of desialylated drug occurs in the kidney, bone marrow, and spleen. Renal failure does not affect the elimination of erythropoietin. Erythropoietin is not hemodialyzable.

Drug Interactions:
There are no known drug interactions of erythropoietin.

Dosage:
The usual dosage in cancer patients is 150 units/kg three times per week for about 8 weeks. If patients do not respond with increasing hematocrit or reducing transfusion requirements in 2 weeks, the dosage may be increased to 300 units/kg three times weekly.

Dose Forms:
Erythropoietin is available in 2,000, 3,000, 4,000, and 10,000 units in 1 mL vials and 20,000 units in 2 mL vials.

Administration:
Erythropoietin may be administered IV over a period of 2 to 3 minutes, or SC.

Compatibilities: Not tested.

Incompatibilities: Not tested.

Adverse Reactions:
There have been no major adverse reactions to erythropoietin noted in cancer patients. While not common in cancer patients, hypertension occasionally occurs and patients' blood pressure should be monitored periodically.

Although seizures and thromboses have been reported in cancer patients receiving erythropoietin, adverse effects may have been attributable to the progression of disease. Local pain on injection is common. Occasionally, patients may complain of nausea, vomiting, diarrhea, fever, asthenia, fatigue, dizziness, and parasthesia. A clear association with these adverse effects has not been established for erythropoietin.

Practitioner Interventions:

1. Monitor patient's complete blood cell count (CBC) weekly. If the hematocrit rises by 4% over a 2-week period, the dose of erythropoietin should be decreased. If the hematocrit reaches 36%, erythropoietin may be discontinued.
2. Monitor patient's blood pressure weekly.

3. Instruct patient about self-injection technique and appropriate needle disposal procedure.
4. Instruct patient to use an injection-site chart and calendar to note site of injection and day of injection.
5. Monitor patient for any signs and symptoms of erythema, pain, or edema at injection sites.

References:
1. Markham A, Bryson HM. Epoetin alfa: A review of its pharmacodynamic and pharmacokinetic properties and therapeutic use in non-renal applications. Drugs 1995;a49:232–254.
2. Oster W, Herrman F, Gamm H, Zeile G, et al. Erythropoietin for the treatment of anemia of malignancy associated with neoplastic bone marrow infiltration. J Clin Oncol 1990;8:956–962.

ESTRAMUSTINE PHOSPHATE

Other Names:
Estracyte®, Emcyt®.

Uses:
Advanced prostate carcinoma.

Mechanism of Antitumor Action:
Estramustine may have estrogenic effects in tissues dependent on hormones. It may also cause anti-microtubule disassembly, as demonstrated by metaphase arrest of tumor cells *in vitro*.

Pharmacokinetics:

Absorption: 75% after oral administration.

Distribution: Unknown, but should be large because of high protein binding of estramustine phosphate.

Protein Binding: Unknown, but probably large because of hormone side chain of estramustine phosphate.

Metabolism: Hepatic metabolism includes glucuronidation and dephosphorylation of the steroid component.

Half-life: 20 to 24 hours.

Elimination: Only 23% of the recovered dose of estramustine phosphate is in the urine. Biliary and fecal excretion of metabolites have been demonstrated.

Drug Interactions:

Vinblastine plus estramustine produce synergistic cytotoxicity in human prostate cancer cells *in vitro.*

Dosage:

The usual oral dose of estramustine phosphate is 560 mg per day in divided doses. The maximum dose is 1,120 mg per day.

Dose Forms:

Emcyt® is available as 140 mg capsules.

Administration:

Oral administration of capsules with meals or with antacids.

Adverse Reactions:

Gastrointestinal: Nausea and vomiting may occur within 2 hours of administration of estramustine phosphate. The severity is mild and the condition responds to conventional antiemetics. Diarrhea has been reported in about 25% of patients.

Gynecologic: A wide range of incidences of gynecomastia have been reported, but the incidence averages about 50% of patients treated, due to the estrogen component of estramustine phosphate.

Cardiovascular: Cardiovascular complications are rare but include congestive heart failure (due to the sodium retention of the estrogen), thromboembolism, and ischemic effects.

Practitioner Interventions:

1. Administer antiemetic therapy 30 minutes prior to estramustine phosphate.

2. Counsel patients about risk of gynecomastia. Instruct patient to notify physician if breast enlargement occurs.
3. Monitor patients for signs and symptoms of heart failure and edema.

References:
1. Stearns ME, Tev KD. Antimicrotubule effects of estramustin, an antiprostatic tumor drug. Cancer Res 1985;45:3891–3897.
2. Yamanaka H, Shimazaki J, Imaik, et al. Effect of Estracyt® on the rat prostate. Invest Urol 1977;14:400–404.

ETOPOSIDE

Other Names:
VePesid®, VP-16.

Uses:
Testicular carcinoma, small-cell lung cancer, non-small-cell lung cancer, lymphoma, Hodgkin's disease, leukemia (nonlymphocytic), multiple myeloma.

Mechanism of Antitumor Action:
Etoposide interacts with topoisomerase-II to stabilize a topoisomerase–DNA complex, blocking strand-passing activity and cell progression out of the G_2 phase of the cell cycle. Thus, DNA breakage occurs, and is characterized by chromatid exchanges.

Pharmacokinetics:

Absorption: The bioavailability of etoposide in gelatin capsules is about 50%.

Distribution: Not fully characterized. Etoposide rapidly distributes into body fluids. The apparent Vd averages 25% of body weight. The major metabolite (the *trans*-hydroxy acid) distributes into the body water.

Protein Binding: 95% of etoposide is protein bound, principally to albumin. The percentage of unbound drug ranges from 6 to 37% among patients. Decreased albumin and bilirubin levels result in higher free fractions and a greater degree of myelosuppression.

Metabolism: Hydroxy acids are formed, but are much less active than the parent compound.

Half-life: The $T_{1/2}\alpha$ is 0.6 to 2 hours. The $T_{1/2}$ terminal $= 3$ to 19 hours. The half-life of etoposide may be prolonged in patients with elevated bilirubin levels.

Elimination: Etoposide undergoes hepatic metabolism and excretion in bile/feces (2%) and urine (about 50%) within 72 hours after IV administration. Between 5 and 25% is excreted in urine after oral administration.

Drug Interactions:

High dose *cyclosporine* (serum concentrations >2000 ng/mL) decreases the clearance and increases the volume of distribution of etoposide leading to increased leukopenia. *Ritovir* increases the serum concentration of etoposide resulting in enhanced toxicity.

Dosage:

Testicular cancer: 50 to 100 mg/m^2 IV daily for 5 days, or 100 mg/m^2 on days 1, 3, and 5. Repeat cycles every 3 weeks.

Small Cell Lung Cancer: 35 to 50 mg/m^2 IV daily for 4 or 5 days.

Oral Dosing: Twice the IV dose, rounded to the nearest 50 mg.

Dosage in Renal or Hepatic Impairment: Criteria for dose adjustment of etoposide are not established. One group suggests a 50% reduction of the dose in patients with a serum bilirubin of 1.5 to 3.0 mg/dL; a 75% reduction with a serum bilirubin of 3.1 to 4.9 mg/dL; and no drug in cases of a bilirubin greater than 5 mg/dL (Perry 1982). In patients with creatinine clearances of 60, 45, and 30 mL/min, etoposide doses may be reduced to 25, 20, and 15%, respectively. (Anderson, 1976; Joel 1991; Joel 1993). The dose may be decreased by 25 to 30% in patients with low serum albumin levels (< 3.5 mg/dL).

Dose Forms:

VePesid® is available in 20 mg/5 mL vials and 50 mg capsules.

Administration:

Do not give etoposide by rapid IV injection. Administer diluted solution over a period of 30 to 60 minutes for usual doses. Concentrations of 0.2 and 0.4 mg/mL are stable for 96 and 48 hours, respectively. Although concentrations > 0.4 mg/mL are not recommended because of instability, some high-dose regimens may require concentrations greater than 0.4 mg/mL, in order to decrease the amount of fluid to administer. These solutions should be made immediately prior to administration.

Undiluted etoposide may be administered over a period of 4 to 6 hours with periodic monitoring of vital signs (i.e. blood pressure, pulse).

Compatibilities: In a concentration of 0.2 to 0.4 mg/mL in NS, etoposide is compatible with carboplatin cisplatin, cyclophosphamide, cytarabine, daunorubicin, floxuridine, fluorouracil, and ifosfamide.

In simulated Y-site infusion of 0.4 mg/mL in NS, etoposide is compatible with allopurinol sodium, melphalan HCl, ondansetron HCl, sargramostim, and vinorelbine tartrate.

In simulated Y-site infusion of 0.4 mg/mL in D5W, etoposide is compatible with fludarabine phosphate, ondansetron HCl, paclitaxel, and piperacillin sodium–tazobactam sodium.

Incompatibilities: Cefepime HCl, filgrastim, gallium nitrate, idarubicin HCl.

Adverse Reactions:

 Hematologic: Bone marrow suppression is dose limiting. Leukopenia is greater than thrombocytopenia. Nadir 14-16 days; recovery by day 21.

 Gastrointestinal: Nausea and vomiting occur in about 35% of patients and are usually mild to moderate.

 Cardiovascular: Hypotension occurs in about 2% of patients during IV infusion.

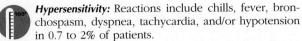 *Hypersensitivity:* Reactions include chills, fever, bronchospasm, dyspnea, tachycardia, and/or hypotension in 0.7 to 2% of patients.

 Alopecia: The average incidence is about 30% (8 to 66%) and the condition appears to be dose related.

 Chemical phlebitis: Rare, although etoposide is not a vesicant. Hyaluronidase has been effective as treatment in an animal model.

Neurologic: Peripheral neuropathy is uncommon (1 to 3% of patients). Peripheral signs include paresthesia. CNS side effects is dose related and includes somnolence, fatigue, headache, and mental confusion.

 Ocular: Transient cortical blindness, and optic neuritis are rare.

Practitioner Interventions:

1. Etoposide must be diluted before administration to a concentration not exceeding 0.4 mg/mL, except in investigational protocols.

2. Administer usual doses over a period of at least 30 minutes. Doses > 200 mg/m^2 may require slower infusion.

3. Monitor patient's blood pressure every 15 minutes for the first 30 minutes of dosing, then every hour.

4. Check injection site for signs of phlebitis.

5. Premedicate patient with antiemetics 30 minutes before start of infusion.

6. Counsel patients regarding risk of second malignancy.

References:

1. Anderson RJ, Gambertoglio JG, Schrier RW. Clinical Use of Drugs in Renal Failure. Charles C Thomas; Springfield, 1976, pp. 15-17.
2. Fleming RA, Miller AA, Stewart CF. Etoposide: An update. Clin Pharm 1989;8:274–293.
3. Joel S, Clark P, Slevin M. Renal function and etoposide pharmacokinetics: Is dose modification necessary? Proc Am Soc Clin Oncol 1991;10–103.
4. Joel SP, Shah R, Slevin ML. Etoposide dosage and pharmacodynamics. Cancer Chemother Pharmacol 1994;34(Suppl):569–575.
5. O'Dwyer RJ, Leyland-Jones B, Alonso MT, et al. Etoposide, current status of an active anticancer drug. N Engl J Med 1985;312:692–700.
6. Perry MC. Hepatotoxicity of chemotherapeutic agents. Semin Oncol 1982;9:65–74.

ETOPOSIDE PHOSPHATE

Other Names:
Etopophos®.

Uses:
Testicular carcinoma and small-cell lung cancer.

Mechanism of Antitumor Action:
Etoposide phosphate is a water-soluble prodrug of etoposide, and must be dephosphorylated to etoposide to become active. After activated, etoposide interacts with topoisomerase-II to stabilize a topoisomerase–DNA complex, blocking strand-passing activity and cell progression out of the G_2 phase of the cell cycle. Thus, DNA breakage occurs, and is characterized by chromatid exchanges.

Pharmacokinetics:

Absorption: Etoposide phosphate is only given IV.

Distribution: Not fully characterized. Etoposide phosphate rapidly distributes into body fluids with a Vd between 7 and 17 L/m^2. The major metabolite (the *trans*-hydroxy acid) distributes into the body water.

Protein Binding: 95% of etoposide phosphate is protein bound, principally to albumin. The unbound drug ranges from 6 to 37% among patients. Decreased albumin and bilirubin levels result in higher free fractions and a greater degree of myelosuppression.

Metabolism: Hydroxy acids are formed, but are much less active than the parent compound. O-demethylation occurs in the liver through cytochrome P450 3A4.

Half-life: The $T_{1/2}\alpha$ is 0.6 to 2 hrs. The $T_{1/2}$ terminal = 3 to 19 hrs. The half-life may be prolonged in patients with elevated bilirubin levels.

Elimination: Etoposide phosphate undergoes hepatic metabolism and excretion in bile/feces (2%) and urine (about 12%) within 72 hours after IV administration.

Drug Interactions:
High dose **cyclosporine** (serum concentrations >2000 ng/mL) decreases the clearance and increases the volume of distribution of etoposide leading to increased leukopenia. **Ritovir** increases the serum concentration of etoposide resulting in enhanced toxicity.

Dose:

Testicular Cancer: 50 to 100 mg/m^2 IV daily for 5 days, or 100 mg/m^2 on days 1, 3, and 5. Repeat cycles every 3 weeks.

Small Cell Lung Cancer: 35 to 50 mg/m^2 IV daily for 4 or 5 days.

Dosage in Renal or Hepatic Impairment: Criteria for dose adjustment are not established. One group suggests a 50% reduction of dose size in patients with a serum bilirubin of 1.5 to 3.0 mg/dL; 75% reduction with serum bilirubin of 3.1 to 4.9 mg/dL; and no drug in cases of a bilirubin greater than 5 mg/dL (Perry, 1982). In patients with a creatinine clearance of >50 mL/min, 100% of the dose is given, and in those with creatinine clearances between 15 and 50 ml/min, 75% of the dose is given.

Dosage Forms:
Vials containing etoposide phosphate equivalent to 100 mg etoposide are available for parenteral use.

Administration:
Unlike etoposide, Etopophos® (etoposide phosphate) is highly water soluble, can be prepared in high concentration, does not precipitate in solution, and may be given by bolus injection. It may be given over a period of 5 to 210 minutes. Solutions of Etopophos® in concentrations ranging from 0.1 to 22 mg/mL in D5W or 0.9% NaCl are stable for 24 hours.

Incompatibilities: Cefepime HCl, filgrastim, gallium nitrate, idarubicin HCl.

Adverse Reactions:

Hematologic: Bone marrow suppression is the dose-limiting toxicity of etoposide phosphate. Leukopenia is more severe than thrombocytopenia, with cell counts reaching a nadir at 14 to 16 days and recovery by day 21.

Gastrointestinal: Nausea and vomiting occur in about 35% of patients, and are usually mild to moderate.

Cardiovascular: Hypotension occurs in about 4% of patients during IV infusion of etoposide phosphate.

Hypersensitivity/anaphylactoid: Reactions, chills, fever, bronchospasm, dyspnea, tachycardia, and/or hypotension occur in 0.7 to 2% of patients.

Alopecia: The average incidence is about 30% (8 to 66%), and appears to be dose related.

Chemical phlebitis: Rare, although etoposide phosphate is not a vesicant. Hyaluronidase has been effective as treatment in an animal model.

Neurologic: Peripheral neuropathy is uncommon (1 to 3% of patients). Peripheral signs include paresthesia. CNS side effects include somnolence, fatigue, headache, and mental confusion.

Ocular: Transient cortical blindness and optic neuritis are rare.

Practitioner Interventions:

1. Initiate a new intravenous site prior to starting infusion of etoposide phosphate.
2. The patient's blood pressure should be checked at 15 to 30 minutes after the start of an infusion of etoposide phosphate. If clinically significant hypotension occurs, appropriate supportive measures should be taken.
3. Hypersensitivity/anaphylactic reactions should be managed with cessation of the infusion. Have an anaphylaxis kit of corticosteroid, antihistamine, an Ambu bag, and volume expanders available at the bedside.
4. Check the injection site for signs of phlebitis.

References:

1. Anderson RJ, Gambertoglio JG, Schrier RW. Clinical use of drugs in renal failure. Charles C Thomas, Springfield, 1976, pp. 15–17.
2. Etopophos® Product Information. Bristol Laboratories, May 1996.
3. Fleming RA, Miller AA, Stewart CF. Etoposide: An update. Clin Pharm 1989;8:274–293.
4. Hainsworth JD, Levitan N, Wampler GL, et al. Phase II randomized study of cisplatin plus etoposide phosphate or etoposide in the treatment of small cell lung cancer. J Clin Oncol 1995;13:1336–1342.

5. Joel S, Clark P, Slevin M. Renal function and etoposide pharmacokinetics: Is dose modification necessary? Proc Am Soc Clin Oncol 1991;10–103.
6. Joel SP, Shah R, Slevin ML. Etoposide dosage and pharmacodynamics. Cancer Chemother Pharmacol 1994;34(Suppl):569–575.
7. O'Dwyer RJ, Leyland-Jones B, Alonso MT, et al. Etoposide, current status of an active anticancer drug. N Engl J Med 1985;312:692–700.
8. Perry MC. Hepatotoxicity of chemotherapeutic agents. Semin Oncol 1982;9:65–74.

FILGRASTIM

Other Names:
Neupogen®, G-CSF.

Uses:
To decrease the incidence of infection in patients who are receiving chemotherapy. Filgrastim may also be effective as a rescue treatment for aplastic anemia, cyclic neutropenia, congenital neutropenia, and myelodysplastic disorders. It also reduces neutropenia following bone marrow transplantation, and is additionally used to augment peripheral-blood stem-cell mobilization.

Mechanism of Antitumor Action:
Filgrastim enhances the proliferation, differentiation, and activation of granulocyte progenitor cells. Both neutrophil chemotaxis and phagocytosis are increased in the presence of filgrastim.

Pharmacokinetics:

Absorption: Filgrastim is not absorbed systemically when given orally. After SC administration, the drug is absorbed systemically and peaks 4 to 8 hours after administration.

Distribution: Filgrastim distributes into blood and bone marrow.

Protein Binding: Unknown.

Metabolism: Filgrastim is metabolized in the liver and kidney, but is unaffected by hepatic or renal dysfunction.

Half-life: The elimination half-life ranges from 3 to 5 hours.

Elimination: Unknown. It is postulated that filgastrim may be cleared by receptor-mediated mechanisms (neutrophilic endocytosis and degradation).

Drug Interactions:
None reported to date.

Dosage
The usual dose of filgrastim for chemotherapy-induced neutropenia is 5 μg/kg daily, given SC, beginning 1 to 5 days after chemotherapy and continuing for 14 days or until the absolute neutrophil count reaches 5,000 to 10,000/mm^3. Some institutions round off the dose to a full vial size (300 μg or 480 μg daily) in order to minimize wastage.

The dose for other indications, such as chronic neutropenia or myelodysplastic disorders, is currently being investigated. In acquired immune deficiency syndrome (AIDS)-related neutropenia, the dose of filgrastim may be as low as 1 μg/kg daily.

Dose Forms:
Neupogen® is available in 300 μg (1 mL) and 480 μg (1.6 mL) vials.

Administration:
Filgrastim is usually given as an SC injection once daily. It has also been given as a 24-hour continuous SC infusion in 10 mL of D5W.

Filgrastim may also be given as an IV infusion over a period of 15 to 30 minutes in D5W. When the drug is diluted to concentrations of 5 to 15 μg/mL, normal serum albumin should be added to a concentration of 2 mg/mL. Filgrastim at concentrations >15 μg/mL does not require the addition of albumin.

Compatibilities: Simulated Y-site infusions of filgrastim at a 30 μg/mL concentration in D5W are compatible with the following:

Cytotoxic drugs: Bleomycin sulfate, carboplatin, carmustine, cisplatin, cyclophosphamide, cytarabine, dacarbazine, daunorubicin HCl, doxorubicin HCl, methotrexate sodium, mitoxantrone HCl, plicamycin, streptozocin, vinblastine sulfate, vincristine sulfate, and vinorelbine tartrate.

Noncytoxic drugs: acyclovir sodium, allopurinol sodium, amikacin sodium, aminophylline, ampicillin sodium, ampicillin sodium-sulbactam sodium, aztreonam, bumetanide, butorphanol tartrate, calcium gluconate, cefazolin sodium, cefotetan disodium, ceftazidime, chlorpromazine HCl, cimetidine HCl, dexamethasone sodium phosphate, diphenhydramine HCl, doxycycline hyclate, droperidol, enalaprilat, famotidine, fluconazole, gallium nitrate, ganciclovir sodium, gentamicin sulfate, haloperidol lactate, hydrocortisone sodium phosphate, hydrocortisone sodium succinate, hydromorphone HCl, hydroxyzine HCl, imipenem-cilastatin sodium, leucovorin calcium, lorazepam, meperidine HCl, mesna, metoclopramide HCl, netilmicin sulfate, ondansetron HCl, potassium chloride, promethazine HCl, ranitidine HCl, sodium bicarbonate, ticarcillin disodium, ticarcillin disodium–clavulanate potassium, tobramycin sulfate, trimethoprim-sulfamethoxazole, vancomycin HCl, and zidovudine.

Incompatibilities: Simulated Y-site infusion of filgrastim in a concentration of 30 μg/mL of D5W is incompatible with amphotericin B, cefepime HCl, cefonicid sodium, cefoperazone sodium, cefotaxime sodium, cefoxitin sodium, ceftizoxime sodium, ceftriaxone sodium, cefuroxime sodium, clindamycin phosphate, dactinomycin, etoposide, fluorouracil, furosemide, heparin sodium, mannitol, methylprednisolone sodium succinate, metronidazole, mezlocillin, mitomycin, piperacillin sodium, prochlorperazine edisylate, sodium chloride 0.9%, and thiotepa.

Adverse Reactions:

Bone Pain: Expansion of neutrophils within the bone marrow may lead to bone pain, particularly in medullary and iliac regions. This occurs in about 20% of patients treated with filgrastim and may be more common after IV dosing.

 Hypersensitivity: Rare cases of anaphylaxis have been reported.

Hepatic: Transient elevation of lactate dehydrogenase and alkaline phosphatase have been reported.

Neutrophilia: High levels of neutrophils ($>40,000/mm^3$) are common in patients receiving continued therapy with filgrastim after attaining normal levels of neutrophils. Fever and chills are occasionally reported.

Practitioner Interventions:

1. Administer SC injections of filgrastim at different sites.
2. Observe patient for bone pain. May use acetaminophen for control of bone pain.
3. Monitor patient's neutrophil count daily.
4. Discontinue filgrastim after neutrophils have attained a level of $5,000/mm^3$. In stem-cell mobilization, higher neutrophil counts are desired.
5. IV solutions of filgrastim should be made up only in D5W.
6. Instruct patient in self injection techniques and appropriate disposal methods.

References:

1. Crawford J, Ozer H, Stoller R, et al. Reduction of granulocyte colony stimulating factor of fever and neutropenia induced by chemotherapy in patients with small cell lung cancer. N Engl J Med 1991;315:164–170.
2. Hollingshead LM, Goa KL. Recombinant granulocyte colony stimulating factor (rG-CSF): A review of its pharmacologic properties and prospective role in neutropenic conditions. Drugs 1991;42:300–330.
3. Morstyn G, Campbell L, Lieschke G, et al. Treatment of chemotherapy-induced neutropenia by subcutaneously administered granulocyte colony-stimulating factor with optimization of dose and duration of therapy. J Clin Oncol 1989;7:1554–1562.
4. Ohno R, Tomonaga M, Robayashi T, et al. Effect of granulocyte-stimulating factor after intensive induction therapy in relapsed or refractory acute leukemia. N Engl J Med 1990;323:871–877.

FLOXURIDINE

Other Names:
FUDR®, fluorodeoxyuridine.

Uses:
The primary indication for floxuridine is in the treatment of gastrointestinal adenocarcinomas metastatic to the liver.

Mechanism of Antitumor Action:

Floxuridine is activated in the liver to FUDR-monophosphate and fluorodeoxyuridine monophosphate (FdUMP). It is also catabolized to fluorouracil. FdUMP binds to the intracellular enzyme thymidylate synthase, which is responsible for the conversion of uridine to thymidine. This effect results in an inhibition of DNA synthesis.

Pharmacokinetics:

Absorption: Floxuridine is poorly absorbed by the oral route.

Distribution: After intravenous infusions, floxuridine primarily stays in the plasma. After hepatic arterial administration, over 90% of the drug is extracted into hepatocytes in one pass through the liver.

Protein Binding: Unknown.

Metabolism: Floxuridine is rapidly converted to fluorouracil by the liver. The primary metabolic products of fluorouracil are CO_2.

Half-life: The elimination half-life of floxuridine is about 15 minutes.

Elimination: About 30% of floxuridine is excreted in urine as inactive metabolites.

Drug Interactions:

Leucovorin: May enhance the cytotoxic effects of floxuridine. No studies have been performed to define appropriate combination regimens of leucovorin and floxuridine.

Cisplatin: Additive cytotoxic effects *in vitro* are known, but no clinical studies have been performed to establish that this combination has synergistic activity in human tumors.

Dosage:

The IV dose of floxuridine is 0.1 to 0.3 mg/kg/day by continuous infusion for 7 to 14 days. The drug is more often given by intraarterial (IA) infusion. The recommended dose for hepatic tumors is 0.1 to 0.2 mg/kg/day for 7 to 14 days. Floxuridine IA has also been combined with fluorouracil IV in doses of 800 mg/m^2/day for 5 days. However, this combination often necessitates dose reductions because of hepatic and gastric toxicity.

Dose Forms:
FUdR® is available as a 500 mg vial for injection.

Administration:
The usual route of administration of floxuridine is intraarterial infusion. The drug may also be given by the IV route. Intraarterial administration is performed through implantable catheters placed surgically into an artery that supplies the tumor with its primary vascular supply. The hepatic artery is most often used for liver tumors, while the carotid artery is used for head and neck tumors.

Compatibilities: In Y-site injection of 3 mg/mL, floxuridine is compatible with carboplatin, cisplatin, etoposide (0.2 mg/mL), fluorouracil, leucovorin calcium, filgrastim, fludarabine phosphate, melphalan HCl, ondansetron HCl, paclitaxel, piperacillin sodium–tazobactam sodium, sargramostim, and vinorelbine tartrate.

Incompatibilities: Allopurinol sodium, cefepime HCl.

Adverse Reactions:

Hepatotoxicity: The dose limiting toxicity of intraarterial floxuridine is hepatic toxicity. It is manifested as sclerosing cholangitis and is dose related. Doses greater than 0.2 mg/kg/day produce more than a 20% incidence of biliary damage. Over 80% of patients will require dose reduction.

Gastrointestinal: Severe gastritis may result from hepatic arterial infusions of floxuridine. A major risk factor for this complication is inadequate gastroduodenal artery ligation during the surgical placement of the intraarterial catheter. Mucositis is less commonly observed during infusion.

Dermatologic: Several skin reactions have been reported, including dermatitis, rash, and pruritis after both intraarterial and IV floxuridine.

Ocular: Dacrocystitis has been reported after both IV and intraarterial administration of fluoxuridine. Topical corticosteroids may be needed for symptomatic control of this condition.

CNS: Rare cases of confusion, disorientation, and seizures have been reported after IV dosing of floxuridine.

Hematologic: Bone marrow suppression is minimal with floxuridine in usual doses. The nadir in cell counts occurs at 7 to 10 days, with recovery by 14 to 17 days.

Practitioner Interventions:

1. Obtain baseline liver function tests prior to therapy and monthly while the patient is receiving floxuridine.
2. Initial doses should not exceed 0.3 mg/kg/day IV × 7 days and 0.2 mg/kg/day IA × 7 days.
3. Monitor patient for signs of gastritis. Decrease dose for grade III toxicity or higher.
4. Monitor patient for signs of ocular toxicity. Decrease the dose of floxuridine or give concurrent ophthalmic corticosteroids if necessary.
5. Administer appropriate medication to treat gastritis.

References:

1. Ensminger WD, Rosowsky A, Raso V, et al. A clinical pharmacological evaluation of hepatic arterial infusions of 5-fluoro-2′-deoxyuridine and 5-fluorouracil. Cancer Res 1978;38:3784–3792.
2. Hohn DC, Melnick J, Stagg R, et al. Biliary sclerosis in patients receiving arterial infusions of floxuridine. J Clin Oncol 1985;3:98–102.
3. Hohn DC, Staggg RJ, Price DC, Lewis BJ, et al. Avoidance of gastroduodenal toxicity in patients receiving intraarterial 5-fluoro-2′-deoxyuridine. J Clin Oncol 1985;3:1257–1260.
4. Kemeny N, Daly N, Reichman B, Geller N, et al. Intrahepatic or systemic infusion of fluorodeoxyuridine in patients with liver metastases from colorectal carcinoma. Ann Intern Med 1987;107:459–465.

FLUDARABINE PHOSPHATE

Other Names:
Fludara®, 2-Fluoro-ara-amp.

Uses:
Chronic lymphocytic leukemia (CLL), low-grade lymphomas, mycosis fungoides (cutaneous T-cell lymphoma).

Mechanism of Antitumor Action:

Fludarabine phosphate suppresses DNA synthesis by inhibition of ribonucleotide reductase.

Pharmacokinetics:

Absorption: Although an oral formulation of fludarabine is unavailable in the United States, the drug is well absorbed after oral administration.

Distribution: Fludarabine is widely distributed and has a Vd of 96 to 98 L/m^2. It concentrates in liver, kidney, and spleen. The drug and one of its metabolites, 2-fluoroadenine, distributes into the extracellular fluid.

Protein Binding: Unknown.

Metabolism: Fludarabine phosphate is rapidly and completely dephosphorylated to fludarabine after IV administration. Fludarabine enters cells and is then rephosphorylated to fludarabine triphosphate, the active metabolite.

Half-life: The half-life in adults is biphasic. An early phase $T_{1/2}\alpha$ is 0.6 hour; $T_{1/2}\beta$ is 9.3 hours. In pediatric patients, the plasma concentration profile is also biphasic, with a slightly longer $T_{1/2}\alpha$ of 1.2 hours and a $T_{1/2}\beta$ of 12 to 19 hours.

Elimination:

Approximately 25% of an IV dose of fludarabine phosphate is excreted in the urine over a period of 5 days.

Drug Interactions:

Fludarabine increases intracellular levels of ***cytarabine.***

Dosage:

In adults, the dose range of fludarabine phosphate is from 18 to 30 mg/m^2/day $\times$ 5 days, given over a period of 30 minutes. The dose for chronic lymphocytic leukemia is 25 mg/m^2/day for 5 consecutive days. Cycles are repeated every 4 to 5 weeks. The efficacy of fludarabine has not been established in children.

Dose Forms:

Fludara® is available in a 50 mg vial to be reconstituted with 2 ml of sterile water for injection.

Administration:

Fludarabine is given as a short IV infusion over a period of 30 minutes. After reconstituted, the solution should be used within 8 hours.

Compatibilities: In a 1:1 mixture at 1 mg/mL in D5W for Y-site simulation, fludarabine is compatible with the following:

Cytotoxic drugs: amsacrine, bleomycin sulfate, carboplatin, carmustine, cisplatin, cyclophosphamide, cytarabine, dacarbazine, dactinomycin, doxorubicin HCl, etoposide, floxuridine, fluorouracil, ifosfamide, mechlorethamine HCl, mesna, methotrexate sodium, mitoxantrone HCl, pentostatin, vinblastine sulfate, vincristine sulfate, vinorebline tartrate.

Noncytotoxic drugs: amikacin sulfate, aminophylline, ampicillin sodium, ampicillin sodium-sulfactam sodium, aztreonam, butorphanol tartrate, cefazolin sodium, cefoperazone sodium, ceforanide, cefotaxime sodium, cefotetan disodium, ceftazidime sodium carbonate, ceftizoxime sodium, ceftriaxone sodium, cefuroxime sodium, cimetidine HCl, clindamycin phosphate, dexamethasone sodium phosphate, diphenhydramine HCl, doxycycline hyclate, droperidol, famotidine, fluconazole, furosemide, gentamicin sulfate, haloperidol lactate, heparin sodium, hydrocortisone sodium phosphate, hydrocortisone sodium succinate, hydromorphone HCl, imipenem–cilastatin sodium, lorazepam, magnesium sulfate, mannitol, meperidine HCl, mesna, methylprednisolone sodium succinate, metoclopramide HCl, mezlocillin, minocycline HCl, morphine sulfate, multivitamins, nalbuphine HCl, netilmicin sulfate, ondansetron HCl, piperacillin sodium, potassium chloride, promethazine HCl, ranitidine HCl, sodium bicarbonate, tetracycline HCl, ticarcillin disodium, ticarcillin disodium–clavulanate potassium, tobramycin sulfate, trimethoprim-sulfamethoxazole, and vancomycin HCl.

Incompatibilities: In a 1:1 mixture at 1 mg/mL in D5W, fludarabine is incompatible with acyclovir sodium, amphotericin B, chlorpromazine HCl, daunorubicin HCl, ganciclovir sodium, hydroxyzine HCl, miconazole, and prochlorperazine edisylate.

Adverse Reactions:

 *Hematologic:* The dose-limiting toxicity of fludarabine phosphate is myelosuppression. Granulocytopenia and thrombocytopenia occur with a nadir in cell counts at 13 days and a range of 3 to 25 days. Recovery occurs within 14 days.

 Neurologic: CNS toxicity may occur, including encephalopathy, seizures, coma, and blindness.

 Gastrointestinal: Transient nausea and vomiting.

 Renal: Hyperuricemia, hyperphosphatemia, hematuria, urate crystals, renal failure, hemorrhagic cystitis.

 *Cardiac:* Rare cases of peripheral edema and pericardial effusion have been reported in patients receiving fludarabine phosphate.

Pulmonary: Toxicity is rare and consists of dyspnea, cough, fever, and hypoxia.

Practitioner Interventions:

1. Monitor patient's complete blood cell count (CBC), along with platelet count, on a weekly basis.
2. Give antiemetics as needed.
3. Administer allopurinol to prevent tumor lysis in patients with bulky disease.
4. In patients with bulky disease, monitor for signs and symptoms of tumor lysis syndrome:
   a. Increasing potassium.
   b. Increasing phosphorus.
   c. Decreasing calcium.
   d. Increasing uric acid, and lactate dehydrogenase.
      If tumor lysis is noted:
   a. Administer fluids at rate of 200–300 mL per hour to keep urinary output at 100–200 mL/h.

b. Check electrolytes, uric acid and lactate dehydrogenase every 6 to 12 hours until levels decrease to normal (usually 48–72 hours).

References:

1. Keating MJ, Kantarjian H, Talpaz M, et al. Fludarabine: a new agent with major activity against chronic lymphocytic leukemia. Blood 1989;74: 19–25.
2. Rodriguez G. Fludarabine phosphate. A new anticancer drug with significant activity in patients with chronic lymphyocytic leukemia and with lymphoma. Invest New Drugs 1994;12:75–92.
3. Tosi P, Visani G, Ottaviami E, Manfori S, et al. Fludarabine + ara-C + GCSF: Cytotoxic effect and induction of apoptosis on fresh acute myeloid cells. Leukemia 1994;8:2076–2082.

FLUOROURACIL

Other Names:

Adrucil®, 5-FU, 5-Fluorouracil.

Uses:

Carcinomas of the colon, rectum, breast, stomach, pancreas, esophagus, head and neck, and prostate, and renal cell carcinoma.

Mechanism of Antitumor Action:

Fluorouracil is an antimetabolite that interferes with pyrimidine synthesis by blocking thymidylate synthase, purine synthesis, and *de novo* protein synthesis, and by interfering with the synthesis of DNA. It is also metabolized to the ribonucleotide triphosphate, fluorouracil triphosphate (FUTP), and is then incorporated into RNA, inhibiting its function.

Pharmacokinetics:

Absorption: Oral absorption of fluorouracil is very erratic after administration of the parenteral form in acidic solutions (orange/apple juice). The bioavailability ranges from 50 to 80%. Patients with bowel metastases may absorb less drug. Absorption is improved in alkaline solution buffered with sodium bicarbonate.

After topical administration, about 5% of the drug is absorbed systemically. Similarly, very little fluorouracil is absorbed after intra-peritoneal (IP) administration. Systemic absorption following intra-pleural administration has not been quantitated but is believed to be minimal because of a low rate of systemic reactions.

Distribution: Fluorouracil diffuses well into extracellular fluids, in-cluding areas of existing effusions, ascites, and cerebrospinal fluid.

Protein Binding: The binding of 5 fluorouracil to serum protein is not well described.

Metabolism: Fluorouracil is anabolized to fluorodeoxyuridine mon-ophosphate (FdUMP) and FUTP. It is catabolized in the liver to carbon dioxide, urea, ammonia, and alpha-fluoro-beta-alanine. Several non-hepatic sites of metabolism have been described for 5 fluorouracil, including conversion to fluorocitrate. Thus, altered liver function does not require dose modification.

Half-life: 10 to 20 minutes.

Elimination: Only a small amount of fluorouracil is excreted un-changed in the urine, with no intact drug detected 3 hours after ad-ministration. Intracellular concentrations of fluorouracil may persist for hours.

Drug Interactions:

Leucovorin potentiates the antitumor activity of fluorouracil by en-hancing the thymidylate synthase-FdUMP–reduced-folate ternary com-plex.

Dipyridamole appears to increase the *in vitro* cytotoxicity of fluo-rouracil by blocking the pyrimidine salvage pathway for nucleoside synthesis.

Dosage:

Intravenous: 500 to 1,000 mg/m^2 given as a 24-hour infusion for 4 or 5 days every 3 weeks.

Bolus IV push: 12 mg/kg (maximum 800 mg) every week.

Dose Forms:

Fluorouracil is available by various manufacturers in 0.5, 1, 2.5 and 5 g vials, and in a 0.5 g ampule.

Administration:

Intravenous: For rapid infusions of fluorouracil over a period of 10 to 15 minutes, dilute in 25 to 50 mL NS or D5W. For continuous infusion, further dilute in 500 to 1,000 mL of D5W or NS.

Bolus Intravenous push: No diluent is required. Administer over a period of 2 to 5 minutes.

Intraperitoneal: Administration is done through an intraperitoneal catheter or an infusion device. A volume of at least 1500 mL is required to adequately bathe the peritoneal surface with fluorouracil if used alone. The solution is instilled into the peritoneal cavity for at least 4 hours, and then may be drained.

Compatibilities: Fluorouracil is compatible with D5LR, NS, D5W, and amino acid solutions. In admixtures of 1 to 100 mg/L in NS, fluorouracil is compatible with cyclophosphamide, methotrexate sodium, etoposide, floxuridine, leucovorin sodium (24 hours only), ifosfamide, prednisolone sodium phosphate and vincristine sulfate.

Syringe compatibility: Although data indicate that fluorouracil is compatible for 5 minutes with several drugs when admixed in a syringe, this method of administration is not recommended because of inconvenience.

Y-site infusions: One-to-one mixtures of fluorouracil (50 mg/mL) are compatible for the following:

Cytotoxic drugs: bleomycin sulfate, cisplatin, cyclophosphamide, doxorubicin HCl, fludarabine phosphate (16 mg/mL fluorouracil), methotrexate sodium, mitomycin, vinblastine sulfate, and vincristine sulfate.

Noncytotoxic drugs: furosemide, heparin sodium, hydrocortisone sodium succinate, leucovorin calcium, metoclopramide HCl, ondansetron HCl (0.8 mg/mL fluorouracil), potassium chloride, sargramostim, and vitamin B complex with vitamin C.

Incompatibilities: Admixtures of fluorouracil are incompatible with carboplatin, cisplatin, cytarabine, diazepam, doxorubicin HCl, methotrexate (200 mg/L methotrexate and 250 mg/mL fluorouracil).

One-to-one mixtures of fluorouracil (50 mg/mL) in simulated Y-site infusions are incompatible with droperidol, ondansetron HCl (16 mg/mL fluorouracil). In spills of fluorouracil, sodium hypochlorite 5% (household bleach) may be used to inactivate the drug.

Adverse Reactions:

 Hematologic: Both the bone marrow and gastrointestinal toxicity of fluorouracil may be dose limiting. Leukopenia, anemia, and thrombocytopenia may all occur. The nadir of the WBC count usually occurs at 9 to 14 days, with recovery by 25 to 30 days. The nadir of the platelets count occurs at 7 to 14 days with recovery by 25 to 30 days.

 Gastrointestinal: Nausea and anorexia are very common but rarely severe. Stomatitis may be significant, causing substantial local discomfort. Diarrhea occurs often and can be life threatening, especially after high-dose continuous infusion regimens.

 Dermatologic: Hair loss occurs frequently but is usually not total. Rash, hyperpigmentation of veins, and nail-bed changes are also seen.

 Neurologic: Disorientation, confusion, euphoria, ataxia, nystagmus, headache, and acute cerebellar dysfunction (dysarthria, altered gait, nystagmus) are rare side effects, but require discontinuation of therapy with fluorouracil.

 Opthalmologic: Tear duct stenosis and dry eyes are infrequent. Dacrocystitis, an inflammation of the tear ducts and lacrimal gland, occurs occasionally. Topical ophthalmic corticosteroids may be helpful for treating fluorouracil-induced conjunctivitis.

Practitioner Interventions:

1. Give antiemetic 30 minutes prior to 5-fluorouracil.
2. Initiate mouth-care regimen for patient.
3. Instruct patient about oral self-examination for stomatitis.
4. Monitor patient daily for mucositis.
5. Change peripheral IV site every 72 hours.
6. Monitor IV site frequently for signs of phlebitis and hyperpigmentation.
7. Instruct patient about possible nail bed changes, probable alopecia and potential eye problems.
8. Monitor patient for signs and symptoms of diarrhea; instruct patient to notify health-care provider if more than three stools are passed per day.

9. Instruct patients about photosensitivity reactions to fluorouracil.

References:
1. Baltzer L, Berkey R. Oncology Pocket Guide to Chemotherapy. CV Mosby, St. Louis, 1994, pp. 80–84.
2. Moertel CG, Fleming TR, Macdonald JS, et al. Levamisole and fluorouracil for adjuvant therapy of resected colon carcinoma. N Engl J Med 1990;322:352–358.
3. Moertel CG, Macdonald JS. Fluorouracil plus levamisole as effective adjuvant after resection of stage III colon carcinoma: a final report. Ann Intern Med 1995;122:321.
4. Preston F, Wilfinger C. Memory Bank for Chemotherapy. Jones & Bartlett, Boston, 1993, pp. 82–84.

FLUTAMIDE

Other Names:
Eulexin®.

Uses:
Metastatic prostate cancer, when used in combination with an inhibitor of gonadotropin-releasing hormone (GnRH) such as leuprolide.

Mechanism of Antitumor Action:
Flutamide is a nonsteroidal antiandrogen that blocks the feedback inhibition of luteinizing hormone production by testosterone.

Pharmacokinetics:

Absorption: Flutamide is absorbed in 2 to 4 hours after oral administration.

Distribution: The distribution of the drug and its metabolites is not well described.

Protein Binding: Flutamide and its metabolites are extensively bound (86 to 94%) to plasma proteins. The hydroxy metabolite, hydroxyflutamide, has a 20-fold binding affinity to the androgen receptor.

Metabolism: Flutamide is converted to several metabolites, the major one being hydroxyflutamide. The half time to formation of the hydroxy metabolite is about 1 hour.

Half-life: Flutamide has half-lives of 0.8 and 7.8 hours, while hydroxyflutamide has a half-life of 8 to 10 hours.

Elimination: Only 4% of flutamide is excreted unchanged in the urine. Most of the drug is metabolized.

Drug Interactions:
No drug interactions have been described for flutamide.

Dosage:
The dose of flutamide is 250 mg orally taken three times daily, preferably at 8-hour intervals.

Dose Forms:
Eulexin® is available in 125 mg capsules.

Administration:
Flutamide should be administered on an empty stomach. In cases of GI intolerance, the drug may be given with food.

Adverse Reactions:

Endocrine: Hot flashes occur in about 60% of patients treated with flutamide. This may be controlled with clonidine 0.1 to 0.2 mg PO daily. Impotence occurs in about one-third of male patients. Gynecomastia, nipple pain, and galactorrhea are also reported.

Gastrointestinal: Nausea, vomiting, and diarrhea may have been reported.

Hepatic: Transient elevations in transaminase enzymes. Hepatitis is rare.

Practitioner Interventions:

1. Use antiemetics as needed.
2. Use antidiarrheals as needed. If diarrhea is severe, flutamide may have to be stopped.
3. Instruct patient about risks of decreased libido, hot flashes, and impotence.
4. Observe patient/family for need to obtain counseling on sexuality.

References:

1. Goldspiel BR, Kohler DR. Flutamide: an antiandrogen for advanced prostate cancer. Drug Intelligence and Clinical Pharmacy 1990;24:616–623.
2. Hillner BF, McLeod DG, Crawford ED, Bennett CL. Estimating the cost effectiveness of total androgen blocking with flutamide in M1 prostate cancer. Urology 1995;45:633–640.
3. Labrie F. Mechanism of action and pure anti androgenic properties of flutamide. Cancer 1993;72:3816–3827.

GALLIUM NITRATE

Other Names:
Ganite®.

Uses:
Cancer-associated hypercalcemia refractory to hydration.

Mechanism of Antitumor Action:
Gallium nitrate inhibits calcium resorption from bone, in addition to complexing to intracellular calcium and magnesium.

Pharmacokinetics:

Absorption: Gallium nitrate is given by the IV route.

Distribution: The Vd of free gallium ranges from 128 to 186 L.

Protein Binding: There is little information on the protein binding of gallium.

Metabolism: Gallium nitrate is not metabolized to any extent.

Half-life: After a bolus dose of gallium nitrate, the $T_{1/2}\alpha$ = 1.5 hours and the $T_{1/2}\beta$ ranges from 6 to 24 hours. After continuous infusion, the $T_{1/2}\alpha$ ranges from 8 to 26 minutes and $T_{1/2}\beta$ ranges from 9 to 196 hours.

Elimination: Recovery of gallium nitrate in urine is approximately 65% within 24 hours after a bolus dose, and between 69 and 91% after continuous IV infusion.

Drug Interactions:

Concurrent use of other nephrotoxic agents e.g. ***aminoglycosides, amphotericin B, cyclosporin, foscarnet***) may increase the risk of renal dysfunction. Concurrent use of ***foscarnet*** and ***gallium nitrate*** may cause additive hypocalcemia.

Dosage:

200 mg/m^2/day continuous IV infusion $\times$ 5 days. The drug should be held if serum creatinine is 2.5 mg/dL or higher.

Dose Forms:

Ganite® is available as 500 mg (25 mg/ml) in a 20 ml single-dose vial.

Administration:

Administer gallium nitrate as a 24-hour continuous infusion for 5 days. The daily dose should be diluted in 1,000 ml of NS or D5W. Gallium nitrate is stable for 48 hours at room temperature and for 7 days under refrigeration.

Compatibilities: In a concentration of 0.4 mg/mL in NS, gallium nitrate is compatible with allopurinol sodium, melphalan HCl, and vinorelbine tartrate.

In a concentration of 0.4 mg/mL in D5W, gallium nitrate is compatible with filgrastim and piperacillin sodium–tazobactam sodium.

In a concentration of 1 mg/mL in NS, gallium nitrate is compatible with acyclovir sodium, aminophylline, ampicillin sodium–sulbactam sodium, cefazolin sodium, ceftazidime, ceftriaxone sodium, cimetidine HCl, ciprofloxacin, cyclophosphamide, dexamethasone sodium phosphate, diphenhydramine HCl, fluconazole, furosemide, heparin sodium, hydrocortisone sodium succinate, ifosfamide, magnesium sulfate, mannitol, meperidine HCl, mesna, methotrexate sodium, metoclopramide HCl, ondansetron HCl, piperacillin sodium, potassium chloride, ranitidine HCl, sodium bicarbonate, ticarcillin disodium-clavulanate potassium, trimethoprim–sulfamethoxazole, and vancomycin HCl.

Incompatibilities: Cefepime HCl, cisplatin, cytarabine, doxorubicin HCl, etoposide, fluorouracil, haloperidol lactate, hydromorphone HCl, imipenem-cilastin sodium, lorazepam, morphine sulfate, and prochlorperazine edisylate.

Adverse Reactions:

Renal: Nephrotoxicity from gallium nitrate has been reported in about 12% of patients. The drug should be withheld if the serum creatinine is 2.5 mg/dL or greater. Hydration with 2 L/day may prevent renal toxicity.

Metabolic: Hypocalcemia may result in up to 38% of patients treated with gallium nitrate. Asymptomatic hypotension may occur with this agent. Alteration in electrolytes, such as hypophosphatemia and hypomagnesemia, may also result. Decreased levels of sodium bicarbonate have also been reported.

Neurologic: Fatigue, lethargy, headache, mood changes, optic neuritis and vision changes, confusion, and dizziness have been rarely reported. Hearing loss and tinnitus have also been reported.

Dermatologic: Skin rash is uncommon.

Hematologic: Bone marrow suppression is uncommon.

Practitioner Interventions:

1. Check patient's baseline serum creatinine level and monitor daily.
2. Do not administer gallium nitrate if creatinine is above 2.5 mg/dL.
3. Adequately hydrate the patient with at least 3 L of fluid per day.

4. Monitor fluid intake and output and weigh patient daily.
5. Monitor electrolytes daily, with special attention to Ca^{++}, $PO_4^{=}$, Mg^{++}, and Na^+.
6. Encourage patient to ambulate during therapy.
7. Monitor for any sign or symptoms of neurotoxicity.

References:
1. Bockman RS. Studies on the mechanism of action of gallium nitrate. Semin Oncol 1991;18(4 Suppl 5):21–25.
2. Mundy GR. Pathophysiology of cancer-associated hypercalcemia. Semin Oncol 1990;17(2, Suppl 5):10–15.
3. Olver IN, Webster LK, Sephton RG, et al. A Phase II study with pharmacokinetics of gallium nitrate in non-small cell lung cancer. Proc Am Assoc Cancer Res 1991;32:1132.
4. Warrell RP, Alcock, NW, Bockman RS. Gallium nitrate inhibits accelerated bone turnover in patients with bone metastases. J Clin Oncol 1987;5:292–598.
5. Warrell RP, Israel R, Frisone M, et al. Gallium nitrate for acute treatment of cancer-related hypercalcemia. Ann Intern Med 1988;108:609–674.
6. Warrell RP, Murphy WK, Schulman P, et al. A randomized double-blind study of gallium nitrate compared with etidronate for control of cancer-related hypercalcemia. J Clin Oncol 1991;9:1467–1475.

GEMCITABINE

Other Names:
Gemzar®.

Uses:
Gemcitabine is approved for the treatment of metastatic pancreatic carcinoma. It also has activity in breast cancer, bladder cancer, small-cell and non-small-cell lung cancer, and ovarian cancer.

Mechanism of Antitumor Cell Cycle Action:
Gemcitabine is a cell cycle phase specific nucleoside analogue that blocks the progression of cells through the G_1/S-phase boundary of the cell cycle. It is a prodrug that is activated by nucleoside kinases to the active diphosphate and triphosphate nucleosides. The diphosphate inhibits ribonucleotide reductase, which is necessary for the formation of deoxycytidine and is important for DNA synthesis. Gemci-

tabine triphosphate also competes with deoxycytidine for incorporation into DNA.

Pharmacokinetics:

Absorption: Gemcitabine is given by the IV route.

Distribution: After a short infusion, gemcitabine has a Vd of 50 L/m². Suggesting a significant degree of intracellular binding to proteins.

Protein Binding: This has not been studied, but gemcitabine is probably highly bound to cellular proteins.

Metabolism: The primary metabolite of gemcitabine is difluorodeoxyuridine (inactive).

Half-life: After short infusions of gemcitabine, the plasma half-life ranges from 30 to 90 minutes. After a long infusion, the half-life is 4 to 10 hours, due to the higher Vd.

Elimination: Plasma clearance of gemcitabine is slower in women than in men, and in elderly persons than in younger ones. The impact of renal or hepatic dysfunction on gemcitabine has not been studied.

Drug Interactions:

No reports of specific drug interactions with gemcitabine have appeared in the literature. No drug interaction studies have been conducted with gemcitabine.

Dose:

The recommended dose of gemcitabine for pancreatic cancer is 1000 mg/m² IV given over a period of 30 minutes once weekly for 7 weeks. After 1 wk of rest, the same dose is resumed once weekly for 3 weeks in a 4-week cycle. Dose adjustment is based on the degree of myelosuppression. Therapy should be adjusted according to the guideline below:

Dose Modification

Absolute Granulocyte Count	Platelet Count	% Full Dose
≥1000	and >100,000	100
500–999	or 50–99,000	75
<500	or <50,000	Hold 1 wk

Dosage Forms:
Gemzar® is available in 200 and 1000 mg lyophilized single-use vials.

Administration:
Gemzar® is reconstituted to concentrations up to 40 mg/mL with non-preserved NS. Shake to dissolve. The drug may be further diluted in 0.9% sodium chloride to concentrations as low as 0.1 mg/mL. Gemzar® solutions are stable at room temperature (20 to 25°C) for 24 hours. Solutions should not be refrigerated because of the potential for crystal formation.

Compatibilities: The compatibility of other drugs with gemcitabine has not been studied.

Incompatibilities: Not determined to date.

Adverse Reactions:

 Hematologic: Myelosuppression is the dose limiting toxicity of gemcitabine. Maximum leukopenia occurs at 10 to 14 days and recovery by day 21. Thrombocytopenia is rarely severe (<50,000/mm^3). About 6% of patients develop a nadir below 500 neutrophils/mL.

 Dermatologic: About 30% of patients may have a maculopapular rash. About 13% will complain of pruritis.

 Gastrointestinal: Mild to moderate nausea and vomiting occur in about 70% of patients treated with gemcitabine. Severe nausea and vomiting occur in less than 15% of patients.

 *Hepatic:* Transient elevations in transaminase enzymes are reported in about two-thirds of patients.

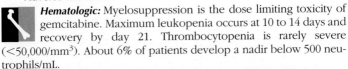 *Pulmonary:* Mild to moderate dyspnea has been reported in about 20% of various patients receiving gemcitabine. However, in patients with pancreatic cancer, the incidence was about 10%, none severe enough to require discontinuing therapy.

 Renal: Mild proteinuria and hematuria are common occurrences. Hemolytic uremic syndrome has been reported in a few cases (0.25%).

Acute infusion-associated reactions: Reactions such as flushing, shortness of breath, facial swelling, headache, chills, back pain, and hypotension occur in about 7% of patients treated with gemcitabine and may be infusion-rate-related. Slowing or discontinuing the infusion results in resolution over the course of several hours to a day.

 Flu-like syndrome: Symptoms of malaise, lethargy, chills, and fever have been reported in about 20% of patients. About 40% of patients develop a fever within 6 to 12 hours of administration of gemcitabine. However, infections are reported in only about 16% of patients.

Edema: Peripheral edema occurs in about 20% of patients.

Practitioner Interventions

1. Monitor patient's complete blood cell count and platelet count on a weekly basis.
2. Obtain baseline liver function tests and check every month for abnormalities.
3. Premedicate patient 30 minutes prior to infusion with conventional antiemetics such as phenothiazines, to prevent nausea and vomiting.
4. Obtain patient's baseline weight and monitor weight and fluid status. Weight gain and edema may be controlled with mild diuretics.
5. Skin reactions may be controlled with topical corticosteroids. Discontinue use of gemcitabine if skin reactions are severe.
6. The infusion of gemcitabine should be given over a minimum of 30 minutes. If the patient experiences flushing, shortness of breath, or facial swelling, the infusion should be discontinued until the symptoms subside, and should be reinstituted at half the infusion rate.
7. Instruct patient regarding the possibility of blood in urine; check for protein in urine on a weekly basis.
8. Instruct patient to contact health care provider with any symptoms of hematuria, change in color of urine, or difficulty in passing urine due to clots.

References:
1. Carmichael J, Fink U, Russell RCG, et al. Phase II study of gemcitabine in patients with advanced pancreatic cancer. Br J Cancer 1996;73:101–105.
2. Kaye SB. Gemcitabine: current status of phase I and II trials. J Clin Oncol 1994;12:1527–1531.
3. Moore M, Anderson J, Burris H, et al. A randomized trial of gemcitabine versus 5-fluorouracil as first-line therapy in advanced pancreatic cancer. Proc Am Soc Clin Oncol 1995;14:473.
4. Pollera CF, Ceribelli A, Crecco M, Calabresi F. Weekly gemcitabine in advanced and metastatic tumors: a clinical phase I study. Invest New Drugs 1994;12:111–119.

GOSERELIN

Other Names:
Zoladex®.

Uses:
Prostate cancer, breast cancer.

Mechanism of Antitumor Action:
Goserelin is an analog of luteinizing hormone-releasing hormone. It is a slow-release form of a potent inhibitor of gonadotropin release from the pituitary gland, resulting in low concentrations of luteinizing hormone (LH), follicle-stimulating hormone (FSH), testosterone, or estrogen.

Pharmacokinetics:

Absorption: Systemic absorption of goserelin occurs over a period of 27 days, but is slower during the first 8 days after depot injection, and decreases 3 weeks after administration.

Distribution: The Vd of goserelin is 13.7 L.

Protein Binding: Protein binding is not well described for goserelin.

Metabolism: Goserelin is not metabolized to any substantial extent.

Half-life: The elimination half-life of goserelin ranges from 4 to 5 hours. The half-life is prolonged to about 12 hours in severe renal dysfunction.

Elimination: Goserelin is almost entirely eliminated unchanged in the urine, and is cleared renally.

Drug Interactions:
None known.

Dosage:
The usual dose of goserelin is 3.6 mg injected SC every 28 days.

Dose Forms:
Zoladex® is available as a 3.6 mg and 10.8 mg syringes for SC implantation.

Administration:
The pellet is injected SC into abdominal body fat. A local topical anesthetic may be given prior to administration to decrease pain on injection.

Adverse Reactions:

 Endocrine: Primary reactions to goserelin are due to its endocrine effects and include hot flashes (50%), decreased libido (9%), and gynecomastia (9%). Goserelin would also stop ovulation and menstruation.

Bone: Bone pain may result during the first week after starting goserelin (17%), and represents a tumor flare. This can be blocked with the concurrent use of flutamide.

Practitioner Interventions:

1. Instruct patients about potential for increased bone pain with goserelin therapy. Prescribe analgesics if necessary.
2. Instruct patients about endocrine side effects of goserelin.

3. Monitor patient for gynecomastia.
4. Counsel patient about potential for decreased libido, and initiate appropriate referral for therapy as necessary.
5. Instruct patient about appropriate injection technique for goserelin and disposal method.

References:

1. Newling DW, Denis L, Veroneylen K. Orchiectomy versus goserelin and flutamide in the treatment of newly diagnosed metastatic prostate cancer. Analysis of the criteria of evaluation used in the European Organization for Research and treatment of Cancer—Genitourinary Group Study 30853. Cancer 1993;72(Suppl 12):3793–3798.
2. Tyrrell CJ, Altwein JE, Klippel F, et al. A multi-center randomized trial comparing the Luteinizing-releasing hormone analogue goserelin acetate alone and with flutamide in the treatment of advanced prostate cancer. The International Prostate Cancer Study Group. J Urol 1991;146: 1321–1326.

HYDROXYUREA

Other Names:
Hydrea®.

Uses:
Chronic phase chronic myelogenous leukemia, myeloproliferative syndrome, refractory ovarian cancer, brain cancer, and in combination with radiation therapy for head and neck cancer.

Mechanism of Antitumor Action:
Hydroxyurea selectively interrupts the conversion of ribonucleotides to deoxyribonucleotides. It also inhibits DNA synthesis by inhibiting thymidine incorporation into DNA. It does not interfere with the synthesis of RNA or protein.

Pharmacokinetics:

Absorption: Hydroxyurea is rapidly and completely absorbed (80%) from the gastrointestinal tract.

Distribution: Rapid passive diffusion into white blood cells and other cells of the hematopoietic system. Hydroxyurea readily crosses the blood–brain barrier. Also, high concentrations are seen in brain, lung, kidney, breast milk, and peritoneal and pleural effusions.

Protein Binding: Unknown.

Metabolism: 50% of hydroxyurea is metabolized in liver to urea, CO_2, and acetohydroxamic acid.

Half-life: 3 to 4 hours.

Elimination: About half of hydroxyurea is excreted in urine as urea and unchanged drug. Carbon dioxide from metabolism of the drug is expired in the lungs.

Drug Interactions:
Hydroxyurea may enhance the neurotoxicity of 5-fluorouracil.

Dosage:
The adult oral dosage of hydroxyurea in leukemias or myeloproliferative syndromes is 10 to 30 mg/kg/day (rounded to the nearest multiple of 500 mg capsules) (1,000 to 3,000 mg/day) in one to three daily doses titrated to the patient's WBC response. In solid tumors, the dose is 80 mg/kg given as a single dose every third day, or 20 to 30 mg/kg daily given continuously. The pediatric dosage ranges from 1,500 to 3,000 mg/m^2 as a single dose in pediatric astrocytoma, medulloblastoma, and neuroectodermal tumors.

Intravenous - (Investigational only) 50 to 75 mg/kg/day IV by slow push or infusion.

Dose Modification in Renal Dysfunction:

CrCl mL/min	% Normal
>50	100
10–50	50
<10	20

Dose Forms:
Hydrea® is available in 500 mg capsules.

Administration:

Hydroxyurea may be given as a single daily dose or in one to three doses. The contents of capsules may be emptied into 4 ounces of water and taken immediately.

Adverse Reactions:

Hematologic: Bone marrow suppression is the common dose limiting side effect of hydroxyurea, and is dose dependent. White blood cell toxicity is seen in 7 days, with a rapid recovery in 7 to 10 days after discontinuing therapy. Bone marrow suppression may be more severe in patients who have received prior radiation or other chemotherapy.

Gastrointestinal: Mild nausea and vomiting occur in most patients treated with hydroxyurea. Nausea and vomiting could be reduced by dividing the dose into two or three doses. Mucositis and diarrhea are seen when large doses (>2 g/day) are given.

Dermatologic: Maculopapular rash, facial erythema, and pruritus may be seen in some patients. Hair loss is rare.

Fever: Fever may occur 2 to 6 hours after administration of hydroxyurea.

Pulmonary: A rare case of pulmonary alveolitis has been reported.

Neurologic: Headache, CNS disorientation, hallucinations, and convulsions have been rarely observed.

Practitioner Interventions:

1. Give antiemetics 30 minutes prior to high-dose hydroxyurea.
2. Order mouth care regimen if high doses of hydroxyurea are to be administered.
3. Instruct patient about self-inspection for mucositis.
4. Instruct patient to notify physician if more than four stools are passed per day.

5. Instruct patient to monitor skin integrity and to contact the physician if significant rash or pruritus develops.

6. If patient is unable to swallow capsules, instruct patient to empty capsules into a glass of water and swallow immediately.

References:

1. Barton Burke M, Wilkes G, Ingeversen K. Chemotherapy Care Plans. Designs for Nursing Care. Jones & Bartlett, Boston, 1992, pp. 204–207.
2. Belt RJ, Hass CD, Kennedy J, Taylor S. Studies of hydroxyurea administered by continuous infusion: toxicity, pharmacokinetics, and cell synchronization. Cancer 1980;46:455–462.
3. Hehlmann R, Heimpel H, Hasford J, et al. Randomized comparison of interferon-alpha with busulfan and hydroxyurea in chronic myelogenous leukemia. Blood 1994;84:4064–4077.
4. Kantarjian HM, Talpaz M. Chemotherapy and bone marrow transplantation in the treatment of chronic myelogenous leukemia. Semin Oncol 1994;21(suppl 6):8–13.
5. Preston F, Silfinger C. Memory Bank for Chemotherapy. Jones & Bartlett, Boston, 1993, pp. 87–88.
6. Rushing D, Goldman A, Gibb G, et al. Hydroxyurea versus busulfan in the treatment of chronic myelogenous leukemia. Am J Clin Oncol 1982;5:307–313.

IDARUBICIN HCl

Other Names:
Idamycin®, Idarubicin.

Uses:
Idarubicin has been shown to have efficacy in acute myelogenous leukemia (AML), in relapsed acute lymphocytic leukemia (ALL), and in the blast phase of chronic myelogenous leukemia.

Mechanism of Antitumor Action:
Idarubicin is an anthracycline, antitumor antibiotic similar to daunorubicin. Its mechanism of action is intercalation into DNA and inhibition of macromolecule synthesis. It may also degrade double-

stranded DNA by inhibiting topoisomerase II enzymes. This interference results in the formation of protein-associated DNA double-stranded breaks, which predominate if drug exposure occurs in the G_2 phase of cell division.

Pharmacokinetics:

Absorption: Studies with orally administered idarubicin show that it is rapidly but erratically absorbed (20 to 30%) from the gastrointestinal tract.

Distribution: The distribution of idarubucin follows a multicompartment disposition pattern, with a long terminal elimination half-life and extensive tissue uptake. The drug distributes into the cerebrospinal fluid.

Protein Binding: Both idarubicin and its metabolite, idarubicinol, are 97% bound to plasma proteins.

Metabolism: The metabolism of idarubicin occurs in the biliary system, yielding an active metabolite, idarubicinol.

Half-life: The half-life of idarubicin is about 18 hours, but its metabolite idarubicinol has a half life of about 50 hours.

Elimination: The primary route of elimination is biliary elimination into feces. The renal system provides only a minor route of elimination or about 15% after an IV dose.

Drug Interactions:
There are no known drug interactions of idarubicin.

Dosage:
The usual dosage of idarubicin for the treatment of acute leukemia in adults is 12 mg/m²/day IV for 3 consecutive days. Dose reduction should be done for patients with severe hepatic dysfunction. The usual dose in children is 10 mg/m²/day IV for 3 days, repeated every 3 weeks.

Renal failure: The dose should be decreased by 25% in severe renal failure (creatinine clearance <25 mL/min).

Liver failure. The dose in hepatic failure is based on serum bilirubin and data for doxorubicin:

Dose Modification:

Bilirubin Level	% of Full Dose
<2-5 mg/dL	100%
2.5-5 mg/dL	50%
>5 mg/dL	none

Dose Forms:
Idarubicin is available in single-dose vials of 5, 10, and 20 mg of lyophilized powder.

Administration:
Idarubicin should be administered IV as a brief infusion over a period of 10 to 15 minutes into the sidearm of a freely running IV of NS or D5W. This agent is a potent vesicant, and appropriate precautions to prevent its extravasation should therefore be implemented. It also should be handled with care in order to avoid skin reactions.

Compatibilities:

Y-site infusion in a concentration of 1 mg/mL in NS: amikacin sulfate, cimetidine HCl, cyclophosphamide, cytarabine, diphenhydramine HCl, droperidol, erythromycin lactobionate, imipenem–cilastatin sodium, magnesium sulfate, mannitol, metoclopramide HCl, potassium chloride, ranitidine HCl, total parenteral nutrition (TPN) solution.
Y-site infusion in a concentration of 0.5 mg/mL in NS: melphalan HCl, sargramostim, vinorelbine sulfate.
Y-site infusion in a concentration of 0.5 mg/mL in D5W: filgrastim.

Incompatibilities: Acyclovir sodium, allopurinol sodium, ampicillin sodium sulbactim sodium, cefazolin sodium, ceftazidime, clindamycin phosphate, dexamethasone sodium phosphate, etoposide, furosemide, gentamicin sulfate, heparin sodium, hydrocortisone sodium succinate, lorazepam, meperidine HCl, methotrexate sodium, mezlocillin sodium, piperacillin sodium–tazobactam sodium, sodium bicarbonate, vancomycin HCl, and vincristine sulfate.

Adverse Reactions:

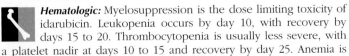

Hematologic: Myelosuppression is the dose limiting toxicity of idarubicin. Leukopenia occurs by day 10, with recovery by days 15 to 20. Thrombocytopenia is usually less severe, with a platelet nadir at days 10 to 15 and recovery by day 25. Anemia is rarely observed with this agent.

Cardiac: Although idarubicin is less cardiotoxic than doxorubicin, cardiomyopathy may occur after a large cumulative dose. In addition, transient arrhythmia (atrial fibrillation) may occur with 24 hours of administration, and lasts 1 to 2 days. Most patients are asymptomatic during atrial arrhythmias.

Gastrointestinal: Mild to moderate nausea and vomiting occur in about 90% of patients treated with idarubicin. The onset is usually within 15 to 30 minutes after infusion. Diarrhea and mucositis occur in about 60% of patients. Anorexia occurs in about 70% of patients, but is usually mild.

Hepatic: Elevated liver function tests may be noted in 20% to 40% of patients receiving both idarubicin and cytarabine.

Dermatologic: Alopecia occurs in about 70% of patients, with complete alopecia noted in 40% of patients. A generalized erythematous rash has been noted to occur in about 50% of patients. Idarubicin is a *potent vesicant* and may cause severe tissue damage if extravasated. If this occurs, treatment with ice and elevation of the affected limb should be initiated. Other therapy should be based on institutional policy.

Practitioner Interventions:

1. Monitor patient's blood cell counts on a weekly basis, including CBC with differential and platelet count.
2. Monitor patient for any signs and symptoms of skin rash and generalized erythema.
3. Premedicate patients with antiemetics at least 30 minutes prior to initiating infusion of idarubicin.

4. Instruct patients about risk of extravasation and methods being undertaken to prevent such an occurrence.
5. Instruct patients in oral care regimen as per institutional policy.
6. Evaluate mouth on a regular basis for stomatitis. Instruct patient about appearance of mouth lesions and when to contact health-care provider.
7. Instruct patient about possibility of diarrhea, and to contact health care provider if more than 3 stools are passed per day.
8. Instruct patient about probable occurrence of alopecia.
9. Monitor liver function tests on a biweekly basis.
10. Have an extravasation kit available at bedside.
11. In the event of an extravasation:
    a. Stop the infusion immediately and do not remove needle.
    b. Aspirate as much vesicant as possible.
    c. Notify physician.
    d. Instill antidote per institutional protocol.

References:

1. Berman E, Heller G, Santorsa J, et al. Results of a randomized trial comparing idarubicin and cytosine arabinoside in adult patients with newly diagnosed acute myelogenous leukemia. Blood 1991;77(8):1666–1674.
2. Berman E, Raymond V, Gee T, et al. Idarubicin in acute leukemia: results of studies at Memorial Sloan-Kettering Cancer Center. Semin Oncol 1989b;16(Suppl 2):30–34.
3. Carella AM, Carlier P, Pungolini E, et al. Idarubicin in combination with intermediate dose citarabine and VP-16 in the treatment of refractory and rapidly relapsed patients with acute myeloid leukemia. The GI-MEMA Cooperative Group. Leukemia 1993;7:196–199.
4. Turowski RC, Durthaler JM. Visual compatibility of idarubicin hydrochloride with selected drugs during simulated Y-site injection. Am J Hosp Pharm 1991;48:2181–2184.

IFOSFAMIDE

Other Names:
Ifex®, isophosphamide.

Uses:
Soft-tissue sarcoma, osteosarcoma, Ewing's sarcoma, non-Hodgkin's lymphoma, small-cell lung cancer, germ-cell testicular cancer, ovarian cancer.

Mechanism of Antitumor Action:

Ifosfamide is an alkylating agent that is metabolically activated in the liver to ifosfamide mustard and acrolein. Cross-linking of DNA strands occurs from ifosfamide mustard. Acrolein binds to bladder epithelia.

Pharmacokinetics:

The pharmacokinetics of ifosfamide are similar to those of cyclophosphamide.

Absorption: Ifosfamide is well absorbed from the GI tract, with a bioavailability close to 100%. However, only the IV form is available commercially.

Distribution: The drug distributes into total body water. Its Vd is about 35 L.

Protein Binding: Protein binding of ifosfamide is not well described.

Metabolism: About 50% of ifosfamide is metabolized. Hydroxylation by the liver is the major metabolic pathway.

Half-life: The half-life of ifosfamide is 3 to 10 hours for low-dose therapy and 13.8 hours for high-dose therapy.

Elimination: Between 70 and 80% of ifosfamide and its metabolites is excreted in urine.

Drug Interactions:

Cimetidine and ***allopurinol*** may increase the generation of ifosfamide alkylating metabolites, and enhance systemic toxicity.

Cisplatin may significantly increase ifosfamide nephrotoxicity.

Dosage:

A variety of dose schedules have been used for ifosfamide. The usual dose is 1,000 to 2,000 mg/m^2 daily for 4 to 5 days, repeated every 3 to 4 weeks. Other schedules have employed 2,400 mg/m^2 daily for 3 days. Single daily doses of up to 5,000 mg/m^2 have also been evaluated, but produce a higher incidence of both bladder toxicity (cystitis) and neurotoxicity (confusion and seizures), and are not recommended. Ifosfamide may be given by slow IV infusion (30 minutes) or continuous IV infusion. An order for mesna (uroprotectant) should accompany all ifosfamide orders.

Special Consideration: Prophylaxis against hemorrhagic cystitis is required. Hyperhydration and mesna must be given concurrently. The IV dose of mesna is 20% of the ifosfamide dose, given before and again at 4 and 8 hours after ifosfamide, or 1 mg for each milligram of ifosfamide if the latter is given as a continuous IV infusion. Mesna may also be given orally at 4 and 8 hours, at 40% of the ifosfamide dose. Oral mesna may be diluted in 4 ounces of juice or water.

Dose Forms:
Ifex® is available in 1 g and 3 g vials.

Administration:
A diluent of 20 ml sterile water or bacteriostatic water should be used for the 1 g vial of ifosfamide, and of 60 ml for the 3 g vial. The resulting solution is stable for 1 week at room temperature and for 3 weeks when refrigerated. If ifosfamide is not reconstituted with bacteriostatic water, solutions should be used within 6 hours. Solutions of ifosfamide in D5W, NS, LR, or sterile water for injection are stable for 1 week at 30°C and for 6 weeks at 5°C.

Compatibilities: Mesna, carboplatin (1 mg/mL), cisplatin (0.2 mg/mL), etoposide (0.2 mg/mL), epirubicin HCl, and fluorouracil (10 mg/mL) are compatible in the same bag with 2 mg/mL ifosfamide in NS. However, ifosfamide is incompatible with mesna plus epirubicin HCl or doxorubicin HCl.

In Y-site infusions of 25 mg/mL NS, ifosfamide is compatible with allopurinol sodium, doxorubicin HCl (2 mg/mL), gallium nitrate, melphalan HCl, sagramostim, and vinorelbine tartrate.

In Y-site infusions of 25 mg/mL D5W, ifosfamide is compatible with cefepine HCl, filgrastim, fludarabine phosphate, ondansetron HCl, paclitaxel, and piperacillin sodium–tazobactam sodium.

Incompatibilities: Epirubicin HCl (admixtures); doxorubicin HCl.

Adverse Reactions:
Hematologic: Myelosuppression with ifosfamide is dose related and dose limiting. It consists mainly of leukopenia and, to a lesser extent, thrombocytopenia. The granulocyte count reaches a nadir in 10 to 14 days, with recovery in 21 days.

Gastrointestinal: Nausea and vomiting are common with ifosfamide, and the drug is moderately emetogenic, depending on the dosage given. The onset of nausea and vomiting is from 3 to 6 hours, and the duration may be up to 3 days. Anorexia occasionally occurs. Mucositis and diarrhea are uncommon but occasionally severe.

 ***Genitourinary:*** Bladder toxicity is common with ifosfamide and consists of hemorrhagic cystitis, dysuria, urinary frequency, and other symptoms of bladder irritation. Mesna plus hydration must be used to prevent bladder toxicity.

 Neurologic: CNS toxicity may occur, especially with single doses of ifosfamide greater than 2500 mg/m^2. Symptoms include lethargy, confusion, seizure, cerebellar ataxia, stupor, and weakness. This toxicity is associated with delayed renal clearance of the metabolite chloracetaldehyde. Thus, patients with decreased renal function are at greater risk for neurotoxicity.

 Hepatic: Liver function test results may be elevated, including those for alkaline phosphatase and serum transaminases, which usually resolve without sequelae.

 Dermatologic: Alopecia is common. Rashes, nail changes, and hyperpigmentation may occur but are rarely dose limiting.

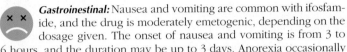 ***Nephrotoxicity:*** Rare cases of acute renal failure have been reported with ifosfamide.

Practitioner Interventions:

1. Give antiemetics 30 minutes prior to ifosfamide.
2. Initiate mesna therapy as ordered.
3. Give IV fluids of at least 2 L/m^2/day during and 6 to 12 hours after the completion of ifosfamide.
4. Monitor patient for blood in urine daily prior to each dose of ifosfamide.
5. Monitor patient for any CNS changes, especially when giving concomitant cisplatinum.
6. Monitor patient's liver and renal function tests.
7. Monitor patient's CBC and platelets on a weekly basis.

References:

1. DeChant KL, Brogden, Pilkington T, et al. Ifosfamide/mesna: a review

of its antineoplastic activity, pharmacokinetics properties and therapeutic efficacy in cancer. Drugs 1991;42:428–467.

2. Goren MP, Wright RK, Pratt CB, et al. Dechlorethylation of ifosfamide and neurotoxicity. Lancet 1986;2:1219–1229.
3. Mesnex® Product Information. Bristol-Myers Squibb, February 1995.
4. Shaw IC, Rose JW. Infusion of ifosfamide plus mesna. Lancet, 1984;1353–54.
5. Zolupski M, Baker LH. Ifosfamide. J Natl Cancer Inst 1988;80:556–566.

INTERFERON ALFA

Other Names:

Alferon®, Intron-A®, Roferon-A®, α-2a-interferon, α-2b-interferon.

Uses:

Hairy cell leukemia, Kaposi's sarcoma, chronic myelogenous leukemia (CML), multiple myeloma, non-Hodgkin's lymphoma, renal cell carcinoma.

Mechanism of Antitumor Action:

Antitumor effects of interferon alfa relate to its direct or indirect regulation of cell growth, and are characterized by activation of other cytokines, such as interleukin-2. Interferon alfa also increases $2'$, $5'$-oligodenylate synthetase and protein kinase activity, downregulates oncogene expression, and inhibits growth signal production.

Pharmacokinetics:

Absorption: Between 80 and 90% of interferon alfa is systemically absorbed after IM or SC administration. The time to maximal concentration is about 4 hours after IM and 7 hours after SC administration.

Distribution: Interferon alfa does not cross the blood–brain barrier even after high IV doses.

Protein Binding: Unknown.

Metabolism: The liver is not involved in metabolism of interferon alfa. Proteolytic degradation occurs in the kidney, catabolizing most of the drug. Some nonrenal metabolism also occurs.

Half-life: The half-life of interferon alfa ranges from 2.3 to 7.3 hours, depending on the route of drug administration.

Elimination: The primary route of elimination of interferon alfa is renal via glomerular filtration, followed by renal tubular reabsorption. Complete proteolysis during tubular reabsorption results in very little systemic drug return and virtually no urinary excretion of the drug.

Drug Interactions:

Many drug interactions with interferon alfa have been limited to *in vitro* cell culture studies or animal studies. Enhanced cytotoxicity has been reported for **carmustine, cisplatin, cyclophosphamide, doxorubicin, fluorouracil,** and **interferon β and γ**. Combination therapy with doxorubicin or cisplatin and interferon alfa has also resulted in increased and often unacceptable toxicity in patients. The mechanism for this interaction is unknown. Since interferon alfa inhibits cytochrome P450 metabolism, the metabolism of drugs such as **cyclophosphamide** and **phenytoin** may be decreased, resulting in increased toxicity. Dexamethasone does not seem to affect the cytotoxicity of interferon alfa. **Zidovudine** increases the hematologic toxicity of interferon alfa.

Dosage

The usual dose of interferon alfa in hairy cell leukemia and chronic myelogenous leukemia is 3 to 5 MU/m^2/day or 2 to 5 MU/m^2 three times a week. For solid tumors and Kaposi's sarcoma, doses of up to 30 MU/m^2 SC given three times a week have been used. In patients receiving zidovudine, a dose of interferon alfa of 9 MU/day is usually the maximum tolerated dose.

Dose Forms:

Interferon alfa is available as a lyophilized powder that is reconstituted with the diluent provided, or with bacteriostatic water for injection. Alferon® is available in vials of 5 million units containing 3.3 mg phenol, 1 mg of albumin, and a phosphate-buffered saline solution. Intron-A® is available as a powder in vials of 3, 5, 10, 18, 25, and 50 million units, and in solution for injection in vials of 3, 5, 10, 18, and 25 million units. Roferon-A® is available as single use injection vials of 3, 9, and 36 million units; multidose injection vials of 9 and 18 million units; and as a powder for injection in vials of 18 million units.

Administration:

Interferon alfa may be administered IV, SC, or IM. IV administration is usually as a short infusion in 50 to 100 mL in NS over a period of 10 to 15 minutes. Do not freeze or shake vials.

Compatabilities: None reported

Incompatibilities: None reported

Adverse Reactions:

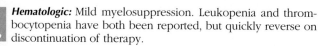

Flu-like syndrome: Fever, chills, slight tachycardia, malaise, myalgias, and headache. Prophylactic acetaminophen may be tried, but often is not effective in preventing symptoms. In this case, indomethacin 25 mg PO given thrice daily should be tried. Fatigue is dose-related and most common after doses of 20 MU or higher. Most patients will experience fatigue after several doses of the drug.

Gastrointestinal: Anorexia is common. Watery diarrhea may occur after high-dose therapy.

Hematologic: Mild myelosuppression. Leukopenia and thrombocytopenia have both been reported, but quickly reverse on discontinuation of therapy.

Hepatic: Mild elevation in transaminase levels.

Neurologic: Somnolence may occur in about one-fourth of patients. Agitation, depression, tremor, dizziness, and seizures have all been reported in patients receiving doses greater than 20 MU/m^2.

Practitioner Interventions:

1. Instruct patient about the management of symptoms of flu-like syndrome.
2. Premedicate patient with acetaminophen to reduce fever and decrease flu-like syndrome. If acetaminophen is ineffective, try indomethacin.
3. Encourage patient to provide for rest periods in the day, owing to fatigue associated with use of interferon alfa.
4. Consult dietician as required for anorexia.
5. Monitor patient's complete blood cell count (CBC) with platelet count on a weekly basis to evaluate neutropenia and thrombocytopenia. Check monthly liver function.

References:
1. Durie BGM, Clouse L, Braich T, et al. Interferon alfa-2b-cyclophospham-

ide combination studies: *In vitro* and phase I-II clinical results. Semin Oncol 1986;13:84–88.

2. Goldstein D, Lazlo J. Interferon therapy and cancer: from imaginon to interferon. Cancer Res 1986;46:4315–4329.

3. Kirkwood JM, Ernstoff MS. Interferons in the treatment of human cancer. J Clin Oncol 1984;2:336–352.

4. Quesada JR, Hersh DM, Reuben J, Gutterman JV. α-Interferon for induction of remission of hairy cell leukemia. N Engl J Med 1984;310: 15–18.

5. Quesada JR, Talpaz M, Rios A, et al. Clinical toxicity of interferons in cancer patients: A review. J Clin Oncol 1986;4:234–243.

IRINOTECAN HCl

Other Names:
Camptosar®, CPT-11.

Uses:
Irinotecan is FDA-approved for colorectal cancer refractory to fluorouracil. Irinotecan also has activity in non-small-cell lung cancer, small-cell lung cancer, squamous-cell carcinoma of the cervix and skin, and cancers of the pancreas, stomach, and ovary.

Mechanism of Antitumor Action:
Irinotecan is a prodrug and is converted by plasma, intestinal mucosa, and hepatic carboxylesterase enzymes to a more active metabolite, SN-38, which is a specific inhibitor of topoisomerase I, resulting in DNA damage and cell death. Colorectal tumors have more topoisomerase I than normal colonic mucosa, and malignant cells in these tumors may be more susceptible to topoisomerase inhibition than normal cells.

Pharmacokinetics:
Studies have noted no correlation of the pharmacokinetic parameters of irinotecan or SN-38 with response to therapy and survival. However, severe diarrhea is associated with higher levels of SN-38 in the bile. Patients with higher levels of SN-38 glucuronide have less frequent severe diarrhea. The kinetics of irinotecan and SN-38 are linear over the dose range of 40 to 180 mg/m^2 IV weekly. Also, no alteration in pharmacokinetic parameters was observed over a 4-week

period, suggesting no metabolic induction. The pharmacokinetics of irinotecan is unknown in pediatric patients.

Absorption: Irinotecan is given by the IV route only, but an oral form is being developed. Mean SN-38 peak levels are observed 1 hour after a 30-minute infusion of the drug.

Distribution: After 24 hours, the mean Vd_{ss} of irinotecan in adults was 150 L/m^2.

Protein Binding: Because of the large Vd of irinotecan, it is expected that there is a high percentage of plasma protein binding of the open-ring carbolyte form of the drug.

Metabolism: Irinotecan is rapidly de-esterfied in plasma, intestinal mucosa, and liver to SN-38, the concentration of which peaks between 30 and 90 minutes after IV administration of the parent drug. SN-38 is also glucuronidated to an inactive metabolite. Both the parent compound and SN-38 exist in either a closed-ring (active) or open-ring (carboxylate, inactive) form depending on pH. An acidic pH drives the equilibrium to a closed-ring form and a basic pH shifts it to the inactive, open-ring form. In the plasma, the closed-ring and lactone forms are present in mean percentages of 34 and 45% for irinotecan and SN-38, respectively.

Half-life: The half-lives of irinotecan and SN-38 are 8 and 13 hours, respectively.

Elimination: Total body clearance of irinotecan is about 14 $L/m^2/hr$. The major route of elimination for irinotecan and SN-38 is in the bile and feces. SN-38 also undergoes extensive enterohepatic recycling. About 70% of the drug is excreted in the feces within 72 hours of administration. In contrast, only about 14% of the drug is recovered in the urine, suggesting that renal clearance is not a major route of elimination.

Drug Interactions:
None reported to date.

Dosage:

Metastatic colorectal cancer: Irinotecan is usually given in a dose of 100 to 125 mg/m^2 IV over a period of 90 minutes once each week for 4 weeks, with the treatment cycle repeated every 6 weeks.

Dose Forms:
Irinotecan is supplied as a 100 mg/5 ml single-use vial.

Administration:
Camptosar® should be diluted in 5% dextrose, (preferred) or normal saline to a concentration range of 0.12 to 1.1 mg/mL and administered by slow IV infusion over a period of 90 minutes. Solutions of Camptosar® are stable for 24 hours at room temperature. Solutions in 5% dextrose may be refrigerated and are stable for 48 hrs. Solutions in normal saline should not be refrigerated because of the potential for particle formation.

Compatibilities: None reported.

Incompatibilities: Normal saline solutions that are refrigerated may result in particle formation.

Adverse Reactions:

 Hematologic: The dose-limiting toxicity of irinotecan has been myelosuppression. Grade 3 or 4 neutropenia occurs in about 20% of patients. The typical neutrophil pattern shows a nadir at days 7 to 10 and recovery by days 21 to 28. Thrombocytopenia and anemia are also noted. Eosinophilia is common occuring in about 22% of patients.

Gastrointestinal: Diarrhea is also a dose-limiting toxicity of irinotecan. It occurs within 6 days of drug administration. Grade 3 or 4 toxicity occurs in over 50% of patients not treated with antidiarrheal medications. **The incidence of grade 3 or 4 diarrhea is about 10% in patients in whom a strict antidiarrheal treatment guideline is followed (see below).** Nausea and vomiting are mild to moderate, and are dose related. Mucositis may be severe in 120-hour infusions of irinotecan.

Renal: Microscopic hematuria has been reported in about 10% of patients.

Hepatic: Occasionally, hepatic enzyme elevation, including elevated alkaline phosphatase and bilirubin, has been reported after treatment with irinotecan. Grade 3 toxicity is reversed after drug discontinuation.

Other: Rarely, shortness of breath has been reported after therapy. Also, a mild hand–foot syndrome has been noted.

Practitioner Interventions:

1. Monitor patient's complete blood cell count (CBC) and platelet counts every week.
2. Monitor patient for fevers and instruct patient to contact health care provider if fever greater than 101°F or 38.5°C occurs.
3. The patient should be instructed on the use of antidiarrheal medication in the event of diarrhea. At the first sign of increase in bowel frequency or loose stools, the patient should begin the following regimen:
   Loperamide 4 mg orally with first loose bowel movement, then 2 mg every 2 hours during the day, 4 mg at bedtime, then 4 mg every 4 hours until baseline bowel function is established for 24 hours. If bowel frequency continues to increase despite treatment, the patient should be seen by a health-care provider to determine if further treatment is necessary.
4. The health-care provider should call the patient starting at day 5 of treatment and follow-up on a daily basis if necessary or the patient to call health care providers so the presence of greater than 3 stools per day.

References:

1. Abigerges D, Armand JP, Chabot GG, et. al. Irinotecan (CPT-11) high-dose escalation using intensive high-dose loperamide to control diarrhea. J Natl Cancer Inst 1994;86:446–449.
2. Camptosar® Product Information. Pharmacia & Upjohn Company, June 1996.
3. Chabot GG, Abigerges D, Catimel G, et. al. Population pharmacokinetics and pharmacodynamics of irinotecan (CPT-11) and active metabolite SN-38 during phase I trials. Ann Oncol 1995;6:141–151.
4. Conti JA, Kemeny NE, Saltz LB, et. al. Irinotecan is an active agent in untreated patients with metastatic colorectal cancer. J Clin Oncol 1996;14:709–715.
5. Greemers GJ, Lund B, Verweij L. Topoisomerase I inhibitors: topotecan and irinotecan. Cancer Treat Rev 1994;20:73–96.
6. Gupta E, Lesting TM, Mick R, et. al. Metabolic fate of irinotecan in humans: correlation of glucuronidation with diarrhea. Cancer Res 1994;54:3723–3725.

7. Rothenberg ML, Kuhn JG, Burris HA, et. al. Phase I and pharmacokinetic trial of weekly CPT-11. J Clin Oncol 1993;11:2194–2204.
8. Slichenmeyer WJ, Rowinsky EK, Donehower RC, Kaufman SH. The current status of camptothecin analogues as antitumor agents. J Natl Cancer Inst 1993;85:271–291.

LEUPROLIDE ACETATE

Other Names:
Lupron®, Lupron Depot®, Lupron Depot-Ped®, Lupron Depot-3 month®.

Uses:
Palliative treatment of metastatic prostate cancer. Leuprolide acetate is effective in both previously treated and untreated patients.

Mechanism of Antitumor Action:
Leuprolide produces a medical castration by acting as a gonadotropin-releasing hormone (GnRH) antagonist. An initial stimulatory effect on follicle stimulating hormone (FSH) is followed by feedback inhibition of the pituitary, which leads to suppression of FSH and luteinizing hormone (LH). The ultimate effect is to produce castrate levels of testosterone in males and low levels of estrogen and progestin in women. After 1 to 2 weeks of continuous therapy with leuprolide or long-acting leuprolide, plasma levels of testosterone and its active metabolite dihydrotestosterone fall to castrate levels.

Pharmacokinetics:
Absorption: After subcutaneous administration of 1 mg, 94% of the dose of leuprolide acetate is absorbed into the systemic circulation. The drug is not absorbed orally.

Distribution: Unknown.

Protein Binding: Only about 10% of leuprolide is bound to plasma proteins.

Metabolism: Unknown in humans.

Half-life: The plasma $T_{1/2}$ of leuprolide is 2.9 hours.

Elimination: Unknown in humans.

Drug Interactions:
None known.

Dosage:
For prostate cancer, the depot form of leuprolide acetate is the most commonly used form, and is given in a dose of 7.5 mg IM once a month or 22.5 mg IM every 3 months.

Dose Forms:
Lupron Depot® is available as single dose vials of 3.75 and 7.5 mg. Lupron Depot-3 Month® is available in a single dose vial of 22.5 mg.

Administration:
Individual daily doses of leuprolide acetate are given SC. The depot suspension should be shaken thoroughly to disperse particles, and should be given IM only.

Adverse Reactions:

Endocrine: Hot flashes, ranging from mild flushing to sweats, are common in patients treated with leuprolide acetate. Decreased libido and impotence have been reported in about one-third of patients treated with the combination of leuprolide and flutamide.

Tumor Flare: Increasing bone pain may occur during the first 2 weeks of administration of leuprolide acetate.

Cardiovascular: Peripheral edema due to sodium retention, increased blood pressure, stroke, myocardial infarction, and arrhythmias are all uncommon with leuprolide acetate.

Other: Other side effects of leuprolide acetate are uncommon and include dysuria, weakness, and lower-extremity numbness. Rare cases of thrombophlebitis and pulmonary emboli have been reported.

Practitioner Interventions:

1. Monitor patient for signs and symptoms of hot flashes.

2. Counsel patient about possibility of transiently increased bone pain.
3. Evaluate patient for peripheral edema.
4. Monitor injection sites for pain, erythema, or infection.
5. Instruct patient about appropriate self injection technique, whether SC or IM.
6. Instruct patient about possibility of decreased libido and erectile impotence. Seek appropriate referrals as necessary for counseling.

References:

1. Barton Burke M, Wilkes G, Ingiversen K. Chemotherapy Care Plans. Jones & Bartlett, Boston, 1993, pp. 228–229.
2. Conn PM, Crowley WF Jr. Gonadotropin-releasing hormone and its analogues. N Engl J Med 1991;324:93–103.
3. Leuprolide Study Group. Leuprolide versus diethylstilbestrol for metastatic prostatic cancer. N Engl J Med 1984;311:1281–1286.

LEVAMISOLE HCl

Other Names:
Ergamisol®.

Uses:
Adjuvant therapy for Duke's stage C colorectal cancer when used together with fluorouracil.

Mechanism of Antitumor Action:
When used alone, levamisole has no antitumor activity. However, its action against colon cancer cells may be due to its ability to enhance the function of T-lymphocytes. In addition, a metabolite, p-hydroxy-tetramisole, may potentiate fluorouracil cytotoxicity by inhibiting tyrosine phosphatase.

Pharmacokinetics:

Absorption: Levamisole is rapidly absorbed.

Distribution: Not studied.

Protein Binding: Not studied.

Metabolism: Levamisole is metabolized in the liver to a glucuronide metabolite.

Half-life: 4 hours.

Elimination: Less than 5% of unchanged drug appears in the urine and feces. About 12% of the hydroxymetabolite is excreted in the urine.

Drug Interactions:
Concurrent ***alcohol*** and levamisole may result in an disulfiram-like reaction. Levamisole may increase ***phenytoin*** levels. The mechanism of this interaction has not been determined. Levamisole may enhance myelosuppression by ***fluorouracil*** and ***carmustine.***

Dosage:
50 mg every 8 hours for 3 days starting 7 to 30 days after primary surgery, followed by 50 mg every 8 hours for 3 days every 2 weeks for 1 year.

Dose Forms:
Levamisole is available in 50 mg tablets.

Administration:
A 50 mg dose of levamisole should be given on an empty stomach every 8 hours around the clock.

Adverse Reactions:

 Gastrointestinal: In patients treated with fluorouracil and levamisole, nausea and vomiting have been reported in 20 to 65% of cases and diarrhea in 52%.

 Dermatologic: Skin rash has occurred in about 25% of patients treated with levamisole. These reactions are more likely due to fluorouracil.

Practitioner Interventions:

1. Premedicate patient with antiemetics 30 minutes prior to dosing with levamisole. Instruct patient to take pills on an empty stomach.

2. Monitor number of patient's stools per day; if more than 3, instruct patient to contact health-care provider.

3. Instruct patient about possibility of skin rash; instruct patient to contact health care provider if rash develops.

References:

1. Grem JL. Levamisole as a therapeutic agent for colorectal carcinoma. Cancer Cells 1990;2:131–137.
2. Moertel CF, Fleming TR, Macdonald JS, et al. Levamisole and fluorouracil for adjuvant therapy of resected colon cancer. N Engl J Med 1990;322:352–358.
3. Moertel CF, Fleming TR, Macdonald JS, et al. Fluorouracil plus levamisole as effective adjuvant therapy after resection of stage III colon carcinoma: a final report. Ann Intern Med 1995;122:321–326.

LOMUSTINE

Other Names:
CeeNu®, CCNU.

Uses:
The uses of lomustine are for the management of primary or malignant brain tumors and advanced Hodgkin's disease.

Mechanism of Antitumor Action:
The cytotoxic effect of lomustine involves the inhibition of both DNA and RNA synthesis through DNA alkylation. The antitumor activity of the drug correlates best with intrastrand crosslinking. Lomustine affects a number of cellular processes including RNA and protein synthesis, and the processing of ribosomal and messenger RNA.

Pharmacokinetics:

Absorption: Lomustine has a high lipid solubility, facilitating its rapid transport across the gastrointestinal mucosa and blood–brain barrier.

Distribution: Lomustine has good penetration of gastrointestinal mucosa, and its penetration into the CNS approximates 15 to 30% of its plasma level.

Protein Binding: Lomustine is highly protein bound.

Metabolism: The metabolism of lomustine is mediated via hepatic microsomal enzymes.

Half-life: The half-life of lomustine is about hours.

Elimination: Lomustine excretion occurs via the renal system and is fairly slow. About 60% of a dose is recovered after 48 hours, with 50% recovered in the first 12 hours.

Drug Interactions:
The H_2 antagonist **cimetidine** has been shown to potentiate lomustine's myelotoxicity in patients being treated for brain tumors.

Dosage:
The dose of lomustine as a single agent is 100 to 130 mg/m^2, given as a single oral dose. This should not be given more frequently than once every 6 weeks.

Dose Forms:
CeeNU® is available in 10 mg, 40 mg, and 100 mg capsules.

Administration:
Administer lomustine orally on an empty stomach. Instruct patients to avoid alcohol for short periods after oral administration of the drug.

Adverse Reactions:
Hematologic: The dose-limiting toxicity of lomustine is delayed and potentially cumulative myelosuppression. Leukopenia occurs with a nadir in the leukocyte count at days 41 to 46 and recovery at days 50 to 55. Thrombocytopenia occurs with a nadir in the platelet count at days 26 to 34 and recovery by days 32 to 44.

Gastrointestinal: Nausea and vomiting are common in patients treated with lomustine and usually occur 2 to 6 hours after dosing. Anorexia may also be present in patients taking lomustine. Stomatitis is uncommon.

 **Neurologic:** Confusion, lethargy, and ataxia are rare.

 Other: Alopecia and transient elevation in hepatic enzymes have occurred.

Practitioner Interventions:

1. Monitor patient's complete blood cell count (CBC) and platelet count weekly.
2. Instruct patient to take lomustine on an empty stomach in the evening before bedtime.
3. Instruct patient to avoid alcohol for at least one hour before and after taking the dose of lomustine.
4. Premedicate patient 30 minutes prior to administering lomustine.
5. Monitor patient for any signs and symptoms of neurotoxicity.
6. Explain to patient the rare possibility of alopecia.
7. Instruct patient on appropriate birth-control methodology, since lomustine is mutagenic and teratogenic.
8. Instruct patient to discontinue taking cimetidine when receiving lomustine unless specifically instructed to do so as part of chemotherapy treatment.
9. Instruct patient to self-monitor for any signs and symptoms of mucositis or stomatitis.

References:

1. Lee FYF, Workman P, Roberts JT, et al. Clinical pharmacokinetics of oral CCNU, lomustine. Cancer Chemother Pharmacol 1985;14:125–131.
2. Oliverio VT. Pharmacology of the nitrosureas: an overview. Cancer Treat Rep 1976;60:703–707.

MECHLORETHAMINE HCl

Other Names:
Mustargen®, Nitrogen mustard.

Uses:
Hodgkin's disease, malignant effusion.

Mechanism of Antitumor Action:

Mechlorethamine is a bifunctional alkylating agent that attaches to guanine in DNA, resulting in DNA miscoding, imidazole ring cleavage; crosslinking of DNA; and DNA strand breakage.

Pharmacokinetics:

Because of the rapid hydrolysis of the drug in plasma, mechlorethamine pharmacokinetics have not been studied.

Absorption: Mechlorethamine is not absorbed orally. It is administered primarily IV. It is sometimes given by the intrapleural route. Systemic absorption probably occurs, since myelosuppression is observed after intrapleural administration.

Distribution: Unknown.

Protein Binding: Unknown.

Metabolism: Mechlorethamine undergoes rapid hydrolysis in plasma to reactive metabolites.

Half-life: The plasma alkylating activity of mechlorethamine has a half-life of 15 to 20 minutes.

Elimination: More than 50% of inactive metabolites of mechlorethamine are excreted in the urine in the first 24 hours after dosing.

Drug Interactions:

Sodium thiosulfate directly neutralizes the activity of mechlorethamine.

Dosage:

The usual IV dose of mechlorethamine as a single agent is 0.4 mg/kg or 0.1 mg/kg daily × 4. In the MOPP regimen, the dose of mechlorethamine is 6 mg/m^2 IV on days 1 and 8. The dose cycle is repeated every 4 weeks.

Dose Forms:

Mustargen® is available in a 10 mg vial.

Administration:

Mechlorethamine must be prepared just prior to administration. It should be administered by IV push in the side arm of a newly placed peripheral IV line or a patent IV central catheter. Spillage of mechlorethamine can be neutralized by soaking with 5% sodium thiosulfate and 5% sodium bicarbonate for 45 minutes.

Compatibilities: In a 1:1 mixture of mechlorethamine at 1 mg/mL in simulated Y-site infusions, the drug is compatible with fludarabine phosphate, ondansetron HCl, and sargramostim.

Adverse Reactions:

Hematologic: Myelosuppression is the dose limiting toxicity of mechlorethamine. Maximum leukopenia and thrombocytopenia occur at days 8 to 14. Recovery of neutrophils and platelets occurs by days 21 to 30.

Gastrointestinal: Nausea and vomiting usually occurs within the first 3 hours and are often severe. Prophylactic antiemetic therapy with a 5HT$_3$ antagonist is recommended.

Dermatologic: Mechlorethamine is a powerful vesicant if extravasated. The approved antidote is 1/6 molar sodium thiosulfate. Alopecia is common.

Endocrine: Reproductive changes including amenorrhea and impaired spermatogenesis will occur with mechlorethamine.

Hypersensitivity: Allergic reactions to mechlorethamine are rare.

Vascular: Phlebitis and thrombosis may occur in veins injected with mechlorethamine. There is no effective prophylaxis for this. The use of implantable vascular devices may avoid phlebitic reactions.

Neurologic: CNS complications consisting of weakness, headache, drowsiness, vertigo, lightheadedness, and convulsions are rare with mechlorethamine. Risk factors for these complications are old age, high dose of mechlorethamine, and concurrent cyclophosphamide or procarbazine.

Other: Other rare reactions to mechlorethamine include jaundice, hearing loss, fever, and metallic taste.

Practitioner Interventions:

1. Premedicate patient with antiemetics (5HT$_3$ antagonist) 30 minutes prior to administration of mechlorethamine.

2. Change or make sure IV site is less than 24 hours old due to vesicant property of drug.

3. Have extravasation kit at patient's bedside with antidote (sodium thiosulfate) available prior to drug administration.

4. Instruct patient about signs and symptoms of infection and when to call health care provider in case these develop.

5. Counsel patient on reproductive issues relating to mechlorethamine. Instruct patient on use of appropriate birth control techniques.

6. Monitor patient's CBC and platelets every week.

7. Monitor for any signs and symptoms of CNS toxicity.

8. In the event of an extravasation, refer to Table 1.2 (pages 223–225) for guidelines on management.

References:

1. Gilman A. The initial clinical trial of nitrogen mustard. Am J Surg 1963;105:574–578.
2. Warwick GP. The mechanism of action of alkylating agents Cancer Res 1963;23:1315–1333.

MEGESTROL ACETATE

Other Names:
Megace®.

Uses:
Megestrol acetate is used in patients who have well differentiated renal carcinoma, endometrial cancer, and breast cancer. It has also been used for patients with cancer cachexia.

Mechanism of Antitumor Action:
The exact mechanism of antitumor action of megestrol acetate is not well known. Megestrol is a synthetic progestogen that has antiestrogenic effects. It works by inducing the enzyme 17-hydroxysteroid dehydrogenase, which oxidizes estradiol to the less potent form, estrone. It also activates estrogen sulfatransferase, which catalyzes the sulfation of estrogens to less active conjugates. Megestrol decreases the number of estrogen receptors, as well as inhibiting the release of luteinizing hormone (LH) receptors. The mechanism by which megestrol increases body weight is unclear.

Pharmacokinetics:

Absorption: Megestrol is rapidly and completely absorbed when given orally. Peak levels are reached in 1 to 3 hours.

Distribution: A large percentage of megestrol is stored in fat.

Protein Binding: Studies of the protein binding of megestrol have not been performed to date. However, natural progesterone is a highly protein-bound (> 95%) product.

Metabolism: Megestrol is about 70% metabolized in the liver in the first pass, and excreted partially in the urine (60 to 80% over a period of 10 days.)

Half-life: Megestrol has a terminal half-life of about 20 hours.

Elimination: Most of a dose of megestrol acetate is metabolized and excreted in the urine as metabolized or inactive products.

Drug Interactions:
The increased weight gain with megestrol acetate has not been shown to change the distribution of any other agent. Megestrol acetate decreases the clearance of ***warfarin***. Prothrombin time and International Normalized Ratio (INR) should be monitored closely in patients on warfarin while they are receiving megestrol acetate.

Aminoglutethimide decreases serum levels of megestrol acetate by about 75%. The mechanism by which this happens is enhanced hepatic metabolism (Lundgren).

Dosage:
The antitumor dose of megestrol acetate is 40 mg PO four times daily. Megestrol acetate may also be given in a dose of 160 mg once daily or 80 mg twice daily. Higher doses (800 mg daily) are used for appetite stimulation.

Dose Forms:
Megace® is available in 20 and 40 mg tablets and as an oral suspension (40 mg/mL in a total volume of 237 mL).

Administration:
Megestrol acetate may be administered via the oral route with or without food, and is usually divided into four daily doses.

Adverse Reactions:

 Genitourinary: Vaginal bleeding, menstrual changes, amenorrhea, and increased urinary frequency are common with megestrol.

 Cardiovascular: Megestrol is generally very well tolerated. Fluid retention is a common complaint, but is usually not clinically significant.

 Gastrointestinal: Nausea, vomiting and abdominal pain may occur in patients receiving megestrol.

 Hepatic: Liver function test abnormalities are rare in patients receiving megestrol. In patients with liver failure, the dose should be reduced.

 Dermatologic: Alopecia may rarely occur. Rash has been reported.

Practitioner Interventions:

1. Instruct patient to monitor for vaginal bleeding, menstrual changes and possibility of amenorrhea.
2. Instruct patients about probable weight gain and fluid retention.
3. Have patients avoid a high-salt diet, since this may contribute to fluid retention.
4. Instruct patients about low probability of alopecia.

References:

1. Allegra JC, Kiefer SM. Mechanics of action of progestational agents. Semin Oncol 1985;12(Suppl 2):3–5.
2. Carpenter JT Jr. Progestational agents in the treatment of breast cancer. Cancer Treat Res 1988;39:147–156.
3. Loprinzi CL, Ellison NM, Schaird DJ, et al. Controlled trial of megestrol acetate for the treatment of cancer, anorexia and cachexia. J Natl Cancer Inst 1990;82:1127–1132.
4. Lundgren SJ, Lonning PE, Aakvaag A, Kvinnsland S. Influence of aminoglutethimide on the metabolism of medroxyprogesterone acetate in postmenopausal patients with advanced breast cancer. Cancer Chemother Pharmacol 1990;27:101–105.
5. Mus HB, Case LD, Capizzi RL, et al. High- versus standard-dose megestrol acetate in women with advanced cancer: A phase III trial of the Piedmont Oncology Association. J Clin Oncol 1990;8:1797–1805.

6. Schacter L, Rozencweig M, Canetta R, et al. Megestrol acetate. Clin Exp Cancer Treat Rev 1989;16:49–63.

MELPHALAN

Other Names:
Alkeran®, L-PAM, phenylalanine mustard, L-sarcolysin.

Uses:
Multiple myeloma, testicular and ovarian cancer, sarcomas, melanoma.

Mechanism of Antitumor Action:
Melphalan is an alkylating agent similar in action to nitrogen mustard. It binds covalently to N-7 guanine residues on DNA and causes rapid destruction of cells.

Pharmacokinetics:

Absorption: Oral absorption of melphalan is poor and erratic. In high oral doses (0.6 mg/kg), the absolute bioavailability has ranged from 25 to 89%. When melphalan is taken with food, its systemic absorption is decreased.

Distribution: The Vd of melphalan appears to approximate total body water (44 L).

Protein Binding: Between 80% and 90% of orally-administered melphalan is bound to plasma proteins (60% to albumin and 20% to α_1-acid glycoprotein).

Metabolism: Melphalan is catabolized in the plasma through spontaneous hydrolysis.

Half-life: The half-life of melphalan is biphasic, with $T_{1/2}\alpha$ of 6 to 8 minutes and a $T_{1/2}\beta$ of about 90 minutes. The hydroxy- metabolites have half-lives two to three times that of the unchanged drug.

Elimination: Between 25 and 30% of a dose of melphalan is excreted in urine within 24 hours. Another 25 to 50% is excreted in feces over a period of about 6 days.

Drug Interactions:
Cyclosporine increases the risk of nephrotoxicity with melphalan. *Misonidazole* increases melphalan cytotoxicity by decreasing its clearance. *Cimetidine* decreases the oral bioavailability of melphalan by approximately 30%. *Corticosteroids* enhance the antitumor effects of melphalan.

Dose:

Oral: Multiple myeloma: 0.25 mg/kg/day or 9 mg/m^2 for 4 to 7 days, repeated every 4 to 6 weeks.

Intravenous: Dose used in bone marrow transplantation is 140 mg/m^2 as a single agent.

The dose of melphalan is reduced in renal failure: If the creatinine clearance <40 mL/min or serum creatinine >2 mg/dL, melphalan should be withheld.

Administration:
Melphalan is usually given orally without food. The parenteral form is given IV by slow infusion in a concentration of < 0.45 mg/mL in NS over a period of 15 to 30 minutes. Melphalan may be an irritant to the vein.

Compatibilities: In Y-site simulation using 0.1 mg/mL melphalan in NS, the drug is compatible with bleomycin sulfate, carboplatin, carmustine, cyclophosphamide, cisplatin, cytarabine, dacarbazine, dactinomycin, daunorubicin HCl, doxorubicin HCl, etoposide, floxuridine, fludarabine phosphate, fluorouracil, gallium nitrate, idarubicin HCl, ifosfamide, mechlorethamine HCl, mesna, methotrexate sodium, metoclopramide HCI, mitomycin, mitoxantrone, ondansetron HCl, pentostatin, plicamycin, streptozocin, thiotepa, vinblastine sulfate, vincristine sulfate, and vinorelbine tartrate.

Incompatibilities: Chlorpromazine HCl, amphotericin B.

Dosage Forms:
Alkeran® is available as 2-mg tablets. An IV form is also available as a 50 mg vial for injection (diluent containing povidone, alcohol, propylene glycol, and sodium citrate).

Adverse Reactions:

 Hematologic: Myelosuppression is the dose-limiting toxicity of melphalan. Leukopenia and thrombocytopenia are maximum at 14 days and 21 days, respectively. The effect may be cumulative, with a nadir of 5 to 6 weeks, in older patients.

 Gastrointestinal. Nausea and vomiting are mild in patients treated with melphalan. Stomatitis and diarrhea are infrequent with usual doses.

 Pulmonary. Fibrosis and interstitial infiltrates are rare.

Dermatologic. Alopecia, except when melphalan is given with other high-dose chemotherapeutic agents, is uncommon.

Hypersensitivity. Hypersensitivity reactions are rare after oral administration of melphalan. After IV administration, less than 10% of patients experience anaphylaxis, diaphoresis, hypotension, tachycardia, bronchospasm, dyspnea, and cardiac arrest. Less than 10% of patients develop secondary neoplasia (acute myelogenous leukemia and myelodysplasias) with chronic long-term oral use of melphalan.

Practitioner Interventions:

1. Instruct patient to take oral dose of melphalan in a single dose on an empty stomach.
2. Make sure antiemetics are given prior to IV dosing with melphalan.
3. Monitor patient's complete blood cell count (CBC) and platelet count every week.
4. Monitor patient for prolonged nadir in blood cells.
5. Initiate treatment with colony stimulating factors to shorten cell count nadir as appropriate.
6. Keep anaphylaxis kit at patient's bedside prior to IV administration of melphalan.
7. Initiate new IV and monitor IV site for signs of erythema, pain, or burning.

8. Evaluate patient's renal function prior to drug administration; decreased renal function may enhance melphalan toxicity.

References:
1. Gera S, Musch E, Osterheld HKO, Loos U. Relevance of the hydrolysis and protein binding of melphalan to the treatment of myeloma. Cancer Chemother Pharmacol 1989;23:76–80.
2. Race PA, Hill HS, Green RM, et al. Renal clearance and protein binding of melphalan in patients with cancer. Cancer Chemother Pharmacol 1988;22:348–352.
3. Sarosy G, Leyland-Jones B, Soochan P, Cheson BD. The systemic administration of intravenous melphalan. J Clin Oncol 1988;6: 1768–1782.

MERCAPTOPURINE

Other Names:
Purinethol®, 6-MP.

Uses:
Acute lymphoblastic leukemia (ALL), chronic granulocytic leukemia (CGL), chronic myelogenous leukemia (CML), non-Hodgkin's lymphomas, immune disorders.

Mechanism of Antitumor Action:
In the cell, mercaptopurine is phosphorylated to a 6-thioribo nucleotide, which acts as a purine antagonist and thus inhibits the synthesis of RNA and DNA.

Pharmacokinetics:

Absorption: Mercaptopurine is erratically and incompletely absorbed, with about 50% of an oral dose absorbed. Food decreases absorption by another 50%. A large amount of intestinal and first-pass metabolism occurs, resulting in even poorer bioavailability (only 5 to 37%).

Distribution: Mercaptopurine and its metabolites are widely distributed in body water. The apparent Vd is 0.9 L/kg.

Protein Binding: About 30% of mercaptopurine is bound to plasma proteins.

Metabolism: Mercaptopurine undergoes hepatic metabolism in two ways: (1) methylation of the sulfhydryl form to an active metabolite; (2) oxidation by xanthine oxidase to 6-thiouric acid. Plasma levels of 6-mercaptopurine reflect several metabolites.

Half-life: After IV administration, the plasma half-life of mercaptopurine ranges between 20 and 50 minutes. The half-life after oral administration is about 1.5 hours.

Elimination: After 24 hours, 50% of mercaptopurine and its metabolites are excreted in the urine (11% in the first 6 hours).

Drug Interactions:

Concomitant use of ***allopurinol*** requires a 75% dose reduction of 6-mercaptopurine. In addition, the anticoagulant effects of ***warfarin*** are antagonized by 6-mercaptopurine by some unknown mechanism.

Dosage:

The usual initial oral dose of mercaptopurine in adults is 80-100 mg/m^2/day or 2.5 mg/kg/day (calculated to the nearest 25 mg), and 50 mg per day in children. If no response is observed after 4 weeks, the dose may be increased to 5 mg/kg daily. After complete remission is obtained, a maintenance dose of 1.5 to 2.5 mg/kg daily may be given along with other agents (usually methotrexate).

In patients with renal failure, the dose of mercaptopurine should be decreased to prevent drug accumulation. Because of the many inactive metabolites of mercaptopurine, it is unclear what the extent of dose reduction should be in the presence of renal dysfunction or with one single daily dose.

Dose Forms:

Purinethol® is available as 50 mg tablets.

Administration:

Because food decreases the absorption of mercaptopurine, the oral dose should be given on an empty stomach. It is appropriate to administer mercaptopurine as a single daily dose at bedtime.

Adverse Reactions:

 Hematologic: Myelosuppression with mercaptopurine is mild; with nadir of leukopenia at 11 days and recovery by about 21 days. Anemia is noted only with high-dose therapy.

 Gastrointestinal: Nausea and vomiting are uncommon and mild in patients treated with mercaptopurine. Mucositis and stomatitis are commonly seen with large doses. Anorexia may also occur.

 Dermatologic: Dry scaling rash, drug fever, eosinophilia, and photosensitivity.

 Hepatic: The usual dose of mercaptopurine rarely causes hepatotoxicity. Jaundice and hepatitis have been observed 1 to 2 months into treatment, and may resolve following drug withdrawal. The most common sign of these hepatic effects is hyperbilirubinemia.

 Kidney: With IV therapy, renal failure is rare and is manifested by hematuria and crystalluria soon after administration on day 2 or 3 of IV treatment. Flank pain may also be noted. Symptoms usually disappear within 24 hours.

Practitioner Interventions:

1. Monitor complete blood cell count (CBC) and platelet count every week.
2. Monitor patient for any signs and symptoms of gastrointestinal effects of mercaptopurine.
3. Instruct patient about oral care regimen if high-dose IV therapy is being given.
4. Instruct patient to take oral drug all at once on an empty stomach.
5. Instruct patient about skin care and avoidance of direct sunlight, which may enhance dry scaling skin.
6. Monitor bilirubin/liver function tests weekly.
7. Monitor patient's renal function daily during IV therapy. Heme-test all urine during IV infusion.
8. Instruct patient to contact health care provider in case of signs or symptoms of decreasing urinary output, blood in urine, or pain or burning upon urination.

References:
1. Grindey GB. Clinical pharmacology of the 6-thiopurines. Cancer Treat Rev 1979;6(Suppl):19–25.
2. Koren G, et al. Systemic exposure to mercaptopurine as a prognostic factor in acute lymphocytic leukemia in children. N Engl J Med 1990;323: 17–22.

MESNA

Other Names:
Mesnex®, 2-mercaptoethanesulfonic acid.

Uses:
Mesna is used to prevent bladder toxicity due to ifosfamide or cyclophosphamide.

Mechanism of Action:
Mesna has no antitumor activity. It is a selective urinary protectant for oxazophosphorine-type alkylating agents. Its effect occurs primarily in renal tissue and bladder.

Pharmacokinetics:

Absorption: About 75% of oral mesna is available as either mesna or dimesna.

Distribution: Mesna distributes well in total body water. Its apparent Vd is 0.65 L/kg.

Protein Binding: Mesna or its metabolite dimesna are not protein bound.

Metabolism: The parent drug dimerizes in plasma to dimesna, which is inactive. Upon exposure to glutathione in renal tissue, it is reconverted to mesna, in which form it then binds to the alkylating metabolites acrolein and hydroxycyclophosphamide, and is excreted in the urine as a soluble complex.

Half-life: After IV administration of mesna, the half-life is only about 20 minutes because of rapid dimerization.

Elimination: After treatment with alkylating agents (e.g. ifosfamide), mesna and its metabolites are rapidly secreted and excreted in urine along with soluble alkylating agent–mesna complexes.

Drug Interactions:
Mesna is physically incompatible with ***cisplatin*** and ***carboplatin*** in solution. It probably inactivates ***mechlorethamine*** due to its thiol side chain.

Dosage:

Intravenous: Mesna is usually given three times daily in a dose that is 20% of the ifosfamide or cyclophosphamide dose. In high-dose therapy, mesna is often given continuously at a dose that is 100% to 200% of the total ifosfamide or cyclophosphamide dose.

Oral: Mesna should be given in a dose that is 40% of the ifosfamide or cyclophosphamide dose. The oral route is not recommended for use with the first dose of these two drugs, and should be used only in patients with good compliance.

Dose Forms:
Mesna is supplied as 200 mg (100 mg/mL) in a glass ampule and as a 1 gram multidose vial. Multidose vials containing 10.4 mg of benzyl alcohol may be used over a period of 8 days.

Administration:

Intravenous: Mesna may be mixed with D5W, D5NS, NS or LR. Because of the benzyl alcohol content, the multidose vial should not be used in neonates or infants. Mesnex® may be given as a bolus over 5 to 15 minutes or diluted in the same solution and given as a continuous infusion. Dilutions of mesna are stable for 24 hours.

Oral: Stable for 8 days in a 1:1 or 1:5 mixture with grape- or orange-flavored syrups.

Compatibilities: In concentrations ranging from 3 to 79 mg/mL, mesna is compatible with hydroxyzine HCl, ifosfamide, fludarabine phosphate, ondansetron HCl, and sargramostim. In a concentration of 20 mg/mL, mesna is compatible with 2 mg/mL doxorubicin HCl.

Incompatibilities: In a concentration of 1 mg/mL, mesna is incompatible with ***carboplatin***. In a concentration ranging from 0.11 to 3 mg/mL, mesna is incompatible with ***cisplatin***. In a concentration of 80 mg/mL, mesna is incompatible with ***epirubicin HCl***. It is unknown whether mesna is compatible with dacarbazine.

Adverse Reactions:

Gastrointestinal: Nausea and vomiting occur with rapid IV administration of mesna.

Practitioner Interventions:

1. Make sure mesna orders are written prior to administration of ifosfamide or cyclophosphamide.
2. If giving mesna by mouth, evaluate patient for nausea.
3. Make sure first dose of mesna is given IV.

References:

1. Andriole GL, Sandlund JT, Miser JS, et al. The efficacy of mesna (2-mercapto-ethane sodium sulfonate) as a uroprotectant in patients with hemorrhagic cystitis receiving further oxazaphosphorine chemotherapy. J Clin Oncol 1987;5:799–803.
2. Brock N. Oxazaphosphorence cytostatics: past-present-future. Cancer Res 1989;49:1–7.
3. Shepherd JD, Pringle LE, Barnett MJ, et al. Mesna versus hyperhydration for the prevention of cyclophosphamide-induced hemorrhagic cystitis in bone marrow transplantation.
4. Vose JM, Reed EC, Pippert GC, et al. Mesna compared with continuous bladder irrigation as uroprotection during high dose chemotherapy and transplantation: a randomized trial. J Clin Oncol 1993;11:1306–1310.

METHOTREXATE

Other Names:
Folex®, Mexate®, MTX, amethopterin.

Uses:
Acute lymphoblastic leukemia (ALL), intrathecal therapy for ALL and acute myelogenous leukemia (AML), trophoblastic tumors, lym-

phomas (both Hodgkin's and non-Hodgkin's); and breast, lung, head and neck, and osteogenic sarcomas.

Mechanism of Antitumor Action:

Methotrexate induces folate depletion, leading to inhibition of purine synthesis, and resulting in an arrest of DNA, RNA, and protein synthesis.

Pharmacokinetics:

Absorption: Oral absorption of methotrexate is rapid but incomplete (30 to 40% bioavailability) at doses greater than 0.1 mg/kg. Peak blood levels are achieved within 2 hours of oral administration. After IM injection, almost 100% of the drug is absorbed.

Distribution: Methotrexate distributes into total body water and has an apparent Vd of 0.6 L/kg. Cerebrospinal fluid (CSF) levels are only 3 to 10% of plasma levels and are not therapeutic after conventional doses. However, high-dose methotrexate (> 500 mg/m^2 IV over a period of 24 hours) results in therapeutic levels in the CSF. After intrathecal administration, methotrexate can diffuse back into plasma, reaching cytotoxic levels. Myelosuppression and mucositis have been reported after intrathecal therapy with methotrexate.

In patients with pleural effusions, methotrexate can accumulate in the effusion fluid, resulting in delayed drug clearance and increased toxicity.

Protein Binding: 50% to 60% of methotrexate is bound to plasma proteins.

Metabolism: A small fraction (about 10%) of methotrexate is metabolized by the liver to a 7-hydroxymetabolite. The rest of the drug is excreted in unchanged form.

Half-life: After rapid IV injection of methotrexate, a triphasic half-life pattern is observed. The $T_{1/2}\alpha = 45$ min; $T_{1/2}\beta = 2$ to 4 hours; and $T_{1/2}\gamma = 8$ to 10 hours. After infusions of 4 hours or longer, the initial distribution half-life is not observed, and only the beta and gamma (terminal) half-lives are seen.

Elimination: Methotrexate is excreted primarily in the urine, with 60 to 90% excreted as unchanged drug. About 10% is excreted as the

7-hydroxymetabolite in the bile, and is reabsorbed. Renal clearance of methotrexate ranges from 70 to 100 mL/m^2/min. Total body clearance of methotrexate is about 1.6-fold greater than renal clearance, suggesting that the drug is secreted by the renal tubules. Thus, other drugs that are secreted by the renal tubules, such as weak acids, may compete with methotrexate for urinary excretion (see drug interaction section below for specific drugs).

Drug Interactions:
Salicylates, sulfonamides, phenytoin, and *penicillins* will decrease the urinary excretion of methotrexate, resulting in its accumulation and subsequent toxicity. *Warfarin* may be potentiated by methotrexate therapy through protein displacement. These drugs should be discontinued 2 days prior to and restarted 2 days after methotrexate therapy.

Dosage:
A variety of doses and schedules have been used for methotrexate. The dosage of sodium methotrexate refers to the methotrexate dose.

Conventional low doses consist of 30 to 50 mg PO or IV weekly or 40 mg/m^2 IV on days 1 and 8, every 4 weeks.

Intermediate IV doses consist of 50 to 150 mg given by IV push every 2 to 3 weeks, or 0.5 to −1 g/m^2 IV given over a period of 24 to 42 hours every 2 to 3 weeks.

High IV doses are used for osteogenic sarcoma, lymphoma, or leukemia, and range from 1 to 12 g/m^2 IV given over a period of 4 to 24 hours every 1 to 3 weeks.

Intrathecal adult dosage (in nonpreserved NS) in adults ranges from 10 to 15 mg/m^2 (maximum 12 mg) twice weekly until the CSF is clear, followed by weekly dosage for 2 to 6 weeks and by monthly dosage.

Intrathecal pediatric dosage. In children ≤3 months: the intrathecal dose is 3 mg; in children of 4 to 12 months it is 6 mg; in children >1 to 2 years it is 8 mg; in children >2 to 3 years, 10 mg; and in children >3 years, 12 mg.

Dose Forms:

Oral: 2.5 mg tablets.

Injectable preparations: Single use powder vials for injection of 20 mg, 50 mg, and 1 g. Single use liquid injections of 50, 100, 200, 250 mg vials (preservative-free). Liquid injections (25 mg/mL) of 50 mg and 250 mg (with preservative).

Administration:

Methotrexate sodium injection maybe given IM, IV, and IA. Intravenous administration may be by IV push, rapid IV infusion (over 15 to 30 min), or a continuous infusion up to 42 hours.

Oral tablets of methotrexate may be taken all at once on an empty stomach. For intrathecal administration, preservative-free saline solutions of sodium methotrexate as 1 mg/mL are given via lumbar puncture or Ommaya® reservoir. Prior to intrathecal administration of methotrexate, a volume of CSF equivalent to the volume of methotrexate solution to be administered (usually 6 to 15 mL) is removed. Methotrexate should only be given intrathecally if the CSF is clear. Prior to high-dose methotrexate regimens, the patient's urine should be alkalinized (usually with 3 to 4 g of sodium bicarbonate every 3 to 4 hours for 8 to 12 hours are needed) to achieve a urine pH > 6.5. Leucovorin rescue is required at methotrexate doses of 240 mg/m^2 and above.

Methotrexate may be frozen at 20°C for 30 days and thawed by microwave radiation for 2 minutes without significant loss of drug. Repeated freezing and thawing five times has resulted in no change in concentration.

Compatibilities: Methotrexate is compatible with total parenteral nutrition (TPN) solutions and solutions of D5W, NS, and 0.05 molar sodium bicarbonate. Y-site administration of methotrexate in a concentration of 25 mg/mL is compatible with several agents including:

Chemotherapy drugs: Bleomycin sulfate, cisplatin, cyclophosphamide, cytarabine, doxorubicin HCl, fludarabine phosphate, fluorouracil, gallium nitrate, leucovorin calcium, melphalan HCl, mercaptopurine IV, mitomycin, paclitaxel, vinblastine sulfate, vincristine sulfate, and vinorelbine sulfate.

Non-chemotherapy drugs: Allopurinol sodium, cefepime HCl, cimetidine HCl, dexamethasone sodium phosphate, famotidine, filgrastim (in D5W), furosemide, ganciclovir sodium (in D5W), heparin sodium, hydromorphone HCl, lorazepam, methylprednisolone sodium succinate, metoclopramide HCl, morphine sulfate, ondansetron HCl, piperacillin sodium-tazobactam sodium, prochlorperazine edisylate, ranitidine HCl, sargramostim, and vancomycin HCl.

Incompatibilities: Methotrexate (15 to 25 mg/mL) is incompatible with chlorpromazine HCl, droperidol, idarubicin HCl, and promethazine HCl.

Adverse Reactions:

 Hematologic: Leukopenia, thrombocytopenia, and anemia occur with methotrexate therapy. The nadir in cell counts occurs at days 4 to 7 and is followed by partial recovery, after which a second nadir occurs at days 12 to 21 and recovery by day 28.

 Gastrointestinal: Nausea, vomiting and diarrhea are common. Nausea and vomiting are easily prevented with conventional antiemetics.

 Hepatic: Acute hepatotoxicity may be seen as an increase in AST usually within the first 12 hours of treatment with high-dose methotrexate. Chronic transaminase elevation and hepatic fibrosis are rare with the use of daily oral therapy.

 Dermatologic: Erythematous rashes, pruritus, urticaria, folliculitis, vasculitis, photosensitivity, depigmentation, and hyperpigmentation.

 Kidney: Renal failure may occur and may be decreased by alkalinization of urine and intense hydration.

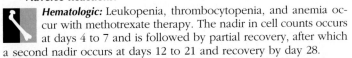 *Pulmonary:* Acute pneumonitis, shortness of breath, and a decreased Po$_2$ are rare with methotrexate and occur within 96 hours of administration. Corticosteroids are effective in rapid reversal of this complication.

Practitioner Interventions:

1. Premedicate patient with antiemetic 30 minutes prior to dosing with methotrexate.

2. Ensure that leucovorin orders are in patient's chart prior to initiating methotrexate therapy.

3. Monitor patient's complete blood cell count (CBC) and platelet count at least every week; in high-dose therapy monitor more frequently.

4. Monitor liver function and renal function tests prior to each course of therapy.

5. Instruct patient to discontinue all medications that may impair methotrexate clearance at least 24 hours before starting dose. (aspirin, cotrimoxazole, nonsteroidal anti-inflammatory drugs, penicillins)

6. Warn patients to stay out of the sun and wear protective clothing and eye wear for at least 1 month after methotrexate therapy. Use sunscreen if out in the sun.

7. Evaluate patient's renal function prior to dosing. If alkalinization is ordered, make sure urine pH is 6.5 or greater prior to starting dose. Check urine pH with each urination.

8. For patients receiving doses $\geq$ 1 g, methotrexate blood levels should be monitored at 24 and 48 hours after the start of drug administration (see section below on methotrexate monitoring).

Methotrexate Level Monitoring

The plasma methotrexate concentration should be monitored in the following patients:

1. Those receiving high-dose methotrexate.

2. Those with renal dysfunction (CrCl of <60 mL/min) regardless of dose.

3. Those who have had excessive toxicity during previous courses of methotrexate.

High-Dose Methotrexate Monitoring:

For patients receiving IV doses of methotrexate at $\geq$ 1 g, serum levels should be monitored to ensure adequate drug clearance. Usually, levels are monitored 24 and 48 hours after the start of the methotrexate infusion. Some institutions obtain serum levels every 12 hours until the methotrexate concentration has fallen to a nontoxic level (< 0.1 micromolar). Patients whose serum half-life of methotrexate (usually determined from an end-infusion level and a 12 hour post-end-infusion level) is greater than 3.5 hours have a greater risk of methotrexate toxicity (usually in patients with creatinine clearance < 70 mL/min). Patients whose 48-hour serum level of methotrexate is greater than 1 micromolar should receive 75 to 100 mg/m^2 of leucovorin IV until the methotrexate level has fallen below 1 micromolar, after which the dose of leucovorin may be decreased to 10 to 15 mg/m^2 IV/PO every 6 hours for 8 to 12 doses. The table below can be used as a guide to leucovorin dosing.

Intrathecal Methotrexate

In patients with meningeal cancer (either from leukemia or lymphoma), intrathecal methotrexate is often prescribed. The usual intrathecal dose ranges from 3 to 12 mg given every 2 to 4 days until the CSF is free of malignant cells. The dosing should be based on age, and not on body surface area (see table). It is recommended that nonpreserved methotrexate solutions be given by the intrathecal route. CSF methotrexate concentrations may be monitored in patients receiving the drug intrathecally twice a week or more often. The chart below may be used to determine if the dose of intrathecal methotrexate should be modified.

Principles of Methotrexate Rescue with Leucovorin:

1. Infusion of methotrexate should not be extended beyond the prescribed duration.
2. Leucovorin orders should be written at the time of a methotrexate order.
3. Leucovorin should be initiated after completion of methotrexate as shown in the table below and continued until the methotrexate concentration has fallen below 0.1 micromolar. The leucovorin delay varies with the duration of methotrexate therapy.

Leucovorin Dosing

Dose of MTX	Infusion time	Leucovorin Delay	Usual Leucovorin Regimen
1-12 g/m² IV	6 hr	2 hr	10-15 mg/m² IV/PO every 6 hours × 12 doses.
240 mg–2.4 g/m² IV	24-36 hr	0-12 hr	50 mg/m² IV every 6 hours × 3, then 10 to 15 mg/m² PO every 6 hours × 9 to 12 doses (or until methotrexate serum level falls below 0.1 μM)
1-3 g/m² IV	4 hr	24 hr	10–15 mg/m² IV/PO every 6 hours × 12 doses.
6-12 mg intra-thecally	3–5 min	24 hr	5 mg PO every 6 hours × 4 doses (if patient at high risk for having systemic toxicity, renal dysfunction or concurrent neutropenia.)

References:

1. Bender JF, Grove WR, Fortner CL. High-dose methotrexate with folinic acid rescue. Am J Hosp Pharm 1977;34:961–965.
2. Bleyer WA. Therapeutic drug monitoring of methotrexate and other antinoplastic drugs. In DM Baer (ed): Interpretations in Therapeutic Drug Monitoring. American Society of Clinical Pathologists, Chicago 1981:pp. 169–186.
3. Bleyer W, Dedrick R. Clinical pharmacology of intrathecal methotrexate. I. Pharmacokinetics in non-toxic patients after lumbar injection. Cancer Treat Rep 1977;61:703–708.
4. Campbell MA, Perrier DG, Dorr RT, et al. Methotrexate: bioavailability and pharmacokinetics. Cancer Treat Rep 1985;69:833–838.
5. Stoller RG, Kaplan HG, Cummings FJ, Calabresi P. A clinical and pharmacological study of high dose methotrexate with minimal leucovorin rescue. Cancer Res 1979;39:908–912.

MITOMYCIN

Other Names:
Mutamycin®, MMC, Mitomycin C.

Uses:
Adenocarcinoma of the stomach, pancreas, colon, and breast. Mitomycin has also been used in head and neck, lung, cervix, and rectal cancers.

Mechanism of Antitumor Action:
Mitomycin is an alkylating agent that crosslinks DNA and causes DNA-strand breakage.

Pharmacokinetics:

Absorption: Since mitomycin is erratically absorbed from the gastrointestinal tract, it is given by the IV route.

Distribution: Mitomycin distributes in total body water plus bile fluids and cervical tissue.

Protein Binding: There is no information on the plasma protein binding of mitomycin.

Metabolism: Mitomycin is bioreduced to an active alkylating species.

Half-life: The plasma half-life of mitomycin is short (less than 1 hour).

Elimination: Less than 10% of the drug is excreted in the urine. About 20% is eliminated by hepatic metabolism through unknown enzymes. Several tissues, including spleen, kidney, and liver, directly inactivate mitomycin. Dose modification in hepatic dysfunction is not necessary.

Drug Interactions:
None known.

Dosage:
As a single agent, the usual dose of mitomycin is 20 mg/m^2 IV every 6 to 8 weeks.

As a combination agent, the dose is 10 mg/m^2 IV every 6 to 8 weeks.

Dose Forms:
Mitomycin is only available for IV administration. It is available as a lyophilized powder in 5, 20 and 40 mg vials. Sterile water is added to result in a concentration of 0.5 mg/mL.

Administration:
Mitomycin is a potent vesicant and care should be taken to avoid its extravasation. Mitomycin is administered by a new IV access device. Serious local ulceration may occur if the drug is delivered outside the vein.

Compatibilities: In Y-site injection of 0.5 mg/mL, mitomycin is compatible with: allopurinol sodium, bleomycin sulfate, cisplatin, cyclophosphamide, doxorubicin HCl, droperidol, fluorouracil, heparin sodium, leucovorin calcium, melphalan HCl, methotrexate sodium, metoclopramide HCll, ondansetron HCl, vinblastine sulfate, and vincristine sulfate.

Incompatibilities: Cefepime HCl, filgrastim, piperacillin sodium–tazobactam sodium, sargramostim, and vinorelbine tartrate.

Adverse Reactions:

Hematologic: Bone marrow suppression is the dose-limiting toxicity of mitomycin. A prolonged nadir in the white blood cell (WBC) count may occur for up to 3 to 8 weeks, with the resulting anemia which may be cumulative. Lifetime doses should be kept under 50 to 60 mg/m^2.

Gastrointestinal: Mild nausea or vomiting may occur within 1 to 2 hours after dosing.

Kidney: Renal toxicity is uncommon and dose related. It usually presents with an increasing blood urea nitrogen (BUN) and serum creatinine level.

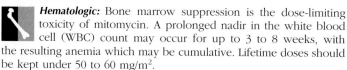*Hemolytic Uremic Syndrome:* Microangiopathic hemolytic anemia is uncommon with mitomycin, but presents with progressive renal failure, hemolysis, and thrombocytopenia.

*Pulmonary:* Cardiopulmonary decompensation may occur with mitomycin. This disease is ultimately fatal within 3 to 4 weeks of diagnosis, although the onset may be delayed for months.

Dermatologic: Severe tissue ulceration and necrosis may be expected if mitomycin leaks out of the vein.

Practitioner Interventions:

1. Initiate a new IV line prior to dosing if giving mitomycin peripherally.
2. Have an extravasation kit available at the patient's bedside.
3. Monitor patient's renal function prior to dosing. Check BUN and creatinine monthly.
4. Premedicate patient with antiemetic 30 minutes before dosing.
5. Monitor patient's complete blood cell count and platelets on a weekly basis. Monitor for significant anemia.
6. Monitor patient for cumulative dose of mitomycin, not to exceed 50 to 60 mg/m^2.

References:

1. Argenta LC, Manders EK. Mitomycin C extravasation injuries. Cancer 1983;51:1080–1082.
2. Crooke ST, Bradner WT. Mitomycin C: a review. Cancer Treat Rev 1976;3:121–139.
3. Doll DC, Weiss RB, Issell BF. Mitomycin: Ten years after approval for marketing. J Clin Oncol 1985;3:276–286.
4. Dorr RT. New findings in the pharmacokinetic, metabolic, and drug-resistance aspects of mitomycin C. Semin Oncol 1988;15(Suppl 3):32–41.
5. Lesesne JB, Rothschild N, Erickson B, et al. Cancer-associated hemolytic-uremic syndrome: Analysis of 85 cases from a national registry. J Clin Oncol 1989;7:781–789.

MITOTANE

Other Names:
Lysodren®, o,p′-DDD.

Uses:
Metastatic adrenocortical carcinoma.

Mechanism of Antitumor Action:
The exact antitumor action of mitotane is unknown, but several effects have been demonstrated, including adrenal atrophy, which results in decreased glucocorticoid and mineralocorticoid production. The onset of these effects occurs about 3 weeks after beginning therapy.

Pharmacokinetics:

Absorption: About 40% of mitotane is absorbed, reaching peak concentrations 3 to 5 hours after a 2 to 4 g dose.

Distribution: Mitotane is very fat soluble and distributes to body fat as well as other tissues.

Protein Binding: Little mitotane is bound to plasma proteins.

Metabolism: Mitotane is metabolized in the liver through oxidative mechanisms.

Half-life: The half-life of mitotane varies widely between 18 and 160 hours.

Elimination: About 10 to 25% of a dose of mitotane appears in the urine as metabolites, while about 15% is exreted unchanged in stool via the biliary tract.

Drug Interactions:
Mitotane induces hepatic microsomal enzymes and may enhance the metabolism of several drugs, including ***barbiturates, phenytoin, cyclophosphamide***, and ***corticosteroids***. Mitotane also appears to enhance the effect of ***warfarin***.

Dosage:
The initial dose for adrenocortical carcinoma is 1 to 6 g/day in three to four divided doses. If the drug is well tolerated, the dose can be titrated to 8 to 10 g daily.

Dose Forms:
Lysodren® is available in 500 mg tablets.

Administration:
Mitotane is given orally in three to four divided doses. It may be given with food, but not with a fatty meal.

Adverse Reactions:

Gastrointestinal: Nausea, anorexia, and vomiting occur frequently; diarrhea may sometimes occur.

Neurologic: About 40% of patients complain of CNS effects of mitotane, including irritability, confusion, sedation, lethargy, and dizziness.

Dermatologic: Skin reactions occur in about 15% of patients and include hyperpigmentation, urticaria, and maculopapular rash.

Endocrine: Adrenocortical insufficiency is common and requires supplemental corticosteroid and mineralocorticoid replacement therapy.

Ocular: Side effects are rare and include visual disturbances, blurred vision, diplopia, lens opacities, and cataracts.

Practitioner Interventions:

1. Replacement hydrocortisone 20 mg PO in the a.m. and 10 mg in the p.m. and fludrocortisone (0.1 mg PO daily) should be prescribed concurrently with mitotane.
2. Monitor patient for neurologic side effects of mitotane, especially during the first 2 weeks of therapy. In patients with lethargy or confusion, decrease the dose of mitotane by 1 g daily and retitrate up slowly.
3. Provide antiemetics during therapy.
4. Instruct patient to contact health care provider if there are more than 3 stools per day.
5. Instruct patient to use moisturizers for itching and dry skin. If unrelieved, contact health care provider.
6. Monitor patient for any vision changes during therapy.

References:

1. Becker D, Schumacher OP. o,p'-DDD therapy in invasive adrenocortical carcinoma. Ann Intern Med 1975;82:677–679.
2. Gutierrez ML, Crooke ST. Mitotane (o,p'-DDD). Canc Treat Rev 1980;7: 49–55.
3. Luton JP, Mahoudreau JA, Bouchard PH, et al. Treatment of Cushing's disease by o,p'-DDD. N Engl J Med 1979;300:459–464.
4. Robinson BG, Hales IB, Henniker AJ, et al. The effect of o,p'-DDD on adrenal steroid replacement therapy requirements. Clin Endocrinol 1987;27:437–344.

MITOXANTRONE HCl

Other Names:
Novantrone®, DHAD, dihydroxyanthracenedione.

Uses:
Acute myelogenous leukemia, breast cancer, ovarian cancer.

Mechanism of Antitumor Action:
Mitoxantrone intercalates with DNA and inhibits the activity of topoisomerase II. Unlike anthracyclines, it does not undergo redox cycling to oxygen free radicals.

Pharmacokinetics:

Absorption: Because mitoxantrone is primarily administered by the IV route, data on its oral absorption are lacking.

Distribution: Mitoxantrone distributes into several tissues including heart, spleen, liver, thyroid, pancreas, and bone marrow.

Protein Binding: Mitoxantrone is 78% bound to plasma proteins.

Metabolism: Mitoxantrone is metabolized via the hepatobiliary system to two inactive, oxidized metabolites.

Half-life: Mitoxantrone plasma clearance follows a triphasic pattern. The $T_{1/2}$ α is 2.4 to 15 minutes; the $T_{1/2}$ β is 17 minutes to 3 hours; and the $T_{1/2}$ γ (terminal) is 3 to 298 hours (mean: 24 hours).

Elimination: Mitoxantrone is eliminated primarily through the hepatobiliary system and, to a lesser extent, by the kidneys. About 25% of drug is found in feces, only 6 to 11% is found in urine. In patients with poor hepatobiliary function, dose adjustment has been recommended.

Drug Interactions:
None reported.

Dosage:
The recommended dose of mitoxantrone is 10 to 12 mg/m² IV daily for 3 consecutive days. For patients with a bilirubin of 1.5 to 3 mg/dL or > 3 mg/dL, the dose should be decreased to 50% and 25% of the full dose, respectively.

Dose Forms:
Novantrone® is available in multidose vials of 10 mg (5 mL), 20 mg (10 mL), 25 mg (12.5 mL), and 30 mg (15 mL).

Administration:
Mitoxantone should be diluted in 50 mL D5W or NS and infused over a period of 15 to 20 minutes.

Compatibilities: In simulated Y-site infusion using a concentration of 0.5 mg/mL, mitoxantrone is compatible with: allopurinol sodium, cefepime HCl, cyclophosphamide, cytarabine, fluorouracil, filgrastim, fludarabine phosphate, hydrocortisone sodium succinate, melphalan HCl, ondansetron HCl, potassium chloride, sargramostim and vinorelbine tartrate.

Incompabilities: Heparin sodium, hydrocortisone sodium phosphate, paclitaxel, piperacillin sodium–tazobactam sodium.

Adverse Reactions:

Hematologic: Myelosuppression is the dose-limiting toxicity of mitoxantrone. The nadir of leukopenia occurs at 10 to 14 days, with recovery by day 21. The degree of myelosuppression is related to the amount of prior therapy, and to the degree of bone marrow involvement with tumor and the performance status of the drug in the particular patient.

 Cardiac: Cumulative exposure to mitoxantrone can result in cardiac injury and congestive heart failure (CHF). The incidence of CHF rises substantially at cumulative doses of 140 to 160 mg/m². Previous anthracycline use is additive in cardiac toxicity.

  Gastrointestinal: Mild nausea and vomiting can occur with mitoxantrone. Antiemetics usually prevent emesis. Stomatitis is common, but is severe in <1% of cases.

 Kidney: Renal excretion of mitoxantrone imparts a blue-green color to the urine that may last for 1 or 2 days.

 Dermatologic: Alopecia occurs in about 25% of patients and is reversible.

Practitioner Interventions:

1. Monitor patient's complete blood cell count and platelet count daily during therapy.
2. Premedicate patient with appropriate antiemetics as needed.
3. Evaluate patient's cardiac function before initiating mitoxantrone therapy and every few treatment cycles during therapy. Discontinue mitoxantrone in case of a left ventricular ejection fraction of less than 50% or a decrease in left ventricular ejection fraction of 15% or greater from baseline.
4. Instruct patient about blue-green urine and possible alopecia.
5. Although mitoxantrone is not a vesicant, monitor the site of its IV infusion for any signs and symptoms of its leaking into tissue, since phlebitis has rarely been reported with the drug.
6. Monitor cumulative dose of drug and any prior anthracycline dose.

References:
1. Faulds D, Balfour JA, Chrisp P, Langtry HD. Mitoxantrone: A review of its pharmacodynamic and pharmacokinetic properties and therapeutic potential in the chemotherapy of cancer. Drugs 1991;41:400–449.

2. Schenkenberg TD, Von Hoff DD. Mitoxantrone: A new anticancer drug with significant activity. Ann Intern Med 1986;105:67–81.

3. Larson RA, Dacy KM, Choi KE, et al. A clinical and pharmokinetic study of mitoxantrone in acute nonlymphocytic leukemia. J Clin Oncol 1987;5: 391–397.

OCTREOTIDE ACETATE

Other Names:
Sandostatin®.

Uses:
Octreotide acetate suppresses the secretory symptoms of neuroendocrine tumors of the gut, such as malignant carcinoid, vasoactive intestinal peptide, insulinoma, glucagonoma, and gastrinoma.

Mechanism of Antitumor Action:
Octreotide is similar in action to endogenous somatostatin, which is a regulatory endocrine and paracrine inhibitor of several hormones and polypeptides, including serotonin, gastrin, insulin, glucagon, luteinizing hormone (LH), gonadotropin releasing hormone, vasoactive intestinal polypeptide (VIP), and somatotropin.

Pharmacokinetics:

Absorption: Octreotide may be given IV or SC. Absorption of the drug following its SC injection is complete within 0.5 hours after administration.

Distribution: Because of its polypeptide structure, octreotide is predicted to distribute in vascular spaces.

Protein Binding: 65% of octreotide is bound to plasma proteins.

Metabolism: Octreotide is catabolized to polypeptide fragments.

Half-life: $T_{1/2}\alpha = 0.2$ hour; $T_{1/2}\beta = 1.5$ hours.

Elimination: About 32% of octreotide is excreted unchanged by the kidney.

Drug Interactions:
Octreotide can cause transient hypo- or hyperglycemia and could therefore alter the response to drugs used to control the blood sugar concentration. It may alter the absorption of ***cyclosporine*** from the gastrointestinal tract.

Dosage:
50 μg given once or twice daily. Dosage of octreotide is titrated over the first 2 weeks to a range of 100 to 600 μg/day in two or three daily fractions.

Administration: Octreotide is usually given by SC injection. Injection sites should be rotated frequently to avoid local site irritation. In emergency situations, very high doses (1,500 to 3,000 μg) of octreotide may be administered IV over an 8-hour period.

Compatibilities: Octreotide at a concentration of 1.5 mg/L in total parenteral nutrition (TPN) solution was compatible with heparin sodium. The drug has not been tested with other drugs in simulated Y-site studies.

Dose Forms:
Sandostatin® is available in ampules of 50, 100, and 500 μg/1 mL of solution. It is also available in multidose vials containing 200 and 1000 μg/5 mL.

Adverse Reactions:

Gastrointestinal: Nausea (8%), abdominal pain (9%), and diarrhea (7%) may occur in patients receiving octreotide.

Dermatologic: Local site reactions, including pain and erythema or a wheal at the injection site, occur in less than 10% of patients treated with octreotide.

Practitioner Interventions:

1. Instruct patient in self-injection technique including injection site rotation.
2. Instruct patient on appropriate disposal of drug vials and sup-

plies after injections. Make sure patient has a needle disposal box.

3. Instruct patient to contact health-care provider for signs and symptoms of diarrhea, nausea, or local injection-site reaction.

References:
1. Dunne MJ, Kutz K. Somatostatin analogues in cancer treatment. In: Stoll BA (ed): Endocrine Management of Cancer. Karger, Basel, 1988, pp. 65–79.
2. Katz MO. Octreotride, a new somatostatin analogue. Clin Pharm 1989;8: 255–273.
3 Kutz K, Nuesch E, Rosenthaler J. Pharmacokinetics of SMS 201-995 in healthy subjects. Scan J Gastroenterology 1986; 21(Suppl 199):65–72.

PACLITAXEL

Other Names:
Taxol®.

Uses:
Ovarian, breast, lung, head and neck cancers.

Mechanism of Antitumor Action:
Paclitaxel promotes the assembly of microtubules, which stabilizes the cell against depolymerization and ultimately blocks cell division.

Pharmacokinetics:

Absorption: Paclitaxel is primarily given by the parenteral route.

Distribution: Paclitaxel has a steady-state Vd of 49 to 180 L/m^2, which is consistent with extensive protein binding. Its initial Vd is 8 to 20 L/m^2. No drug is identified in the cerebrospinal fluid (CSF) after drug administration.

Protein Binding: Paclitaxel is 98% bound to plasma proteins.

Metabolism: Paclitaxel is rapidly metabolized in the liver to 6-hydroxypaclitaxel (6-HT) by the cytochrome P450 enzyme system. 6-HT is equipotent to paclitaxel in effects on tubulin and mitotic arrest (apoptosis).

Half-life: Paclitaxel displays nonlinear elimination, with its clearance decreasing with increasing dose size. On average, paclitaxel plasma elimination follows a biphasic pattern with $T_{1/2}\alpha$ of about 30 minutes and a longer $T_{1/2}\beta$ ranging from 4 to 9 hours.

Elimination: Biliary secretion is probably a primary route of elimination of paclitaxel and accounts for 25% of the administered dose. Renal excretion accounts for only 4 to 8% of administered drug.

Drug Interactions:
Paclitaxel should be given prior to cisplatin to decrease toxicity and enhance the clearance of paclitaxel.

Dosage:
In ovarian cancer, the recommended dose of paclitaxel is 135 mg/m^2 IV every 3 weeks. However, other dosage schedules are being evaluated. In breast cancer, the recommended dose is 175 mg/m^2 IV every 3 weeks. In lung cancer, the dose may range from 175 to 225 mg/m^2 IV over 3 hours every 3 weeks. Longer infusions are more toxic to bone marrow.

Dose Forms:
Paclitaxel is available for IV use in 30 mg/5 mL and 100 mg/16.7 mL vials.

Administration:
Paclitaxel may be administered by IV infusion over a period of 1 hour, 3 hours, or 24 hours. Dilute in NS or D5W or D5NS to a final concentration of 0.3 to 1.2 mg/mL. These solutions are stable for 27 hours at room temperature.

Compatibilities:

Non-Chemotherapy Compatibility: In simulated Y-site infusion with 1.2 mg/mL in D5W, paclitaxel is compatible with acyclovir, amikacin, aminophylline, ampicillin-sulfactam sodium, butorphenol tartrate, calcium chloride, cefepime HCl, cefotetan disodium, ceftazidime, ceftriaxone sodium, cimetidine HCl, dexamethasone–sodium phosphate, diphenhydramine HCl, droperidol, famotidine, fluconazole, furosemide, ganciclovir sodium, gentamicin sulfate, haloperidol lactate, heparin sodium, hydrocortisone sodium phosphate and succinate, hydromorphone HCl, lorazepam, magnesium sulfate, mannitol, meperidine HCl, metoclopramide, morphine sulfate, nalbuphine HCl, ondansetron HCl, potassium chloride, prochlorperazine edisylate, ranitidine HCl, sodium bicarbonate, vancomycin HCl, and zidovudine.

Chemotherapy Compatibility: Bleomycin sulfate, carboplatin, cisplatin, cyclophosphamide, dacarbazine, doxorubicin HCl, etoposide, floxuridine, fluorouracil, ifosfamide, mesna, methotrexate sodium, and pentostatin.

Incompatibilities: Amphotericin B, chlorpromazine HCl, hydroxyzine HCl, methylprednisolone sodium succinate, mitoxantrone HCl, and plasticized PVC equipment.

Adverse Reactions:

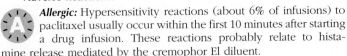 **Allergic:** Hypersensitivity reactions (about 6% of infusions) to paclitaxel usually occur within the first 10 minutes after starting a drug infusion. These reactions probably relate to histamine release mediated by the cremophor El diluent.

Hematologic: Bone marrow suppression is related to the duration of dosing above a threshold concentration (0.05 micromolar) of paclitaxel. Doses >190 mg/m^2 usually exceed the threshold and are particularly myelosuppressive. Leukopenia occurs in more than 60% of patients, with a leukocyte nadir at day 10 and recovery by day 15. Anemia and thrombocytopenia occur in 90% and 27% of patients, respectively. Severe anemia (Hgb <8 g/dL) occurs in about 25% of patients. Red blood cell transfusion may be needed for severely anemic patients.

Neurologic: The dose limiting toxicity of paclitaxel is neurologic. It presents as peripheral neuropathy manifested by numbness, tingling, pain, impairment of fine motor skills, and difficulty in ambulating, with loss of deep tendon reflexes. Neuropathy is reversible over several months after the drug is discontinued.

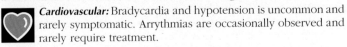 **Cardiovascular:** Bradycardia and hypotension is uncommon and rarely symptomatic. Arrythmias are occasionally observed and rarely require treatment.

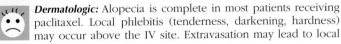 **Dermatologic:** Alopecia is complete in most patients receiving paclitaxel. Local phlebitis (tenderness, darkening, hardness) may occur above the IV site. Extravasation may lead to local

pain, edema, and erythema at the infusion site, but not to skin necrosis. These symptoms resolve over a period of several days.

 Flulike symptoms: Arthralgias, myalgias, fever, headache, and fatigue are common symptoms in patients receiving paclitaxel.

Practitioner Interventions:

1. Keep anaphylaxis kit at patient's beside before initiating treatment, - including Ambu bag, Benadryl (diphenydramine), hydrocortisone, and epinephrine.
2. Premedicate patient with an H₁ blocker, diphenhydramine, and an H₂ blocker such as cimetidine/ranitidine 30 minutes before giving dose of paclitaxel. Give dexamethasone 20 mg IV PO 30 minutes before dose.
4. Monitor patient's vital signs every 15 minutes for first hour of dosing with paclitaxel.
5. Have a physician available on patient's unit for first 15 minutes of dosing with paclitaxel.
6. Administer paclitaxel in either glass, polyolefin, or polypropylene containers, using a 0.22 μ filter and a polyethylene-lined administration set.
7. Monitor patient's complete blood cell count (CBC) and platelet count weekly.
8. Monitor patient for signs and symptoms of peripheral neuropathy. Have patient inform health-care provider in case of significant burning and tingling in hands and feet.
9. Instruct patient that alopecia will be almost total, and give information about obtaining wigs, scarves, etc.
10. Have patients report any change in pulse rate to health-care provider, and warn patient that bradycardia may occur.

References:
1. Greco FA, Hainsworth JD. Paclitaxel (Taxol®). Phase I/II trial comparing 1-hour infusion schedules. Semin Oncol 1994;21(Suppl 8):3–8.
2. Kearns CM, Gianni L, Egorin MJ. Paclitaxel pharmacokinetics and pharmacodynamics. Semin Oncol 1995;22(Suppl 6):16–23.
3. National Cancer Institute. NCI Investigational Drugs. NIH Publication 91-2141. US Department of Health and Human Services, Bethesda, 1990, pp. 151–153.
4. Rowinsky E, Gilbert M, McGuire W, et al. Sequences of taxol and cisplatin: a phase I and pharmacologic study. J Clin Oncol 1991:1692–1703.

5. Schiller JH, Storer B, Tutsch K, Arzoomanian R, et al. A Phase I Trial of 3-hour Infusions of Paclitaxel (Taxol) with or without granulocyte colony-stimulating factor. Semin Oncol 1994;21(Suppl 8):9–14.
6. Weiss RB, Donehower RC, Wiernik PH, et al. Hypersensitivity reactions from Taxol. J Clin Oncol 1990;8:1263–1268.

PAMIDRONATE DISODIUM

Other Names:
Aredia®.

Uses:
Pamidronate is approved for the treatment of hypercalcemia of malignancy in patients >18 years old. It has also been approved for the treatment of malignant bone pain.

Mechanism of Action:
Pamidronate is a more potent bisphosphonate than etidronate, and inhibits bone resorption through its effect on osteoclast precursors. It also binds to bones, inhibiting cytokine-induced osteoclastic activity. The onset of its calcium-lowering effect is 3 days, and the effect is maximal between days 7 and 10.

Pharmacokinetics:

Absorption: The absorption of oral pamidronate is poor (about 1%), and is further impaired when the drug is given with food.

Distribution: Pamidronate is rapidly and widely distributed in body tissues. It concentrates in bone, liver, and spleen. The Vd is about 1 L/kg.

Protein Binding: The extent of plasma protein binding of pamidronate is unknown but probably minimal.

Metabolism: Very little pamidronate is metabolized.

Half-life: Pamidronate has a half-life of about 24 hours, but its release from skeletal bone is very slow, with an estimated $T_{1/2}$ of 300 days.

Elimination: From 10 to 50% of pamidronate is excreted unchanged in the urine 48 hours after a dose.

Drug Interactions:
None reported.

Dosage
The recommended dose of pamidronate is 60 to 90 mg in an IV infusion over a period of 2 to 24 hours once every 1 to 2 weeks, depending on the degree of hypercalcemia. For a serum Ca^{2+} >13.5 mg/dL, 90 mg of pamidronate should be given, and for serum Ca^{2+} of 12 to 13.5 mg/dL, 60 mg should be given. For the treatment of bone pain, the recommended dose is 60 mg IV every 2 to 4 weeks or 90 mg IV over 2 hour monthly.

Dose Forms
Acredia® is available in vials of 30, 60, and 90 mg of lyophilized powder.

Administration:
Pamidronate is administered in 1,000 mL of NS, 0.45% sodium chloride or 5% dextrose over a period of 2 to 24 hours. The shorter infusion time allows for outpatient treatment. The infusion solution is stable for 24 hours at room temperature.

Compatibilities: NS, D5W.

Incompatibilities: Pamidronate has not been studied for compatibility with other drugs in simulated Y-site infusions.

Adverse Reactions:

 Gastrointestinal. After a 90 mg dose of pamidronate, the incidence of nausea is about 20%, of vomiting 15%, and of abdominal pain 2%.

 Cardiac. Tachycardia, atrial fibrillation, hypertension, and syncope have been reported in up to 6% of patients treated with a 90 mg dose of pamidronate.

 Electrolyte. Hypocalcemia, hypokalemia, and hypomagnesemia occur in about 10% of patients given pamidronate; hypophosphatemia occurs in about 15%.

Neurologic. Insomnia, sleepiness, or abnormal vision occurs in about 2% of patients treated with pamidronate.

Practitioner Interventions:

1. Prior to dosing with pamidronate evaluate hydration status.
2. Infuse pamidronate over a period of 2 to 24 hours. If patient complains of nausea or vomiting, the drug should be given more slowly.
3. Monitor patient's daily serum calcium concentration for the first 3 days after pamidronate administration. The hypocalcemic effect of pamidronate occurs in about 72 hours.
4. Instruct patient regarding side effect potential when using for bony pain relief.

References:

1. Fitton A, McTavish D. Pamidronate: A review of its pharmacological properties and therapeutic efficacy in resorptive bone disease. Drugs 1991;44:289–318.
2. Fleisch H. Bisphosphonates. Pharmacology and use in the treatment of tumor-induced hypercalcemia and metastatic bone disease. Drugs 1991;42:919–944.
3. Glover D, Lipton A, Keller A, et al. Intravenous pamidronate disodium treatment of bone metastases in patients with breast cancer. Cancer 1994;74:2949–55.
4. Gucalp R, Theriault R, Gill I, et al. Treatment of cancer-associated hypercalcemia. Double-blind comparison of rapid and slow intravenous infusion regimens of pamidronate disodium and saline alone. Arch Intern Med 1994;154:1935–1944.
5. Hortobagy GN, Theriault RL, Porter L, et al. Efficacy of pamidronate in reducing skeletal complications in patients with breast cancer and lytic bone metastases. Protocol 19 Aredia Breast Cancer study group. New Engl J Med 1996;335:1785–1791.
6. Kellihan MJ, Mangino PD. Pamidronate. Ann Pharmacother 1992;26:1262–1269.
7. Leyvraz S, Hess H, Flesch G, et al. Pharmacokinetics of pamidronate in patients with bone metastases. J Natl Cancer Inst 1992;84:788–792.
8. Warrell RP. Etiology and current management of cancer-related hypercalcemia. Oncology 1992;6:37–43, 47–50.

PEGASPARAGINASE

Other Names:
Oncaspar®, PEG-L-asparaginase.

Uses:
Acute lymphoblastic leukemia (ALL) and refractory non-Hodgkin's lymphoma in patients who have developed hypersensitivities to the native forms of L-asparaginase (*Escherichia-coli* derived).

Mechanism of Antitumor Action:
Pegasparaginase exerts its antitumor effect by depleting asparagine, which is essential for cellular protein biosynthesis.

Pharmacokinetics:

Absorption: Pegasparaginase is given by the IM or IV route. Oral absorption is poor.

Distribution: Pegasparaginase is mainly localized in plasma.

Protein Binding: Unknown

Metabolism: Pegasparaginase is rapidly cleared.

Half-life: Pegasparaginase has a longer half-life (5.7 days) than *E.-coli*-derived asparaginase (~1.3 days).

Elimination: Pegasparaginase is eliminated from the body by proteolysis or removal through tissue metabolism.

Drug Interactions:
Pegasparaginase may enhance the anticoagulant effect of ***warfarin, heparin, dipyridamole***, or ***aspirin***.

Dosage:
The dose of pegasparaginase in children or young adults with a BSA ≤0.6 m^2 is 2,500 units/m^2 IM or IV given every 14 days. In patients with a BSA ≤0.6 m^2, the dose is 82.5 units/kg every 14 days.

Dose Forms:

Oncaspar® is available as a 3750 IU (750 IU/mL) vial. Solutions of pegasparaginase are deactivated by freezing, and should be kept refrigerated at 2 to 8° C. Avoid excessive agitation. Do NOT shake. Do not use if cloudy.

Administration:

Intravenous: Dilute dose in 100 mL NS or D5W and give over a period of 1 to 2 hours.

Intramuscular: Not to exceed 2 ml in any one area.

> *Compatibilities:* None reported.

> *Incompatibilities:* None reported.

Adverse Reactions:

The IM route is preferable because toxicities to liver, GI, and coagulopathy are less than that when using the IV route.

Hypersensitivity: About one-third of patients given pegasparaginase develop skin reactions (mild urticaria).

Pancreatitis: Hyperglycemia requiring insulin therapy may occur with pegasparaginase, due to pancreatic islet cell damage.

Liver: Hypoalbuminemia. Coagulation defects are rare and are due to decreased fibrinogen, and factors II, VI, VII, VIII, X and protein C deficiencies, resulting in bleeding and thrombosis.

Neurologic: CNS changes with pegasparaginase include lethargy and somnolence in a small number of patients.

Practitioner Interventions:

1. During IV administration of pegasparaginase, make sure that an anaphylaxis kit is at the patient's bedside, including epinephrine, hydrocortisone, diphenhydramine and an Ambu bag.
2. Use caution against accidental exposure to pegasparaginase, since skin rashes in health-care personnel have been reported.
3. Monitor fibrinogen, glucose, prothrombin time (PT), partial thromboplastin time (PTT), amylase, and liver function at least twice weekly.

4. If giving pegasparaginase IM, monitor injection sites.
5. Instruct patient to report any CNS changes to health care providers.

References:

1. Asselin BL, Whitin JC, Coppola DJ, et al. Comparative pharmacokinetic studies of three asparaginase preparations. J Clin Oncol 1993;11:1780–1786.
2. Ettinger LV, Jurtzberg J, Voute PA, et al. An open-label, multicenter study of polyethylene glycol-L-asparaginase for the treatment of acute lymphoblastic leukemia. Cancer 1995;75:1176–1181.
3. Keating MV, Holmes R, Lorner S, Ho DH. L-asparaginase and PEG asparaginase—past, present, and future. Leukemia Lymphoma 1993; 10(Suppl):153–157.
4. Pegasparaginase in acute lymphoblastic leukemia. Medical Letter 1995;37:23–24.

PENTOSTATIN

Other Names:
Nipent®, 2′-Deoxycoformycin.

Uses:
Hairy-cell leukemia, chronic lymphocytic leukemia, acute lymphoblastic leukemia (ALL), adult T-cell leukemia, lymphoblastic lymphoma.

Mechanism of Antitumor Action:
Pentostatin inhibits the enzyme adenosine deaminase. It also depletes nicotinamide adenine dinucleotide, thus blocking DNA repair.

Pharmacokinetics:

Absorption: Pentostatin is typically given by IV infusion.

Distribution: The Vd of pentostatin is about 20 L/m² of body water.

Protein Binding: Only 4% of pentostatin is bound to plasma proteins.

Metabolism: Very little pentostatin is metabolized.

Half-life: Pentostatin plasma clearance follows a biphasic pattern. The $T_{1/2}\alpha$ ranges from 9 to 85 minutes. The longer, terminal $T_{1/2}\beta$ ranges from 5 to 14 hours.

Elimination: Most of a dose of pentostatin is cleared unchanged in the urine.

Drug Interactions:

Allopurinol may enhance the therapeutic toxicity of pentostatin. The combination of pentostatin and *fludarabine* may result in fatal pulmonary toxicity and should be avoided. The metabolism of *vidarabine* is inhibited, leading to increased toxicity.

Dosage:

The usual dose of pentostatin for the treatment of hairy cell leukemia is 4 mg/m^2/week given every other week. The dose should be modified in patients with renal dysfunction according to the guideline below.

Dose Modification

CrCl *(mL/min)*	% of *Normal Dose*
120	100
100	80
80	70
60	60
50	40
<50	0

Modified from Dorr and Von Hoff. Cancer Chemotherapy Handbook. Appleton & Lange; East Norwalk, 1994; pp 776.

Dose Forms

Nipent® is available as a 10 mg lyophilized powder vial.

Administration:

Pentostatin is typically administered as a short IV infusion in 50 to 100 mL of D5W or NS over a period of 20 to 60 minutes. Reconstituted or diluted solutions should be used within 8 hours.

Compatibilities: NS, D5W (20 mg/L), LR, fludarabine phosphate, melphalan HCl, ondansetron HCl, paclitaxel, and sargramostim.

Incompatibilities: None reported.

Adverse Reactions:

Pentostatin causes substantial toxicities. Many of the toxicities are dose-related, but dose alone cannot predict toxicity. Other factors include performance status, age, renal function, and existing CNS disease. Initial studies with higher doses (10 mg/m^2/day × 5 days) than the currently recommended dose (4 mg/m^2/day × 5 days) have found frequent and sometimes fatal toxicities with pentostatin.

 Dermatologic: Rash and dry skin occur in about one-fourth of patients treated with pentostatin.

 Hematologic: The dose limiting toxicity of pentostatin is myelosuppression. Neutropenia occurs by day 15 and recovery is seen by days 21 to 27. Thrombocytopenia occurs infrequently.

 Hepatic: Liver function tests are occasionally elevated, but this is reversible. Severe hepatitis is rare.

 Kidney: Elevated serum creatinine and renal dysfunction occur in about 5% of patients treated with pentostatin. Most cases are reversible.

Lymphocytopenia: Lymphocytopenia is common in patients treated with pentostatin; both T cells and B cells are suppressed. Thus, the incidence of infections is increased, especially pneumonias, gram-negative and gram-positive infections, and viral infections by herpes simplex and zoster.

 **Neurologic:** Lethargy and fatigue are common and dose related. There have been rare cases of coma.

  Ocular and Ototoxicity: Occasional keratoconjunctivitis, ear pain, ocular, blepharitis, diplopia, photophobia, lacrimal disorder, labrinthitis, optic neuritis, and tinnitus have occurred in patients treated with pentostatin.

 Other: Fever, chills, arthralgia, and myalgias have been reported.

Gastrointestinal: Nausea and vomiting are mild to moderate.

Practitioner Interventions:

1. Monitor patient's renal function prior to administering pentostatin. Adjust dose based on creatinine clearance.
2. Premedicate patient with conventional antiemetics 30 minutes prior to dose of pentostatin.
3. Monitor patient's complete blood cell count (CBC) and platelet count weekly.
4. Instruct patient about signs and symptoms of infection and when to call health-care provider.
5. Instruct patient on possibility of developing fatigue and lethargy from agent.
6. Instruct patient regarding possible ototoxicity and opthalmic toxicities and when to call a health care provider.
7. Instruct patient on use of moisturizing cream for dry skin care.

References:

1. Brogden RN, Sovkin EM. Pentostatin. A review of its pharmacodynamic and pharmacokinetic properties, and therapeutic potential. Drugs.
2. Cheson BD. New antimetabolites in the treatment of human malignancies. Semin Oncology 1992;19:695–706.
3. Saven A, Piro L. Newer purine analogs for the treatment of hairy cell leukemia. New Engl J Med 1994;330:691–697.
4. Smyth JF, Paine RM, Jackman AL, et al. The clinical pharmacology of the adenosine deaminase inhibitor deoxycoformycin. Cancer Chemother Pharmacol 1980;5:93–101.

PLICAMYCIN

Other Names:
Mithracin®, Mithramycin.

Uses:
Plicamycin is approved for the treatment of hypercalcemia unresponsive to other methods of treatment. It may also be useful for blast crisis of chronic myelogenous leukemia (CML).

Mechanism of Antitumor Action:
Plicamycin inhibits osteoclasts and blocks the action of parathyroid hormone, reducing the serum calcium concentration. Its antitumor action is probably due to its binding to DNA.

Pharmacokinetics:

Absorption: Plicamycin is given only by the IV route. It is not absorbed well when given orally.

Distribution: Plicamycin is distributed into hepatocytes, bone marrow, and renal tubules. It readily crosses the blood–brain barrier, achieving cerebrospinal fluid (CSF) concentrations equivalent to that in the plasma.

Protein Binding: Unknown

Metabolism: Plicamycin is metabolized by the liver to unknown inactive metabolites.

Half-life: The half-life of plicamycin is not well-defined, but ranges from 2 to 24 hours.

Elimination: Metabolites of plicamycin appear in the urine within 15 hours after dosing.

Drug Interactions:
None are known, but there is reason for concern about drug metabolism, owing to the hepatotoxic properties of plicamycin.

Dosage:
For hypercalcemia, 25 μg/kg IV daily for 3 days. For tumors, 25 to 30 μg/kg IV for 8 to 10 days. Plicamycin should be avoided in patients with moderately severe impairment of renal function (creatinine clearance < 50 mL/min).

Dose Forms
Mithracin® is available in 2,500 μg vials. The vials are stable for 2 years if stored under refrigeration. Unused solution should be discarded.

Administration:
Plicamycin should be given as a slow IV infusion in 100 to 500 mL of NS or D5W over a period of 30 to 60 minutes or in 1 liter of D5W or NS and given over 4 to 6 hours via a central line.

Compatibilities: In simulated Y-site infusion, plicamycin is compatible with: allopurinol sodium, filgrastim, melphalan HCl, piperacillin sodium–tazobactam sodium, and vinorelbine tartrate.

Incompatibilities: In simulated Y-site infusion, plicamycin is incompatible with cefepime HCl.

Adverse Reactions:
In general, intermittent weekly doses of plicamycin used for the treatment of hypercalcemia cause fewer side effects than doses given on a daily basis.

 Gastrointestinal: Nausea, vomiting, anorexia, and diarrhea occur in patients treated with plicamycin. A metallic taste and stomatitis also occur.

Hypocalcemia: Hypocalcemia may occur after achieving normocalcemia with plicamycin.

 Hematologic: Myelosuppression is uncommon at the doses of plicamycin used for the treatment of hypercalcemia, but may include leukopenia or thrombocytopenia.

 Renal: Proteinuria, azotemia, and elevated serum creatinine.

 Hepatic: Elevated transaminase levels, hyperbilirubinemia. Hypoprothrombinemia occurs in about 20% of patients treated with antitumor doses of plicamycin, and may lead to severe bleeding diathesis, epistaxis, and ecchymoses.

 Dermatologic: Skin rash, facial flushing, skin thickening, and hyperpigmentation.

 *Neurologic:* Lethargy, weakness, and malaise may occur.

Practitioner Interventions:
1. Premedicate patient with antiemetic 30 minutes prior to dosing with plicamycin.

2. Monitor patient's serum calcium level before administration and every 24 to 48 hours after dosing with plicamycin.
3. Monitor patient's complete blood cell count (CBC) and platelet count every week.
4. Patient should have received 2 to 3 L of NS plus furosemide to replenish fluid loss and ensure diuresis.
5. Check patient's serum creatinine concentration. If > 2 mg/dL, plicamycin should be withheld.
6. Monitor patient's coagulation parameters if treatment is for antitumor use.

References:

1. Godfrey TE. Mithramycin for hypercalcemia of malignant disease. Calif Med 1971;115:1–4.
2. Koller CA and Miller DM. Preliminary observations on the therapy of the myeloid blast phase of chronic granulocytic leukemia with plicamycin and hydroxyurea. N Engl J Med 1986;315:1433.
3. Perlia CP, Gubisch NJ, Wolter J, et al. Mithramycin treatment of hypercalcemia. Cancer 1970;25:289–394.

PROCARBAZINE HCl

Other Name:
Matulane®, PCR, N-methylhydrazine.

Uses:
Hodgkin's disease, non-Hodgkin's lymphoma, mycosis fungoides, brain tumors, and small-cell lung cancer.

Mechanism of Antitumor Action:
The mechanism of action of procarbazine is unclear; it inhibits preformed DNA and RNA, and protein synthesis. It directly damages DNA, causing chromosomal breakage. It also inhibits methylation of transfer RNA.

Pharmacokinetics:

Absorption: Procarbazine is rapidly absorbed from the gastrointestinal tract, reaching a peak concentration in 1 hour similar to that following its IV administration.

Distribution: Procarbazine distributes into liver, kidney, intestine, and skin. The drug equilibrates between the blood and the CNS. Peak cerebrospinal fluid (CSF) levels occur 30 to 90 minutes after dosing.

Protein Binding: Data on the protein binding of procarbazine are lacking.

Metabolism: Procarbazine is rapidly metabolized in the liver to azo-procarbazine by cytochrome P-450 enzymes. Monoamine oxidase accounts for about 40% of procarbazine oxidation.

Half-life: The plasma half-life of procarbazine is 1 hour after oral administration and 7 minutes after IV administration.

Elimination: From 25 to 70% of a dose of procarbazine is recovered in urine after 24 hours, primarily as metabolites. Only 5% of the drug is eliminated in unchanged form.

Drug Interactions:

The concurrent use with procarbazine of the drugs listed in the table below may cause clinically important adverse reactions:

Drug	Reaction
Alcohol- or Tyramine-containing foods	Nausea, vomiting, increased CNS depression, hypertensive crisis, headache
Sympathomimetics (ephedrine, norepinephrine, phenylpropanolamine, amphetamine, methylphenidate)	Hypertension, tremors, palpitations
Levodopa	Hypertension
Meperidine	Hypertension
Tricyclic antidepressants (imipramine, nortriptyline, desipramine)	CNS excitation, hyperpyrexia, mania
Dextromethorphan (present in Robitussin-DM and other generic cough preparations)	Hyperpyrexia, coma, death
Fluoxetine	Coma, death

Drug	Reaction
Antidiabetic agents	Possible hypoglycemia
Antihistamines (Diphenhydramine, hydroxyzine)	CNS depression, respiratory depression
Barbiturates, narcotic analgesics	Respiratory depression, CNS depression

Dosage:

The usual dose of procarbazine in the methotrexate, Oncovin®, procarbazine, prednisolone (MOPP) regimen for Hodgkin's disease is 100 mg/m² (rounded to the nearest 50 mg) PO daily for 14 days.

When procarbazine is used as a single agent, the dose is 50 to 200 mg/day given for 10 to 20 days.

Dose Forms

Matulane® is available in capsules of 50 mg.

Administration:

Capsules of procarbazine are given in one dose on an empty stomach. If the patient exhibits nausea or vomiting after the total dose is given, the dose may be subdivided into two or three daily doses.

Adverse Reactions:

Hematologic: The dose limiting toxicity of procarbazine is myelosuppression. Myelosuppression may be protracted, especially producing profound thrombocytopenia. The nadir in cell counts is usually 4 weeks; white cells and red cells decrease after platelets and cell counts usually return to normal numbers in 4 to 6 weeks.

Gastrointestinal: Nausea, vomiting, and diarrhea usually develop in the first few days of treatment.

Flulike syndrome: Fever, chills, sweating, lethargy, myalgias and arthalagias may occur.

Dermatologic: Skin reactions are rare and may include alopecia, pruritus, and allergic drug rash.

Carcinogenic: Secondary neoplasia, especially leukemia, has been reported with procarbazine. The drug is a teratogen, mutagen, and carcinogen.

Endocrine and Reproductive: Azoospermia and amenorrhea are noted with high doses of procarbazine. These effects may reverse after the drug is discontinued. Gynecomastia and atrophy of the testes may be noted.

Neurologic: High doses of procarbazine (>300 mg/day) have been associated with paresthesias, neuropathies, ataxia, weakness, lethargy, hallucinations, and seizures.

Practitioner Interventions:

1. Antiemetics such as $5HT_3$ antagonists should be given 30 minutes prior to administration of procarbazine.
2. Obtain patient's complete blood cell count (CBC) and platelet count on a weekly basis.
3. Instruct patient that nausea will decrease with continued treatment.
4. Instruct patient to notify physician if fever or chills are present.
5. Counsel patients about temporary azoospermia and potentially premature menopause.
6. Instruct patient not to take any medications—including over-the-counter medications—without checking with physicians or pharmacists.
7. Instruct patient about foods to avoid during therapy with procarbazine (dark beer, wine, cheese, bananas).

References:

1. Andrieu JM, Ifrah N, Payen C, et al. Increased risk of secondary acute non-lymphocytic leukemia after extended field radiation therapy combined with MOPP chemotherapy for Hodgkin's disease. J Clin Oncol 1990;8:1148–1154.
2. Black DJ, Livingston RB. Antineoplastic drugs in 1990. A review (part 1). Drugs 1990;39:489–501.
3. Levine EG, Bloomfield CD. Leukemias and myelodysplastic syndromes secondary to drug, radiation, and environmental exposure. Semin Oncol 1992;79:47–84.

SARGRAMOSTIM

Other Names:
Leukine®, Prokine®, Granulocyte–macrophage colony-stimulating factor, GM-CSF.

Uses:
Sargramostim is approved for use in bone marrow transplantation in patients with non-Hodgkin's lymphoma, acute lymphoblastic leukemia (ALL), and Hodgkin's disease who are undergoing autologous bone marrow transplantation. Sargramostim is also approved for failure of bone marrow transplantation or engraftment delay after allogeneic or autologous bone marrow transplantation, myelodysplastic syndromes, aplastic anemia, congenital anemias, and human immunodeficiency virus (HIV)-associated neutropenia and/or drug-associated neutropenia from zidovodine or interferon alfa (α-IFN). It has also been useful in promoting granulocyte expansion of peripheral blood progenitor cells prior to apheresis for autologous stem-cell rescue. It has recently been approved for use following induction therapy in patients aged >55 to 70 years with acute myelogenous leukemia (AML), in order to shorten the time to neutrophil recovery and reduce the incidence of severe or life-threatening infections.

Mechanism of Action:
Sargramostim has no antitumor activity. It promotes granulocyte proliferation and function through its effects on partially committed progenitor cells in the granulocyte–macrophage pathways.

Pharmacokinetics:
Absorption: Sargramostim is readily absorbed after SC administration. Peak levels are observed 2 hours after injection, and the drug remains detectable in the blood for 6 hours.

Distribution: Sargramostim enters various tissues, especially liver, spleen, and kidney. It is unknown whether it enters the cerebrospinal fluid.

Protein Binding: Sargramostim is highly protein bound.

Metabolism: The metabolic fate of sargramostim is not well established.

Half-life: The α half life of sargramostim is 12 to 17 minutes, with a terminal half life of 10 to 15 hours.

Elimination: Very little sargramostim is excreted intact in the urine, although catabolism to inactive fragments in the renal tubule may constitute a major route of elimination of the drug.

Drug Interactions:
Sargramostim increases the percentage of leukemia blast cells in the S phase of the cell cycle, which further enhances ***cytarabine*** cytotoxicity.

Dosage:
Stem Cell Transplant (Allogeneic or autologous). The recommended dosage of sargramostim in bone marrow transplant patients is 250 μg/m^2/day (about 5 μg/kg/day) until the peripheral neutrophil count is 5,000/mm^3 for 1 day or >1500/mm^3 for 3 consecutive days. Treatment should begin 2 to 4 hours after marrow reinfusion and not less than 24 hours after the last dose of chemotherapy. Some institutions round the dose to the nearest 250 or 500 μg depending on body weight. Patients weighing 70 kg and over would receive 500 μg, while those <70 kg would receive 350 μg.
Neutophil recovery following chemotherapy in AML. The recommended dose is 250 μg/m^2/day IV over 2 hours starting 4 days after chemotherapy until the ANC is >1500/mm^3 for 3 consecutive days.
Mobilization of Peripheral Blood Progenitor Cells. The recommended dose is 250 μg/m^2/day IV over 24 hours or SC once daily until protocol amounts of cells have been collected.

Dose Forms
Prokine® and Leukine® (sargramostim) is available in 250- and 500-μg vials.

Administration:
Sargramostim may be administered by IV infusion over a period of 30 to 120 minutes, or by rapid SC injection depending on the indication for use. Reconstituted solutions may be further diluted in NS or D5W. If the final concentration is less than 10 μg/mL, albumin should be added to a concentration of 1 μg/mL. Reconstituted solutions of Leukine® prepared with bacteriostatic water are stable for 20

days in the refrigerator. Solutions prepared with non-preserved sterile water should be used within 6 hours.

Compatibilities: In Y-site infusion with a dose of 10 µg/mL, sargramostim is compatible with the following:

Chemotherapy: bleomycin sulfate, carboplatin, carmustine, cisplatin, cyclophosphamide, cytarabine, dacarbazine, dactinomycin, doxorubicin HCl, floxuridine, fluorouracil, idarubicin HCl, ifosfamide, mechlorethamine HCl, mesna, methotrexate sodium, mitoxantrone HCl, pentostatin, teniposide, vinblastine sulfate, vincristine sulfate and vinorelbine taxtrate.

Non-Chemotherapy: Amikacin sulfate, aminophyllin, amphotericin B, aztreonam, butorphanol tartrate, calcium gluconate, cefazolin sodium, cefepime HCl, cefotaxime sodium, cefotetan sodium, ceftazidime (for 2 hours only), ceftizoxime sodium, ceftriaxone sodium, cefuroxime sodium, cimetidine HCl, clindamycin phosphate, cyclosporine (2 hours), dexamethasone sodium phosphate, diphenhydramine HCl, dopamine HCl (2 hours), doxycycline hyclate, droperidol, famotidine, fentanyl citrate (2 hours), fluconazole, furosemide, gentamicin sulfate, heparin sodium, IV immune globulin, magnesium sulfate–mannitol, meperidine HCl, metoclopramide HCl, metronidazole, mezlocillin, miconazole, minocycline HCl, netilmicin sulfate, piperacillin sodium–tazobactam sodium (D5W), potassium chloride, prochlorperazine edisylate, promethazine HCl, ranitidine HCl, ticarcillin disodium, icarcillin disodium-clavulanate potassium, TPN, trimethoprim-sulfamethoxazole, vancomycin (sargramostim with no albumin), and zidovudine.

Incompatibilities: In Y-site infusion with a dose of 10 µg/mL, sargramostin is incompatible with:

Chemotherapy: Mitomycin.

Non-Chemotherapy: Acyclovir sodium, amphotericin, ampicillin sodium, ampicillin sodium-sulbactam sodium, chlorpromazine HCl, ganciclovir sodium, haloperidol lactate, hydrocortisone sodium phosphate or succinate, hydromorphone HCl, hydroxyzine HCl, imipenem-cilastatin sodium, lorazepam, methylprednisolone sodium succinate, morphine sulfate, nalbuphine HCl, ondansetron HCl, piperacillin sodium, sodium bicarbonate, tobramycin sulfate, and vancomycin (sargramostim with albumin).

Adverse Reactions:

Vascular: Higher doses of sargramostim (>30 µg/kg) may produce capillary leak syndrome, pericarditis, and fluid retention.

Flulike syndrome: Usual doses of sargramostim of 250 µg/m²/d may produce side effects such as a flulike syndrome, characterized by lethargy, malaise, fever, and headache.

Bone pain: (substernum, shoulder, or hip) may occur, especially in patients whose bone marrow is engrafting. This can be controlled with acetaminophen.

Hypersensitivity: Mild local reactions at injection sites may also occur.

Practitioner Interventions:

1. Monitor patient's white blood cell (WBC) on a daily basis.
2. Instruct patient about usual side effects of sargramostim, including flulike syndrome, malaise, fever, and bone pain.
3. If fever is present, premedicate patient with acetaminophen on a daily basis.
4. Instruct patient in appropriate self-injection technique if sargramostim is to be given SC.
5. Instruct patient about needle disposal and injection site rotation if sargramostim is being given SC.
6. Premedicate patient with acetaminophen for bone pain.
7. Instruct patient to notify health care provider if any erythema, pain, or edema occur at injection sites.

References:

1. Brandt SJ, Peters WP, Atwater SK, et al. Effect of recombinant human granulocyte-macrophage colony-stimulating factor on hematopoietic reconstitution after high dose chemotherapy and autologous bone marrow transplantation. N Engl J Med 1988;318:869–876.
2. Neumanitis J, Singer JW, Buchner CD, et al. Use of recombinant human granulocyte macrophage colony-stimulating factor in autologous marrow transplantation for lymphoid malignancies. Blood 1988;72:834–836.
3. Trissel LA, Bready BB, Kwan VW, Santiago NM. Visual compatibility of sargramostim with selected antineoplastic agents, anti-infectives, or other

drugs during stimulated Y-site injection. Am J Hosp Pharm 1992;49:402–406.

STREPTOZOCIN

Other Names:
Zanosar®, Streptozotocin.

Uses:
Islet-cell pancreatic carcinoma, carcinoid tumor, non-small-cell lung cancer.

Mechanism of Antitumor Action:
Streptozocin selectively inhibits DNA synthesis without significantly affecting RNA or protein synthesis.

Pharmacokinetics:

Absorption: Streptozocin is administered only by the IV route.

Distribution: Streptozocin metabolites cross the blood–brain barrier and appear to concentrate in the liver and kidney. The parent compound concentrates in pancreatic beta cells.

Protein Binding: There is no information on the protein binding of streptozocin.

Metabolism: The liver is the primary site of metabolism of streptozocin. After IV administration, the drug is rapidly and extensively metabolized. All of the drug is rapidly converted to active metabolites.

Half-life: The half-life of streptozocin is only 15 minutes. The half-lives of the metabolites are unknown.

Elimination: Only 10% of streptozocin or its metabolites is excreted in the urine.

Drug Interactions:

Glucocorticosteroids and streptozocin may cause severe hyperglycemia. *Phenytoin* may antagonize the effect of streptozocin.

Dosage:
The usual dose of streptozocin is 1-1.5 g/m^2 IV weekly.

Dose Forms:
Zanosar® is available in 1 g vials. It should be diluted with 9.5 mL of NS or sterile water for injection.

Administration:
Zanosar® is given IV either as a short infusion in 5% dextrose or NS over a period of 10 to 15 minutes or as a slow infusion over a period of 6 hours. In patients complaining of local burning, the infusion should be slowed.

Compatibilities: In simulated Y-site infusions, streptozocin is compatible with filgrastim, melphalan HCl, ondansetron HCl, and vinorelbine trtrate.

Incompatibilities: Allopurinol sodium, cefepime HCl, and piperacillin sodium–tazobactam sodium.

Adverse Reactions:

Hematologic: Myelosuppression and leukopenia may occur in 20% of patients treated with streptozocin and are usually mild.

Renal: Nephrotoxicity is common in patients receiving streptozocin (40 to 60%) and usually manifests as transient proteinuria and azotemia; however, permanent tubular damage has been seen.

Gastrointestinal: Severe nausea and vomiting may occur. 5-HT$_3$ antagonists are recommended for antiemetic prophylaxis.

Hepatic: Mild and transient increases in serum glutamic oxaloacetic transaminase (SGOT), alkaline phosphatase, and bilirubin may be observed 2 to 3 weeks after beginning streptozocin.

Endocrine: Hyperglycemia may occur from damage of pancreatic beta cells, but this effect is not predictable.

Vascular: Local burning may occur during infusion of streptozocin, and may diminish if the infusion rate is slowed.

Practitioner Interventions:

1. Premedicate patient with antiemetics 30 minutes prior to administration of streptozocin.
2. Monitor patient's complete blood count (CBC) and platelet counts every week.
3. Monitor patient's renal function and liver function tests on a weekly basis.
4. Send patient's urine weekly for sugar and protein evaluation.
5. Start new IV if streptozocin is given peripherally, to reduce risk of phlebitis.
6. Instruct patient to recognize signs of hyperglycemia polyuria and polydipsia.

References:
1. Broder LE, Carter SK. Pancreatic islet cell carcinoma II. Results of streptozotocin in 52 patients. Ann Intern Med 1973;79:108–118.
2. Junod A, Lamber AE, Orci K, et al. Studies of the diabetogenic action of streptozotocin. Proc Soc Exp Biol Med 1967;126:201–205.
3. Weiss RB. Streptozocin: A review of pharmacology, efficacy, and toxicity. Cancer Treat Rep 1982;66:427–438.

TAMOXIFEN CITRATE

Other Names:
Nolvadex®, TAM.

Uses:
Breast and endometrial carcinomas, melanoma, prostate-stage D and renal-cell carcinomas.

Mechanism of Antitumor Action:
Tamoxifen blocks estrogen receptors in most, but not all, hormonal tissues. It is a mixed estrogen antagonist/agonist.

Pharmacokinetics:

Absorption: Tamoxifen is completely absorbed when given orally. Peak concentrations occur 6 hours after administration. No data are available on the effect of food on the bioavailability of the drug.

Distribution: Tamoxifen and its metabolites distribute in most tissues, especially those with known estrogen receptors.

Protein Binding: Tamoxifen binds to estrogen receptors.

Metabolism: Most of the dose of tamoxifen is metabolized by hepatic microsomes to the conjugated active metabolites N-desmethyltamoxifen and the N-oxide metabolite.

Half-life: The parent compound and its metabolites have terminal half-lives of 7 to 20 days.

Elimination: After enterohepatic circulation, about 75% of a dose of tamoxifen is eliminated in feces. Renal dysfunction does not lead to drug accumulation. In patients with hepatic obstruction, the drug and its metabolites may accumulate, but the clinical significance of such accumulation is unknown.

Drug Interactions:
Tamoxifen modulates a multidrug resistance phenomenon in tumor cells treated with natural-product antineoplastic agents.

Dosage:
The dosage of tamoxifen citrate is expressed in terms of tamoxifen. The dose of tamoxifen is 10 mg PO twice daily or 20 mg PO daily.

Dose Forms:
Tamoxifen comes in 10 and 20 mg tablets.

Administration:
Tablets of tamoxifen should be administered orally once or twice a day on an empty stomach.

Adverse Reactions:
Severe reactions to tamoxifen are rare.

 Endocrine: Menopausal symptoms, hot flashes, nausea, occasional vomiting can occur with tamoxifen. Gynecologic problems, such as vaginal bleeding and menstrual irregularities, can also occur.

Other: Acute flare of breast cancer symptoms, bone pain, and hypercalcemia. General reactions include lassitude, headache, leg cramps, dizziness, slight peripheral edema, and a distaste for food. Thrombosis has been rarely reported.

Hepatic: Elevated serum glutamic oxaloacetic transaminase (SGOT), alkaline phosphatase, and bilirubin levels are uncommon.

Second malignancy: A very slight increase in the incidence of endometrial cancer has been reported among patients treated with tamoxifen.

Hematologic: Myelosuppression is rare.

Practitioner Interventions:

1. Instruct premenopausal patients about probability of menopausal symptoms with tamoxifen therapy.
2. Counsel breast cancer patients that they may notice an increase in bone pain during the first few weeks of therapy.
3. Monitor patient's complete blood count (CBC) on a monthly basis for possibility of myelosuppression.
4. Liver function tests should be performed on patient as a baseline procedure, and should be monitored periodically.
5. Counsel patients about the possible risk of second malignancy.

References:

1. Jaiyesimi IA, Buzdar AU, Decker DA, Hortobagyi GN. Use of tamoxifen for breast cancer: twenty-eight years later. J Clin Oncol 1995;13:513–29.
2. Jordan VC. Tamoxifen: toxicities and drug resistance during the treatment and prevention of breast cancer. Ann Rev Pharmacol Toxicol 1995;35:195–211.
3. Legha SS. Tamoxifen in the treatment of breast cancer. Ann Intern Med 1988;109:219–228.
4. Nayfield SG, Karp JE, Ford LG, et al. Potential role of tamoxifen in prevention of breast cancer. J Natl Cancer Inst 1991;83:1450–1459.

TENIPOSIDE

Other Names:
Vumon®, VM-26.

Uses:
Teniposide is approved for the treatment of children with relapsed or refractory acute lymphocytic leukemia (ALL), Kaposi's sarcoma, and cutaneous T-cell lymphoma.

Mechanism of Antitumor Action:
Teniposide is an inhibitor of topoisomerase II. It does not bind
to DNA, but inhibits the strand-passing and DNA ligase activities of
topoisomerase II enzymes in the cell nucleus.

Pharmacokinetics:

Absorption: Teniposide is administered primarily by the IV route.

Distribution: Teniposide is distributed throughout the body, but
tends to concentrate in lymphoid tissue. It does not readily cross the
blood–brain barrier.

Protein Binding: Teniposide is highly bound to albumin
(~99.4%).

Metabolism: Most of teniposide is metabolized in the liver, probably by the cytochrome P450 system. It is thus subject to potential
interactions with other drugs metabolized by cytochrome P450.

Half-life: The average terminal half-life of teniposide is 20 hours.

Elimination: About 40% of teniposide and its metabolites are excreted in the urine. Only 14% is excreted unchanged in the urine.
Another 10% of the drug appears in the bile. Only 10% of the drug is
excreted via feces.

Drug Interactions:
Teniposide enhances the intracellular accumulation of ***methotrexate.***

Dosage:

ALL: 165 mg/m^2 twice weekly for 4 weeks.

Lymphoma: 45 to 160 mg/m^2 every 3 days or weekly.

Dose Forms:
Vumon® is available in a 50 mg ampule (10 mg/mL).

Administration:

Teniposide is given only by IV infusion in 5% dextrose or NS (concentration 0.1 to 1 mg/mL) and given over a period of at least 30 minutes, or as a continuous infusion. It should not be given by IV push, since this may induce severe hypotension. In patients with local burning or pain, slowing the infusion rate may decrease symptoms. Diluted solutions (0.1 to 1.0 mg/mL) are stable for 96 and 48 hours at room temperature, respectively. Avoid extravasation of the drug, since severe burning of skin may occur.

Compatibilities: In simulated Y-site infusion of 0.1 mg/mL in D5W, teniposide is compatible with acyclovir sodium, allopurinol, amikacin sulfate, aminophylline, amphotericin B, ampicillin sodium, ampicillin sodium-sulbactam sodium, aztreonam, bleomycin sulfate, bumetanide, buprenorphine HCl, butorphanol tartrate, cefoperazone sodium, cefotaxime sodium, cefotetan disodium, cefoxitin sodium, ceftazidime, ceftizoxime sodium, ceftriaxone sodium, cefuroxime sodium, chlorpromazine HCl, cimetidine HCl, ciprofloxacin, cisplatin, clindamycin phosphate, cyclophosphamide, cytarabine, dacarbazine, dactinomycin, daunorubicin HCl, dexamethasone sodium phosphate, diphenhydramine HCl, doxorubicin HCl, doxycycline hyclate, droperidol, enalaprilat, etoposide, famotidine, floxuridine, fluconazole, fludarabine phosphate, fluorouracil, furosemide, gallium nitrate, ganciclovir sodium, gentamicin sulfate, haloperidol lactate, heparin sodium, hydrocortisone sodium phosphate, hydrocortisone sodium succinate, hydromorphone HCL, hydroxyzine HCl, ifosfamide, imipenem–cilastatin sodium, leucovorin calcium, lorazepam, mannitol, mechlorethamine HCl, melphalan HCl, meperidine HCl, mesna, methotrexate sodium, methylprednisolone sodium succinate, metoclopramide HCl, metronidazole, mezlocillin sodium, miconazole, minocycline HCl, mitomycin, mitoxantrone HCl, morphine sulfate, nalbuphine HCl, netilmicin sulfate, ondansetron HCl, piperacillin sodium, plicamycin, potassium chloride, prochlorperazine edisylate, promethazine HCl, ranitidine HCl, sodium bicarbonate, streptozocin, thiotepa, ticarcillin disodium, ticarcillin disodium-clavulanate potassium, tobramycin sulfate, trimethoprim-sulfamethoxazole, vancomycin HCl, vinblastine sulfate, vincristine sulfate, vinorelbine tartrate, and zidovudine.

Incompatibilities: In simulated Y-site infusion of 0.1 mg/mL in D5W, teniposide is incompatible with idarubicin HCl.

Adverse Reactions:

 Hematologic: Myelosuppression is the dose-limiting side effect of teniposide. Leukopenia is generally maximum at 7 days, and recovery is noted by day 21. Thrombocytopenia may also occur.

 Cardiovascular: Hypotension may occur if teniposide is given over a period of less than 30 minutes. Chemical phlebitis is frequently noted and related to the infusion rate.

 Hypersensitivity: Reactions are common and are characterized by urticaria, angioedema, flushing, rashes, and hypotension.

 Gastrointestinal: Nausea and vomiting are relatively uncommon and easily controlled with conventional antiemetics.

 Neurologic: Paresthesias, fatigue, somnolence, and seizures have been rarely reported.

 Hepatic: Hyperbilirubinemia and elevated transaminase concentrations may be seen.

 Other: Fever is occasionally reported. Also, secondary acute leukemia has been associated with teniposide use.

Practitioner Interventions:

1. Monitor patient's complete blood cell count (CBC) and platelet count at least every 3 days.
2. Make sure infusion is delivered over a period of at least 30 minutes to prevent hypotension.
3. Premedicate patient with antihistamine to mediate hypersensitivity reactions. Patient may also require acetaminophen if they become febrile during infusion.
4. Have anaphylaxis kit at patient's bedside prior to dosing with teniposide. The kit should include diphenhydramine, hydrocortisone, epinephrine, and an Ambu bag.
5. Start a new IV infusion prior to administration of teniposide.
6. Monitor liver function prior to therapy and every month.
7. Counsel patient regarding possibility of secondary malignancy.

References:
1. Clark, PI, Slevin ML. The clinical pharmacology of etoposide and teniposide. Clin Pharmacokin 1987;12:223–252.
2. Holthuis JJ, de Vries, LG, Postmus, PE, et al. Pharmacokinetics of high-dose teniposide. Cancer Treat Rep 1987;71:599–603.

THIOGUANINE

Other Names:
6-TG

Uses:
Acute myelogenous leukemia (AML), acute lymphocytic leukemia (ALL), chronic myelogenous leukemia (CML).

Mechanism of Antitumor Action:
Thioguanine is converted to an active nucleotide that substitutes for natural purine bases, inhibiting the formation of DNA.

Pharmacokinetics:

Absorption: Only about 30% of a dose of thioguanine is absorbed after oral administration. Peak blood levels are achieved about 12 hours after ingestion and vary widely among patients. In animals, thioguanine does not appear in the cerebrospinal fluid. However, no data have been presented about the metabolites of thioguanine.

Protein Binding: It is unknown how much of a dose of thioguanine is bound to plasma protein.

Metabolism: One hour after IV administration, about 70% of a dose of thioguanine is found in the plasma in unchanged form along with several metabolites, including thioxanthine (13%), thiouric acid (11%), methylthioguanine (1%), and methylthioxanthine. In contrast, 13 hours after IV injection, thioguanine has been metabolized by the liver such that the plasma contains 34% methylthioxanthine, 24% thiouric acid, 12% methylthioxanthine, 10% thioxanthine, and 2% thioguanine. The methylated metabolites are not affected by xanthine oxidase activity. Thus, allopurinol does not significantly affect thioguanine metabolism.

Half-life: Thioguanine has biphasic elimination with a rapid distribution phase ranging from 3 to 40 minutes and a longer terminal half-life of 6 to 29 hours.

Elimination: From 40 to 80% of a dose of thioguanine is excreted in the urine as intact drug and metabolites. Although the liver and kidney are important routes of elimination of thioguanine, a guideline for dose adjustment in hepatic or renal dysfunction has not been established.

Drug Interactions:
Allopurinal does not interact with 6-thioguanine.

Dosage:
In both children and adults, the usual oral dose of thioguanine is 2 to 2.5 mg/kg/day. An investigational IV does is 700 mg/m^2 every 3 weeks.

Dose Forms:
Thioguanine is supplied as 40-mg tablets.

Administration:
Administer thioguanine orally between meals to facilitate complete absorption. The total daily dose may be taken all at one time.

Adverse Reactions:

Hematologic: Myelosuppression is the dose limiting toxicity of thioguanine; leukopenia precedes thrombocytopenia; and anemia occurs to a lesser extent. The nadir in cell counts occurs at 10 to 14 days, with recovery by days 17 to 21.

Gastrointestinal: Nausea, vomiting, and anorexia. Mild stomatitis and severe diarrhea may occur and may necessitate dose reduction.

Hepatic: Hyperbilirubinemia and elevated transaminase concentrations may occur. Jaundice is rare. Veno-occlusive disease has also been rarely reported.

Practitioner Interventions:

1. Monitor patient's complete blood cell count (CBC) on a weekly basis.

2. Instruct patient in oral-care regimen and how to evaluate for stomatitis.

3. Instruct patient to contact a health-care provider if having more than 3 stools per day.

4. Monitor patient's liver function prior to drug administration and on a weekly basis.

5. Administer antiemetic 30 minutes before dosing with thioguanine.

6. Instruct patient to take thioguanine between meals.

Selected References:

1. Brox LW, Birkett L, Belch A. Clinical pharmacology of oral thioguanine in acute myelogenous leukemia. Cancer Chemother Pharmacol 1981;6: 35–38.

2. Grindley GB. Clinical pharmacology of the 6-thiopurines. Cancer Treat Rev 1979;6:19–25.

3. Zimm S, Ettinger LJ, Holcenberg JS, et al. Phase I and clinical pharmacological study of mercaptopurine administered in a prolonged intravenous infusion. Cancer Res 1985;45:1869–1873.

THIOTEPA

Other Names:

Thioplex®, triethylene thiophsphoramide, TSPA.

Uses:

Hodgkin's disease, leukemia, breast cancer, ovarian cancer, malignant effusions, and superficial bladder cancer. Thiotepa may also be given intrathecally for meningeal cancer.

Mechanism of Antitumor Action:

Thiotepa is a polyfunctional alkylating agent similar to the nitrogen mustard compounds. The drug is activated *in vivo* to ethylamine free radicals, which bind to DNA. The activation of thiotepa may be mediated by cytochrome P450 metabolism.

Pharmacokinetics:

Absorption: Oral absorption of thiotepa is incomplete and erratic. Thiotepa is also given by intravesical (bladder instillation), intrathecal, and intraperitoneal routes. The absorption from the bladder may range from 10 to 100% of the administered dose.

Distribution: Thiotepa is widely distributed throughout the body. In adults, the Vd increases with increasing IV doses, and ranges from 0.25 to 1.6 L/kg. After intrathecal administration, distribution outside the cerebrospinal fluid is low.

Protein Binding: About 40% of thiotepa is bound to plasma proteins.

Metabolism: Thiotepa is extensively metabolized to aziridine and desulfurated products. The aziridine metabolites are further hydrolyzed to ethyanolamines, which appear to have cytotoxic properties. Thiotepa is also converted to triethylenephosphoramide and other alkylating metabolites.

Half-life: The half-life of thiotepa may increase with increasing dose. At doses of 30 to 75 mg/m^2, the half-life of the parent compound has been found to range from 1 to 2.5 hours and the active metabolite TEPA from 3 to 21 hours. The pharmacokinetics of high-dose thiotepa (6 or 7 mg/kg) (as used in bone marrow transplant regimens) results in a disproportionate increase in the area under the serum concentration curve, suggesting hepatic saturation. The $T_{1/2}$ in children is about 1.3 hours and does not vary with dosage.

Elimination: About 60% of an IV dose of thiotepa is excreted in the urine within 72 hours. Only a small amount appears as unchanged thiotepa or TEPA. The remainder is excreted as nontoxic metabolites.

Drug Interactions:

Cyclophosphamide does not alter the pharmacokinetics of thiotepa. Since thiotepa decreases pseudocholinesterase levels, muscle relaxants such as ***succinylcholine*** should be avoided during its use.

Dosage:

A variety of dosage regimens have been used with thiotepa. The usual dose is 10 to 20 mg/m^2 IV given every 3 to 4 weeks. One regimen uses 0.5 mg/kg repeated at 1- to 4-week intervals. Doses of up to 65 mg/m^2 have been given without bone marrow or stem cell support. High doses used in bone marrow transplantation range from 180 to 1,100 mg/m^2 IV. The usual intravesical dose for bladder tumors is 60 mg, and the usual intrathecal dose is 15 mg.

Dose Forms:
Thioplex® is available as 15 mg vials. Reconstituted solutions in NS should be filtered through a 0.22-micron filter prior to administration. NS solutions of thiotepa should be used immediately.

Administration:
Thiotepa is given by IV push or as an infusion diluted in 5% destrose, NS, or LR over a period of 15 to 30 minutes. Intravesical administration is usually performed over a 2-hour dwell time. Intrathecal administration should be done with nonpreserved NS.

Compatibilities: In simulated Y-site infusion of 1 mg/mL, thiotepa is compatible with allopurinol sodium, cefepime HCl, and piperacillin-tazobactam sodium. In simulated Y-site infusion of 10 mg/mL, thiotepa is compatible with melphalan HCl.

Incompatibilities: In simulated Y-site infusion, thiotepa is incompatible with filgrastim and vinorelbine tartrate.

Adverse Reactions:
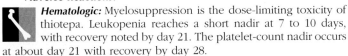
Hematologic: Myelosuppression is the dose-limiting toxicity of thiotepa. Leukopenia reaches a short nadir at 7 to 10 days, with recovery noted by day 21. The platelet-count nadir occurs at about day 21 with recovery by day 28.

Gastrointestinal: Side effects of thiotepa are dose-dependent. Higher doses yield more nausea and vomiting. Mucositis may be dose limiting with high doses.

Dermatologic: Integumentary side effects, including rash and bronzing of skin, occur after doses of thiotepa used for bone marrow transplantation. Erythema and desquamation of the hands and feet may occur after high-dose therapy, requiring topical care.

Practitioner Interventions:
1. Monitor patient's complete blood-cell count (CBC) and platelet count.

2. Premedicate patient with antiemetics at least 30 minutes prior to administering high-dose therapy with thiotepa.
3. Instruct patient to take showers twice daily to prevent skin toxicity if giving transplant doses of thiotepa.
4. Monitor patient for skin changes, rashes, areas of urticaria, and hives.
5. For skin bronzing, flaking, desquamation, initiate skin care protocol (i.e. moisturizers). If skin condition progresses treat with agents such as Burrow's *soalis* and silver *sulfadiazine*.

References:
1. Antman K, Avash L, Elias A, et al. High dose cyclophosphamide, thiotepa, and carboplatin alone with autologous bone marrow support in women with measurable advanced breast cancer responding to standard dose therapy; analysis by age. National Canc Inst Monogr 1994;16:91–94.
2. Hagan B. Pharmacokinetics of thio-tepa and Tepa in the conventional dose-range and its correlation to myelosuppressive effects. Cancer Chemother Pharmacol 1991;27:373–378.
3. Hagan B, Walstad RA, Nilsen OG. Pharmacokinetics of thio-tepa at two different doses. Cancer Chemother Pharmacol 1988;22:356–358.
4. Kletzel M, Kearns GL, Wells TG, Thompson HC Jr. Pharmacokinetics of high dose thiotepa in children undergoing autologous bone marrow transplantation. Bone Marrow Transplant 1992;10:171–175.
5. O'Dwyer PJ, LaCreta F, Engstrom PF, et al. Phase I/II pharmacokinetic re-evaluation of thiotepa. Cancer Res 1991;51:3171–3176.
6. Trissel LA, Martinez JF. Compatibility of thiotepa (lyophilized) with selected drugs during simulated Y-site administration. Amer J Health-system Pharm 1996;53:1041–5.

TOPOTECAN HCl

Other Names:
Hycamtin®, 10-dimethylaminomethyl-9-hydroxy-camptothecin.

Uses:
Non-small-cell lung cancer, ovarian cancer, Ewing's sarcoma.

Mechanism of Antitumor Action:
Topotecan is a specific inhibitor of topoisomerase I, which results in DNA damage during the course of DNA replication.

Pharmacokinetics:

Absorption: Topotecan is given by the IV route only.

Distribution: After 24 hours, the mean Vd_{ss} of topotecan in adults was 560 L/m^2. The Vd in the central compartment ranges from 3.4 to 67 L/m^2 (mean = 22 L/m^2) in children.

Protein Binding: Because of its large Vd, it is expected that topotecan has a high percentage of plasma protein binding of the open-ring carbolyte form of the drug.

Metabolism: Topotecan is rapidly converted in plasma to the open carboxylate form. The drug is also demethylated to an inactive metabolite.

Half-life: The half-life of topotecan in adults increases with continuous infusion. This was not observed after bolus doses. $T_{1/2}$ ranges from 9 to 120 minutes; the $T_{1/2}\beta$ ranges from 80 to 480 minutes. In pediatric patients, the half-life ranges from 1.5 to 4.7 hours.

Elimination: Renal excretion is the major route of elimination of topotecan, and accounts for 50 to 70% of total body clearance of the drug.

Drug Interactions:

Concurrently administered ***filgrastim*** enhances topotecan-induced neutropenia. Potential synergy of topotecan with ***etoposide*** has been observed in a human tumor cloning assay.

Dosage:

Rapid IV infusion: 1.5 mg/m^2/day $\times$ 5 days. The cycle is usually repeated every 3 weeks. A 24-hour continuous infusion of 1.0 to 1.5 mg/m^2/day for 5 days is under investigation.

Dose Forms:

Topotecan is supplied as a 4 mg single-use vial.

Administration:

Topotecan is administered via the IV route by bolus dosing, rapid infusion, or continuous infusion. The optimal method of administration (bolus, push, or continuous infusion) has yet to be determined.

Compatibilities: none reported.

Incompatibilities: non reported

Adverse Reactions:

 Hematologic: The dose-limiting toxicity of topotecan is myelo-suppression. Neutropenia may be significant, with a nadir in the neutrophil count at days 7 to 10 and recovery by days 21 to 28. Thrombocytopenia and anemia are also noted.

 Gastrointestinal: Nausea and vomiting are mild to moderate and are dose related. Mucositis may be severe with 120-hour infusions of topotecan.

 Renal: Microscopic hematuria has been reported in about 10% of patients.

 Other: Fever and flulike symptoms have been noted in patients receiving topotecan.

Practitioner Interventions:

1. Monitor patient's complete blood cell count (CBC) and platelet count every week.
2. Monitor patient for fevers, and instruct patient to contact health-care provider for fever above 101° F or 38.5° C.
3. Premedicate patient with antiemetics 30 minutes prior to dosing with topotecan.
4. If cell count nadir is significant, granulocyte- or granulocyte–macrophage colony-stimulating factors may be used to decrease the depth and duration of the nadir. These drugs should not be given concomitantly with topotecan.
5. Instruct patient on signs and symptoms of hematuria and when to contact health care provider.

References:
1. Gottleib JA, Guarino AM, Call JB, et al. Preliminary pharmacologic and clinical evaluation of camptothecin sodium. Cancer Chemother Rep 1970;54:461–470.
2. Greemers GJ, Lund B, Verweij L. Topoisomerase I inhibitors: topotecan and irinotecan. Cancer Treat Rev 1994;20:73–96.

3. Hycamtin® Product Information. Smith Kline-Beecham, May 1996.

4. Pratt CB, Stewart C, Santana VM, et al. Phase I study of topotecan for pediatric patients with malignant solid tumors. J Clin Oncol 1994;12:539–543.

5. Slichenmeyer WJ, Rowinsky EK, Donehower RC, Kaufman SH. The current status of camptothecin analogues as antitumor agents. J Natl Cancer Inst 1993;85:271–291.

6. Van Warmedam LJ, Verweij J, Schellens JH, et al. Pharmacokinetic and pharmacodynamics of topotecan administered daily for 5 days every 3 weeks. Cancer Chemother Pharmacol 1995;35:237–245.

7. Van Warmerdam W, ten Bokkel Huinink WM, Rodenhuis S, et al. Phase I clinical and pharmacokinetic study of topotecan administered by a 24 hour continuous infusion. J Clin Oncol 1995;13:1768–1776.

VINBLASTINE SULFATE

Other Names:
Velban®, vinblastine, VBL.

Uses:
Hodgkin's disease, non-Hodgkin's lymphoma, testicular carcinoma, choriocarcinoma, and breast cancer

Mechanism of Antitumor Action:
Vinblastine is a vinca alkaloid that binds to tubulin, thereby inhibiting microtubule assembly during mitosis, thus preventing polymerization and causing metaphase arrest.

Pharmacokinetics:

Absorption: Vinblastine is absorbed erratically from the gastrointestinal tract. It is primarily given IV.

Distribution: Vinblastine is widely distributed into most body tissues, except the cerebrospinal fluid, because of poor penetration across the blood–brain barrier. The Vd of vinblastine is very large (about 27 L/kg).

Protein Binding: The plasma protein binding of vinblastine is not reported, but is apparently very high, as indicated by the drug's large Vd.

Metabolism: Vinblastine is cleared very quickly from the plasma. It is partially metabolized in the liver to an active metabolite, deacetylvinblastine. The remainder of the drug is not metabolized and is excreted in unchanged form.

Half-life: Vinblastine has a triphasic half-life of 25 minutes, 52 minutes, and 19 to 25 hours, respectively.

Elimination: About 20% of a dose of vinblastine is excreted intact via the biliary tract and 33% by the kidney. About 70% of the drug is retained in the body over a period of 6 days. Biliary obstruction delays excretion and increases the toxicity of the drug. Doses must be modified in patients with elevated serum bilirubin levels.

Drug Interactions:
Vinblastine is a vesicant agent if extravasated. The antidote is hyaluronidase (Wydase®) plus warm compresses.

Dosage:
The usual dose of vinblastine ranges from 6 to 10 mg/m^2 IV every 2 to 4 weeks. Vinblastine has also been given as a continuous infusion of 1.7 to 2.0 mg/m^2/day for 4 days.

Dose Forms:
Velban® is available as a 10 mg powder vial.

Administration:
Vinblastine is usually given by IV push. The drug is very irritating and is not a vesicant given IM or SC. The dose of vinblastine should be withdrawn into a syringe and given over 1 minute via the side port of a freely flowing IV.

Compatibilities: In simulated Y-site infusion of 1 mg/mL, vinblastine is compatible with bleomycin sulfate, cisplatin, cyclophosphamide, doxorubicin HCl, droperidol, fluorouracil, leucovorin calcium, methotrexate sodium, metoclopramide HCl, and mitomycin HCl.

In simulated Y-site infusion of 0.12 mg/mL in D5W, vinblastine is compatible with ondansetron HCl, piperacillin sodium–tazobactam sodium, and teniposide.

In simulated Y-site infusion of 0.12 mg/mL in NS, vinblastine is compatible with allopurinol sodium, melphalan HCl, paclitaxel, sargramostim, and vinorelbine tartrate.

Incompatibilities: Furosemide, heparin sulfate.

Adverse Reactions:

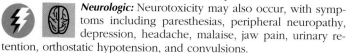

Hematologic: The dose-limiting toxicity of vinblastine is bone marrow suppression. Leukopenia reaches a maximum in 4 to 10 days, with recovery after days 17 to 24. The duration of neutropenia is dose related. Thrombocytopenia is also produced, but is usually mild.

Gastrointestinal: Nausea and vomiting occur rarely. Other gastrointestinal side effects include constipation, adynamic ileus, and abdominal pain. A stimulant laxative (senna) and stool softener (docusate) should be given if constipation occurs.

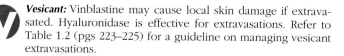

Neurologic: Neurotoxicity may also occur, with symptoms including paresthesias, peripheral neuropathy, depression, headache, malaise, jaw pain, urinary retention, orthostatic hypotension, and convulsions.

Dermatologic: Alopecia with vinblastine is usually mild and is reversible. Photosensitivity reactions may also occur.

Vesicant: Vinblastine may cause local skin damage if extravasated. Hyaluronidase is effective for extravasations. Refer to Table 1.2 (pgs 223–225) for a guideline on managing vesicant extravasations.

Practitioner Interventions:

1. Monitor patient's complete blood cell count (CBC) and platelet count every week.
2. If significant neutropenia is noted, colony stimulating factor may be ordered.
3. Premedicate patient with antiemetics as needed.
4. Initiate bowel regimen when vinblastine is started.
5. Vinblastine is a vesicant and should not be allowed to extravasate; the antidote is hyaluronidase (Wydase®). Warm compresses should be applied at the site of extravasation.

References:

1. Frei III E, Franzino A, Schnider BI, et al. Clinical studies of vinblastine. Cancer Chemother Rep 1961;12:125–129.
2. Nelson RL. The comparative clinical pharmacology and pharmacokinetics of vindesine, vincristine, and vinblastine in human patients with cancer. Med Pediatr Oncol 1982;10:115–127.

VINCRISTINE SULFATE

Other Names:
Oncovin®, Vincasar®, Vincristine, VCR.

Uses:
Acute lymphocytic leukemia (ALL), Hodgkin's disease, non-Hodgkin's lymphoma, rhabdomyosarcoma, neuroblastoma, Wilm's tumor, medulloblastoma, and breast cancer.

Mechanism of Antitumor Action:
Vincristine binds to microtubules during mitosis, leading to metaphase arrest, which results in interruption of DNA, RNA, and protein synthesis.

Pharmacokinetics:

Distribution: Vincristine is rapidly distributed to body tissues, with a large Vd especially in blood elements (8 to 27 L/kg). Vincristine penetrates poorly into the CSF.

Protein Binding: Vincristine shows strong tissue binding, but the percent bound to serum albumin is unknown.

Metabolism: Several vincristine metabolites are formed through hepatic metabolism, including deacetylvincristine, which is active.

Half-Life: Vincristine elimination follows a triphasic pattern similar to that of other vinca alkaloids. The terminal half-life is long (about 85 hours). In adults, the $T_{1/2}\alpha = 0.8$ minute, $T_{1/2}\beta = 7$ minutes, and $T_{1/2}\alpha = 164$ minutes. In children, $T_{1/2}\alpha = 2.6$ minutes, $T_{1/2}\beta = 41$ minutes, and $T_{1/2}\gamma = 1531$ minutes.

Elimination: Vincristine is eliminated primarily by the liver, with approximately 69% of a dose found in feces, and 10 to 20% found in urine.

Drug Interactions:
Vincristine has additive neurotoxicity with other neurotoxic agents, notably ***paclitaxel*** and ***cisplatin***.

Dosage:

Intravenous: Single dose. The usual adult dose is 1 to 1.4 mg/m^2 once weekly. Most doses should not exceed 2 mg as a single dose, except as ordered per protocol. For children who weigh <10 kg or having a BSA <1 m^2, the manufacturers recommend that therapy be initiated at 0.05 mg/kg once weekly.

Continuous IV infusion: In the VAD regimen, vincristine 0.4 mg/day continuous IV infusion for 4 days.

Dose modification:
If bilirubin > 3mg/dL, decrease dose of vincristine by 50%.

Dosage Forms
Oncovin® and Vincasar® are available in 1, 2, and 5 mg (1 mg/mL) vials.

Administration:
The drug is usually given as a rapid IV bolus in the side arm of a newly initiated IV line. It has also been given as a 24-hour continuous infusion via a central IV line. *Vincristine should never be given inthrathecally, since this is uniformly fatal.*

Compatibilities: In simulated Y-site infusion of 1 mg/mL, vincristine is compatible with bleomycin sulfate, cisplatin, cyclophosphamide, doxorubicin HCl, droperidol, fluorouracil, heparin sodium, leucovorin calcium, methotrexate sodium, metoclopramide HCl, and mitomycin HCl.

In simulated Y-site infusion of 0.12 mg/mL in D5W, vincristine is compatible with ondansetron HCl, piperacillin sodium–tazobactam sodium, and teniposide.

In simulated Y-site infusion of 0.12 mg/mL in NS, vincristine is compatible with allopurinol sodium, melphalan HCl, paclitaxel, sargramostim, and vinorelbine tartrate.

Incompatibilities: Cefepime HCl, furosemide, idarubicin HCl.

Adverse Reactions:

  *Neurologic:* The dose-limiting toxicity of vincristine is neurotoxicity. This toxicity is manifested primarily as reduced or absent deep tendon reflexes bilaterally, and by numbness, weakness, myalgias, cramping, and foot drop. Sev-

eral months must be allowed after discontinuing therapy for the symptoms to improve or disappear. CNS toxicity is less common, but consists of cranial neuropathy, jaw pain, parotid pain, and facial palsies.

Gastrointestinal: Constipation, abdominal cramps, nausea, vomiting, paralytic ileus, intestinal necrosis, and oral ulceration. Metoclopramide 10 to 20 mg IV or PO every 4 to 6 hours may reverse vincristine-induced paralytic ileus. A stool softener (docusate) plus a stimulant laxative (i.e., senna) should be used to prevent constipation, especially in elderly patients.

Genitourinary: Reactions occur in <10% of patients and have included dysuria, polyuria and urinary retention due to bladder atony.

Hematologic: Vincristine has few or no myelosuppressive effects.

Dermatologic: Alopecia may occur.

Vesicant: Vincristine is a vesicant and will cause local slim veciosis if extravasated. Hyaluronidase is an effective antidote. Do not use ice on vincristine extravasation, apply dry heat to area. Refer to Table 1.2 (pgs 223–225) for a guideline on managing VCR extravasations.

Practitioner Interventions:

1. Monitor patient's liver function prior to administration of vincristine.
2. Monitor patient for signs and symptoms of constipation and paralytic ileus.
3. Set up bowel regimen for patient.
4. Monitor patient for signs of urinary retention.
5. Avoid concurrent use of drugs that cause urinary retention or neurologic toxicity.
6. Antiemetics are usually not needed. Vincristine is rarely emetogenic.
7. Monitor patient for signs and symptoms of neurotoxicity (e.g., stocking–glove paresthesias).
8. Avoid extravasation. Have an extravasation kit available at the bedside. Apply warm compresses to area of extravasation.

References:

1. Barlogie B, Smith L, Alexanian R. Effective treatment of advanced multiple myeloma refractory to alkylating agents. N Engl J Med 1984;310: 1353–1356.
2. Desai ZR, Van der HW, Bridges JM, et al. Can severe vincristine neurotoxicity be prevented? Cancer Chemother Pharmacol 1982;8:211–214.

VINORELBINE TARTRATE

Other Names:
Nalvelbine®.

Uses:
Non-small-cell lung cancer, breast cancer.

Mechanism of Antitumor Action:
Vinorelbine blocks polymerization of microtubules, which leads to impaired formation of the mitotic spindle and DNA synthesis.

Pharmacokinetics:

Absorption: An oral formulation of vinorelbine is available in Europe. Oral absorption is rapid (by 2 hours) and amounts to 27% as compared to an IV dose. The bioavailability ranges from 24% in liquid-filled capsules to 80% in a liquid formulation.

Distribution: Vinorelbine shows extensive tissue binding to various tissues. The Vd is > 30 L/kg.

Protein Binding: Like other vinca alkaloids, vinorelbine binds avidly to protein. About 80% is bound to plasma proteins. The drug is highly bound to platelets, erythrocytes, lipoproteins, and albumin.

Metabolism: Vinorelbine is metabolized by the liver to two metabolites, vinorelbine-N-oxide (inactive) and deacetylvinorelbine (active.)

Half-life: Triphasic: $T_{1/2}\alpha$ = 2 to 6 minutes; $T_{1/2}\beta$ = 1.9 hours; $T_{1/2}\gamma$ = 40 hours.

Elimination: Vinorelbine elimination is primarily nonrenal: up to 25% of the drug is recovered in human feces within 72 hours. About 15% of a dose is excreted in the urine, mostly as unchanged drug.

When vinorelbine is combined with cisplatin, no change in its pharmacokinetics is observed.

Drug Interactions:
Avoid extravasation of vinorelbine, since leakage may cause soft-tissue necrosis.

Dosage:
The dose of vinorelbine is 27.5 to 35.4 mg/m^2 IV per week. A typical dose is 30 mg/m^2 IV weekly.

Dose Forms:
Nalvelbine® is available as a 10 mg/mL solution in 1 or 5 mL single-use vials.

Administration:
Vinorelbine is usually administered IV as a rapid push or in an IV solution (0.5 to 2 mg/mL) of 5% dextrose or NS over a period of 20 to 30 minutes in the side arm of a newly placed IV line.

Compatibilities: In Y-site injection of 1 mg/mL in NS, vinorelbine is compatible with amikacin sulfate, aztreonam, bleomycin sulfate, buprenorphine HCl, butanide, butorphanol tartrate, calcium gluconate, carboplatin, carmustine, cefotaxime sodium, ceftazidime, ceftizoxime sodium, ceftriaxone sodium, chlorpromazine HCl, cimetidine HCl, cisplatin, clindamycin phosphate, cyclophosphamide, cytarabine, dacarbazine, dactinomycin, daunorubicin HCl, dexamethasone sodium phosphate, diphenhydramine HCl, doxorubicin HCl, doxycline hyclate, droperidol, enalaprilat, etoposide, famotidine, filgrastim, floxuridine, fluconazole, fludarabine phosphate, gallium nitrate, gentamicin sulfate, haloperidol lactate, heparin sodium, hydrocortisone sodium phosphate, hydrocortisone sodium succinate, hydromorphone HCl, hydroxyzine HCl, idarubicin HCl, ifosfamide, imipenem–cilastatin sodium, lorazepam, mannitol, mechlorethamine HCl, melphalan, Meperidine HCl, mesna, methotrexate sodium, metoclopramide HCl, metronidazole, minocycline HCl, mitoxantrone, morphine sulfate, nalbuphine HCl, netilmicin sulfate, ondansetron HCl, plicamycin, streptozocin, teniposide, ticarcillin disodium, ticarcillin disodium–clavulanate potassium, tobramycin sulfate, vancomycin HCl, vinblastine sulfate, vincristine sulfate, and zidovudine.

Incompatibilities: Acyclovir sodium, allopurinol sodium, aminophylline, amphotericin B, ampicillin sodium, cefazolin sodium, cefoperazone sodium, cefotetan disodium, cefuroxime sodium, fluorouracil, furosemide, ganciclovir sodium, methylprednisolone sodium succinate, mitomycin, piperacillin sodium, thiotepa, trimethoprim–sulfamethoxazole.

Adverse Reactions:

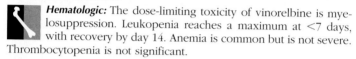 *Hematologic:* The dose-limiting toxicity of vinorelbine is myelosuppression. Leukopenia reaches a maximum at <7 days, with recovery by day 14. Anemia is common but is not severe. Thrombocytopenia is not significant.

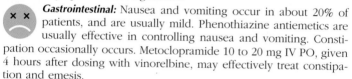 *Gastrointestinal:* Nausea and vomiting occur in about 20% of patients, and are usually mild. Phenothiazine antiemetics are usually effective in controlling nausea and vomiting. Constipation occasionally occurs. Metoclopramide 10 to 20 mg IV PO, given 4 hours after dosing with vinorelbine, may effectively treat constipation and emesis.

 Neurologic: Neurotoxicity is noted through decreased deep tendon reflexes, and is reported in up to one-third of patients receiving vinorelbine.

 Dermatologic: Alopecia occurs in only 25% of patients receiving vinorelbine.

 Vesicant: This agent can produce severe tissue damage if extravasated. Hyaluronidase (Wydase®) can be used to reduce vesicant-related reactions to vinorelbine. See Table 1.2 (pgs 223–225) for a guideline on managing vesicant extravasation.

Practitioner Interventions:

1. Monitor patient's complete blood cell count (CBC) and platelet count weekly.
2. If blood cell nadir is significant (<1,000 neutrophils/mm^3), colony stimulating factor may be used to decrease and shorten the duration of the nadir.
3. Monitor patient's deep tendon reflexes and any other signs of neurotoxicity on a regular basis.
4. Initiate new peripheral line before administering vinorelbine.

Vinorelbine Tartrate

Take extravasation kit to patient's bedside while administering drug. Have Wydase® (hyaluronidase) available.

5. Avoid extravasation, since leakage of vinorelbine may cause soft tissue necrosis. If extravasation is noted, apply heat to site.

References:

1. Cross S, Wright M, Marimato M, et al. Experimental antitumor activity of Navelbine. Semin Oncol 1989;16:15–20.
2. Cvitkovic E, Izzo J. The current and future place of vinorelbine in cancer therapy. Drugs 1992;44(Suppl 4):36–45.
3. Toso C, Lindley C. Vinorelbine: A novel vinca alkaloid. Am J Health Syst Pharm 1995;52:1287–1304.
4. Wargin WA, Lucas VS. The clinical pharmacokinetics of vinorelbine. Semin Oncol 1994;21(5 Suppl 10):21–27.

Table 1-1. DOSAGE MODIFICATION OF CHEMOTHERAPY IN PATIENTS WITH RENAL OR LIVER DYSFUNCTION

Drug	% Excreted in the urine	% of Dose relative to CrCl*		
		>50 mL/min	10–50 mL/min	10 mL/min
Azathioprine	50	100	100	50–75
Bleomycin	50	100	45–75	40
Carboplatin	65	**	**	**
Carmustine	65	100	100	25–50
Cisplatin	20–75	100	50	0
Cyclophos-phamide	10–15	100	100	50
Cytarabine***	10 (90% of AraU)	100	50	25–50
Etoposide	30–40	100	75	50
Ifosfamide	70–80	100	75	50
Lomustine	60	100	100	25–50
Methotrexate	90	100	25–50	0
Mitomycin	11	100	100	75
Plicamycin	50	100	50–75	0
Streptozocin	15	100	100	25–50

Drug	Serum Bilirubin		
	<1.2 mg/dL	1.2–3.0 mg/dL	>3.0 mg/dL
Dactinomycin	100	100	50
Daunorubicin	100	75	50
Doxorubicin	100	50	25
Idarubicin	100	50 (>2.5–5 mg/dL)	0 (>5 mg/dL)
Etoposide	100	50	0
Fluorouracil	100	100	50
Mitoxantrone	100	100	75
Vinblastine	100	50	25
Vincristine	100	50	25
Vinorelbine	100	50	25

* Adjustments based on: (1) Manufacturer's recommendations; (2) dose adjustment formula of Anderson in *Clinical Use of Drugs in Renal Failure*. Charles Thomas Springfield, IL. 1976; pp. 15–17; (3) Stewart CF, Fleming RA, Madden T *in* (RW Schrier, JG Gambertoglio, (eds) *Handbook of Drug Therapy in Liver and Kidney Disease*. Little Brown 1991, pp. 156–183.

** Use the Calvert Formula: Dose = AUC (4 to 9) × (CrCl + 25)

CrCl = creatinine clearance (estimated from Cockroft and Gault formula)

$$= \frac{(140 - \text{age}) \times \text{Wt (in kg)}}{\text{Serum Creatinine (in mg/dL)} \times (72)} \times 0.85 \text{ (if female)}.$$

*** High doses of cytarabine (>1,000 mg/m^2) require dose adjustment because of accumulation of the metabolite AraU.

Data from Bender JF, Grove WR, Fortner CL, (ref 1) Stoller (ref 5), and Bleyer (2, 3).

Table 1-2. PROCEDURES FOR MANAGEMENT OF ANTINEOPLASTIC EXTRAVASATIONS (*continued*)

A. COMMON VESICANT ANTINEOPLASTIC DRUGS

Dactinomycin (Actinomycin)	Mitomycin C (Mutamycin®)
Daunorubicin (Cerubidine®)	Vinblastine (Velban®)
Doxorubicin (Adriamycin®)	Vincristine (Oncovin®)
Idarubicin (Idamycin®)	Vindesine
Mechlorethamine (nitrogen mustard, Mustargen®)	Vinorelbine (Nalvelbine®)

RARE VESICANT ANTINEOPLASTIC DRUGS

Cisplatin (Platinol®)#	Paclitaxel (Taxol®)
Mitoxantrone (Novantrone®)	

IRRITANT ANTINEOPLASTIC DRUGS

Carmustine	Etoposide (Vepesid®)
Dacarbazine (DTIC®)	Plicamycin

Only a few rare case reports.

B. SIGNS AND SYMPTOMS OF A LOCAL EXTRAVASATION REACTION
  1. Patient complaints of local pain, burning, or any acute change at the injection site or proximal to the site if drug is given at a previous site of venipuncture.
  2. Induration or swelling at the injection site.
  3. Lack of blood return during a direct peripheral injection.
  4. Resistance in injecting the drug during peripheral administration, or decrease in IV infusion rate.

C. PROCEDURES FOR MANAGING EXTRAVASATIONS
  At the first sign of extravasation, the following procedures should be performed in the following order:
  1. Stop the injection or infusion, but do not remove the catheter.
  2. Request assistance, notify physician, and obtain order for treatment.

continued

Table 1-2. PROCEDURES FOR MANAGEMENT OF ANTINEOPLASTIC EXTRAVASATIONS (*continued*)

C. PROCEDURES FOR MANAGING EXTRAVASATIONS *continued*

3. Aspirate as much blood or solution from the injection site as possible, in order to remove the extravasated drug.

4. After aspiration, disconnect the syringe from the catheter and inject the antidote through the needle.

5. (Optional) Inject the specific antidote via the same injection needle in which the infiltrated drug was administered (see Table below).

6. If unable to use the existing catheter/needle, give the antidote via a pincushion technique intradermally or subcutaneously (a new 27-gauge needle is used for each injection).

7. Remove the catheter/needle.

8. Apply ice packs (or dry heat for vinblastine, vincristine, and vinorelbine) for at least 30 minutes four times a day to the infiltrated site for at least 24 hours.

9. Complete an incident report with documentation of the site of extravasation and the approximate amount of drug extravasated.

10. Document the occurrence and the measures initiated in the nursing notes.

D. FOLLOW-UP CARE

1. In the inpatient setting, observe the extravasation site every 2 hours and document the condition of the patient.

2. In the outpatient setting, instruct the patient about (a) topical care of the site; (b) individuals to call if needed, and (c) signs and symptoms of worsening of the condition. Call the patient daily to determine the progress of the infiltration.

continued

Table 1-2. PROCEDURES FOR MANAGEMENT OF ANTINEOPLASTIC EXTRAVASATIONS (*continued*)

E. LOCAL ANTIDOTES RECOMMENDED FOR CHEMOTHERAPY EXTRAVASATIONS

Antineoplastic Drug	Antidote	Amount
Cisplatin Dactinomycin, Mechlorethamine, Mitomycin C,	Ice + sodium thiosulfate (4 mL of 25% concentration diluted to 25 mL with sterile water)	2 mL
Daunorubicin, Doxorubicin, Idarubicin	Ice + hydrocortisone PO4 50 mg/mL	0.5 mL diluted with 2 mL normal saline
Vinblastine, Vincristine, Vinorelbine	Dry heat + hyaluronidase 150 Units/mL (obtain from refrigerator)	1 mL

CHAPTER II

Use of Hematopoietic Growth Factors

Hope S. Rugo

Hematopoietic growth factors (including colony-stimulating factors) are proteins that influence the proliferation, differentiation, and survival of specific hematopoietic cells (Figure 2-1). These growth factors promote:

1. *Differentiation* of pluripotent stem cells to committed progenitor cells giving rise to different cell lineages.
2. *Proliferation* and further differentiation of developing cells within a specific lineage.
3. *Stimulation* of the functions of mature myeloid cells, including chemotaxis and phagocytosis.

Three recombinant hematopoietic growth factors are commercially available for clinical use in the United States:

1. Granulocyte-colony stimulating factor: G-CSF (Filgrastim).
2. Granulocyte/macrophage-colony stimulating factor: GM-CSF (Sargramostim).
3. Erythropoietin: EPO (Epoietin)

Many more growth factors are in clinical trials, including interleukin-3 (IL-3), PIXY321, and thrombopoietin (TPO).

The primary use of hematopoietic growth factors is to prevent and/or treat chemotherapy-induced cytopenias in cancer patients and patients with acquired immune deficiency syndrome (AIDS). A major exception is erythropoietin, which was initially approved to treat the anemia associated with renal failure, and has had the broadest use outside of oncology.

227

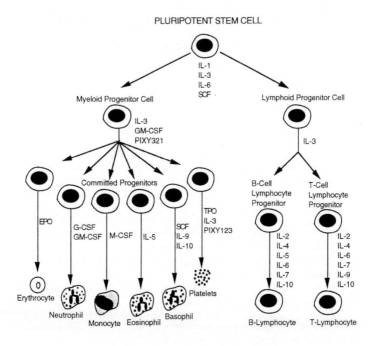

PLURIPOTENT STEM CELL

FUNCTIONAL PROPERTIES OF HEMATOPOIETIC GROWTH FACTORS

G-CSF:

1. Lineage-specific growth factor for granulocyte colony growth and expansion.
2. Regulates the production and function of neutrophils.
3. Results in a dose-related increase in the neutrophil count.

Initial FDA approval: to reduce the incidence of febrile neutropenia in patients receiving myelosuppressive chemotherapy for nonmyeloid malignancies.

Also, reduced length of hospital stay and days of intraveneous antibiotic use.

Current FDA-approved indications for use:

1. Decrease the incidence of febrile neutropenia in cancer patients with nonmyeloid malignancies who are receiving myelosuppressive chemotherapy.
2. Reduce the duration of neutropenia in cancer patients with nonmyeloid malignancies who are receiving bone marrow transplants (BMTs).
3. Mobilization of peripheral blood progenitor cells (PBPCs) for use in hematopoietic progenitor-cell transplantation.
4. Reduce the incidence and duration of neutropenia in patients with severe chronic neutropenia (SCN).

GM-CSF:

1. Regulates earlier, intermediate stages of hematopoiesis.
2. *In vitro:*
   a. Stimulates expansion and growth of granulocyte/macrophage colony-forming units (CFU-GM)
   b. In combination with EPO, stimulates expansion and growth of multipotential colonies containing myeloid, erythroid, and megakaryocytic cells (CFU-GEMM).
   c. Enhances the functional properties of neutrophils and macrophages, including phagocytic and chemotactic responses.
3. Increases neutrophil, eosinophil, and monocyte counts.

Initial FDA approval: to reduce the length of neutropenia in patients with lymphoma following autologous bone marrow transplantation (ABMT).

It also reduces hospital stays, days of IV antibiotic use, and incidence of documented infections.

Current FDA approved indications for use:

1. Shorten time to neutrophil recovery following induction chemotherapy in older patients (> 55 years) with acute myelogenous leukemia (AML).
2. Reduce the duration of neutropenia in cancer patients with nonmyeloid malignancies receiving ABMT.

3. Prolong survival in patients with engraftment delay or failure following BMT.

Note that in current clinical use, G-CSF and GM-CSF are essentially interchangeable (see specific clinical use section below). No large-scale prospective comparative trials exist to assess differences in the clinical efficacy or toxicity of these two factors in specific clinical situations.

EPO

1. First commercially available hematopoietic growth factor.
2. Regulates the production of the red cell line, especially mature red cells.
3. Increases the reticulocyte count.
4. **Initial FDA approval:** to treat the anemia associated with chronic renal failure.
5. **Current FDA-approved indications for use** include the treatment of anemia associated with:
   a. Chronic renal failure
   b. Chemotherapy-induced anemia
   c. Zidovudine-induced anemia
6. Also stimulates red cell production in low-erythropoietin states:
   a. Anemia of chronic disease and in normal individuals:
   b. Replace lost blood volume.
   c. Allows repeated autologous donation.

HEMATOPOIETIC GROWTH FACTORS NOT YET AVAILABLE FOR GENERAL CLINICAL USE:

IL-3 (Multi-CSF)

1. Multilineage hematopoietic growth factor.
   a. Regulates early and intermediate stages of hematopoiesis.
   b. Promotes growth and differentiation of multipotential progenitor and committed myeloid, erythroid, and megakaryocyte cell lineages.
2. Benefit on platelet recovery following chemotherapy not yet clear, but appears minimal.
3. Sequential IL-3 followed by GM-CSF after intensive chemother-

apy may increase the yield of progenitor cells collected for subsequent transplantation.
4. Role following transplantation is unclear.

PIXY321 (GM-CSF/IL-3 fusion protein)

1. Genetically engineered molecule combining effects of the two proteins GM-CSF and IL-3.
2. *In vitro:*
   a. Supports sustained megakaryopoiesis and retains myeloid effects of GM-CSF.
3. *In vivo:*
   a. May reduce cumulative thrombocytopenia associated with multiple cycles of chemotherapy.
   b. May decrease the time to platelet independence following ABMT.
   c. Use as progenitor-cell-mobilizing agent under investigation.
   d. Phase III studies are ongoing.

Thrombopoietin (TPO)

1. Megakaryocyte growth factor.
2. *In vitro:*
   a. Supports megakaryocyte proliferation and growth.
3. *In vivo:*
   a. Stimulates platelet production and megakaryocyte proliferation.
4. Phase I/II clinical trials are in progress.
5. Most exciting and promising new agent available to possibly treat thrombocytopenia (currently only treatable with transfusions) from a wide variety of causes.

SPECIFIC GUIDELINES FOR CLINICAL USE (Table 2-1)

G-CSF/GM-CSF

Chemotherapy-induced neutropenia:

1. Used as **prophylaxis** and as **treatment** for established neutropenia in conjunction with antibiotics.

**Table 2-1. GUIDELINES FOR USE OF HEMATOPOETIC GROWTH
            FACTORS**

Growth Factor	Indication	Dosage	Length of Therapy
G-CSF **GM-CSF**	Chemotherapy induced neutropenia (nonmyeloid malig.) Prophylaxis Treatment	**G-CSF:** 5 μg/kg/day SC or IV. **GM-CSF:** 250 μg/m^2/day SC or IV.	Begin no earlier than 24 hours after chemotherapy, usually 4–7 days after completion. Stop when ANC > 1000/mm^3 for 3 days or >10,000/mm^3.
	AML induction ($\geq$55 yrs)	Begin 4 days after completion of chemotherapy, when hypoplastic BM documented (days 10–14) or following second course of induction. Stop when ANC > 1000/mm^3 for 3 days or > 10,000/mm^3.	
	BMT Reduce duration of neutropenia Treatment engraftment delay or failure: (ANC < 100 by 28 days after BMT or by 21 days with active infection)	**G-CSF:** 5–10 μg/kg/d SC or IV **GM-CSF:** 250– 500 μg/m^2/d SC or IV	Begin 0–6 days following BMT, same stopping rules as above. Start at lower dose, escalate after 2 weeks if NR.
	PBPC mobilization: Growth factor alone with chemotherapy	Use higher dose unless intolerable side effects occur. Begin at least 4 days prior to first leukapheresis and continue through last leukapheresis. *continued*	

Table 2-1. GUIDELINES FOR USE OF HEMATOPOETIC GROWTH FACTORS *(Continued)*

Growth Factor	Indication	Dosage	Length of Therapy
G-CSF **GM-CSF**	Bone marrow failure: Myelodysplasia (MDS) Aplastic anemia (AA) Drug-induced agranulocytosis Severe chronic neutropenia	**G-CSF:** 5 μg/kg/day SC or IV. **GM-CSF:** 250 μg/m²/day SC or IV.	Adjust dose to maintain ANC > 1,500/mm³ and for clinical course. For MDS and AA, discontinue if NR in 2–4 weeks.
	AIDS Drug-induced NTP NTP with infections AIDS-related lymphoma on chemotherapy	Drug induced neutropenia/infections: adjust dose to maintain ANC > 1,500/mm³ and for clinical course. Chemotherapy: follow guidelines for chemotherapy above.	
EPO	Anemia associated with: cancer chemotherapy	50–300 IU/kg thrice weekly SC	Treat at lower dose for 4 weeks, if NR increase dose by 50 IU/kg to achieve desired Hct. Stop if NR by 3 months.
	Chronic inflammatory conditions/Anemia of chronic disease	50–150 IU/kg thrice weekly SC	*continued*

Table 2-1. GUIDELINES FOR USE OF HEMATOPOETIC GROWTH FACTORS *(Continued)*

Growth Factor	Indication	Dosage	Length of Therapy
EPO	Allogeneic BMT	150–200 IU/kg/day or thrice weekly SC	Use during the first 3 months following BMT to reduce the need for red cell transfusions.
	HIV-associated anemias	100 IU/kg thrice weekly SC or IV	Treat for 4 wks, if NR then increase dose by 50–100 IU/kg to achieve desired Hct
	Myelodysplasia	100–1000 IU/kg thrice weekly to daily SC	Begin at lower dose, adjust dose monthly or biweekly to acheive desired Hct. Stop if NR at 3 months.
	Reduce transfusions in surgical patients (high risk who cannot receive transfusions)	300 IU/kg/day SC	Begin 5–10 days before and continue for 3 days after surgery
	Facilitate autologous blood donation for surgery	200–400 IU/kg once weekly SC or IV	For 3–4 weeks. Allows collection of 1–2 additional units of blood

2. Goals of therapy are to:
   a. Prevent or reduce the incidence and severity of neutropenia.
   b. The end result should be a decrease in the complications associated with febrile neutropenia: severe or life-threatening infections, days of hospitalization, use of IV antibiotics, and death.
3. Additional beneficial effects in patients receiving chemotherapy or radiation therapy:
   a. Eliminate or reduce the need for treatment delay and dose reductions.
   b. Allow the use of dose intensification without prohibitive marrow toxicity.
   c. Reduce non-marrow toxicity:
      Reduce the severity and duration of chemotherapy-induced oral mucositis.
4. Used in patients with both nonmyeloid and myeloid malignancies.
   a. There does not appear to be significant stimulation of leukemic cells or a decrease in remission rates when myeloid growth factors are used following induction chemotherapy for AML.
      Survival benefit has been shown only in older patients ($\geq$ 55 years)

Bone Marrow Transplantation

1. Primary use is to reduce the duration of neutropenia:
   a. Marked reduction in time to neutrophil engraftment, infections, and hospital days has been demonstrated.
   b. These beneficial effects have been seen after ABMT, but not after allogeneic BMT.
2. Usually begin therapy on the day of transplant; however, preliminary data suggest that it may be possible to begin as late as day 6 following ABMT and still maintain the beneficial effects noted above.
3. Improves survival and reduces infectious complications in patients with engraftment delay or failure to engraft following ABMT or allogeneic BMT.

PBPC mobilization

1. Significantly increases the concentration of circulating hematopoietic progenitor cells available for transplantation.

2. Chemotherapy mobilization added to growth factors markedly increases the number of circulating progenitor cells. However, additional toxicity from chemotherapy and timing of PBPC collection increases the complexity of this approach.

Reduce the duration and/or severity of neutropenia in acquired or congenital bone marrow failure states:

1. Myelodysplasia
   a. Reduces complications associated with severe neutropenia.
   b. Continued therapy required to sustain improved neutrophil counts.
   c. Decreased red cell or platelet transfusion requirement rarely seen.
2. Aplastic anemia.
   a. Patients with mild to moderate disease have higher response rates.
3. Drug-induced agranulocytosis.
   a. May shorten the time to neutrophil recovery.
4. SCN and cyclic neutropenia.

AIDS/HIV Infection

1. Zidovudine or other drug-induced neutropenia
   a. Allow use of effective medications with otherwise intolerable marrow suppression.
2. Neutropenia associated with serious or repeated infections.
3. AIDS-related lymphoma undergoing chemotherapy.

General dosing guidelines

1. **G-CSF**
   a. 5–10 µg/kg given by SC injection daily. IV route less common.
2. **GM-CSF**
   a. 250–500 µg/m^2 SC or IV daily.
3. **G/GM-CSF** General Comments
   a. Begin at lower dose level. Dose escalation is usually reserved for prolonged severe neutropenia or life-threatening complications associated with neutropenia.
   b. Begin growth-factor therapy at least 24 hours after the last dose of chemotherapy or radiation therapy (existing data suggests that between 24 and 72 hours may be optimal).

    c. Discontinue therapy when the absolute neutrophil count (ANC) is $> 10,000/mm^3$ or when the ANC is $> 1,000/mm^3$ for three consecutive days.

    d. Reduce dose or discontinue therapy if the white blood cell (WBC) count is $> 100,000/mm^3$ during PBPC mobilization.

    e. Stop at least 24 hours before next scheduled cycle of chemotherapy or radiation therapy, since growth factors may enhance the myelosuppressive or other effects of treatment.

EPO (nonrenal applications)

Anemia of chronic disease (ACD)

1. ACD is associated with inappropriately low levels of circulating erythropoietin for the degree of anemia seen.
2. Goal of therapy is to reduce the degree of anemia but, more importantly, to improve quality of life.
3. Documented effectiveness in treating anemia has been reported in the following disease states:

    a. *Malignancy and/or chemotherapy.*
    Reported response rates range from 50 to 85%.
    Decreases or eliminates transfusion requirement.
    Improves energy level and overall quality of life.

    b. *Chronic inflammatory conditions.*
    Use evaluated formally for patients with rheumatoid arthritis, juvenile rheumatoid arthritis, and inflammatory bowel disease.

    c. *Allogeneic BMT.*
    Inadequate production of endogenous erythropoietin for the first 6 months after transplantation.
    Use of EPO during this period, especially the first 3 months following transplantation, reduces the number of required red blood cell transfusions and duration of transfusion dependence.
    No benefit shown following ABMT.

Anemia associated with AIDS/HIV Infection

1. Associated with inappropriately low endogenous erythropoietin levels.

2. Reduced transfusion requirements and improved quality of life.
3. Effective in zidovudine-induced anemia when endogenous erythropoietin levels are ≤ 500 IU/L.

Myelodysplasia (MDS)

1. Transfusion-dependent anemia is often the initial symptom of this disease, and transfusions may be required on a very frequent basis.
2. Response rates are extremely variable and limited, ranging from ~10 to 25%.
3. Very high doses of EPO may be required, resulting in high costs.
4. Patients with lower endogenous erythropoietin levels (<1,000 IU/ml) may have a better chance of responding.
5. Combinations of EPO with myeloid growth factors have been used with limited success.

To reduce transfusion requirements in surgical patients.

1. Given perioperatively for hip replacement surgery, reduces but does not eliminate the need for blood transfusions.

To facilitate autologous blood donation.

1. Reduces or eliminates anemia associated with preoperative blood donation.
2. Increases capacity for blood donation.
3. May not reduce the need for allogeneic blood transfusions following surgery.

Other

1. Sickle cell anemia.
2. Thalassemia.
3. Anemia associated with prematurity.

General dosing guidelines:

1. *Treat only patients with symptomatic or transfusion-requiring anemia*
2. The typical dose range is 50 to 150 IU/kg by SC or IV administered three times a week.
3. Begin at lower dose level and evaluate the reticulocyte count and hemoglobin biweekly.

4. If no response is seen at 4 weeks, raise the dose by 50 to 100 IU/kg and continue to evaluate response at 4-week intervals.
5. Titrate dose to maintain desired hematocrit (usually 30 to 35%).
6. If no response is seen after 3 months, consider discontinuing therapy.

*****Maintain iron stores** Functional iron deficiency is a major cause of failure to respond to EPO. In general, concurrent iron supplementation should be considered with EPO therapy unless a contraindication exists (iron overload in MDS or after BMT).

TOXICITIES

G-CSF/GM-CSF

1. The currently available forms of G-CSF and GM-CSF appear to have relatively similar toxicities occuring with a similar rate of frequency. **Side effects are dose related.**
2. The most frequently reported side effects are:
   a. Bone pain and myalgias.
      • Most severe at the time of rapid neutrophil recovery, often just precedes actual rise in WBC count.
      • Usually responds well to analgesics and/or dose reduction.
   b. Fever.
      • Responds well to acetaminophen.
   c. Mild nausea and headache.
3. Less common side effects:
   a. Spleen pain or splenomegaly.
      • Resolves with cessation of growth-factor therapy.
   b. Injection site erythema, swelling, pain.
      • Alternating sites, application of ice to site usually helps.
4. Rare side effects:
   a. Vasculitis or exacerbation of pre-existing inflammatory conditions (G-CSF).
   b. Dyspnea, capillary leak syndrome, hypotension (GM-CSF).
   c. Acute febrile neutrophilic dermatosis (Sweet's syndrome).
   d. Allergic reaction. These reactions resolve with cessation of growth-factor therapy. Premedication or dose reduction may also be used.
5. In patients treated chronically for SCN with G-CSF, a 3% inci-

dence of MDS/myeloid malignancy has been reported, as well as the development of abnormal cytogenetics. This is thought to be due to the underlying disease rather than the growth-factor therapy. A registry has been established for long-term follow-up of SCN patients.

EPO

1. Toxicities reported in patients with renal failure (hypertension, seizures, thromboembolic events) are not seen in general when EPO is used for other indications.
2. Injection-site pain with SC administration (due to citrate buffer) may be managed by:
   a. Application of ice to site before injection.
   b. Dilution with saline or reduction of injection volume.

MECHANISMS TO PROMOTE COST EFFECTIVE USE OF MYELOID GROWTH FACTORS

Specific guidelines have been proposed by the American Society of Clinical Oncology (ASCO) as well as individual hospitals to promote more cost-effective use of the myeloid growth factors.

1. Limit use in specific situations:
   a. To reduce likelihood of febrile neutropenia:
      • When expected incidence is ≥ 40%.
      • After documented febrile neutropenia in a prior chemotherapy cycle.
      • When the ANC is expected to fall to $< 100/mm^3$ or severe neutropenia is expected to last longer than 7 days.
      • In patients with other high risk features such as compromised immune function.
   b. To reduce the duration of febrile neutropenia:
      • In patients with prognostic factors predictive of clinical deterioration, including pneumonia, hypotension, multiorgan dysfunction (sepsis syndrome), or fungal infection.
   c. Avoid use in *low risk* patients with afebrile neutropenia.
   d. To increase the neutrophil count in myelodysplasia in patients with severe neutropenia and recurrent infection.
   e. Dose escalation is not usually beneficial.

Standardized dosing:

1. Weight-based dosage approximated for vial size.
   a. G-CSF (~5 μg/kg): ≤75 kg: 300 μg/day
      >75 kg: 480 μg/day
   b. GM-CSF (~5 μg/kg): ≤60 kg: 250 μg/day
      >60 kg: 500 μg/day
2. Dose titration may be used for neutropenia unresponsive to initial dose of growth factor, when the time normally required for neutrophil recovery has been exceeded. Increase to next vial size to a maximum of 10 μg/kg/day.

References

Review

1. American Society of Clinical Oncology. Recommendations for the use of hematopoietic colony-stimulating factors: Evidence-based clinical practice guidelines. *J Clin Oncol* 1994;12:2471.
2. Appelbaum FR. Allogeneic marrow transplantation and the use of hematopoietic growth factors. *Stem Cells* 1995;13:344.
3. Lieschke MB, Burgess AW. Granulocyte colony-stimulating factor and granulocyte-macrophage colony-stimulating factor. *N Engl J Med* 1992;327:28.
4. Lieschke MB, Burgess AW. Granulocyte colony-stimulating factor and granulocyte-macrophage colony-stimulating factor. *N Engl J Med* 1992;327:99.
5. Vose JM, Armitage JO. Clinical applications of hematopoietic growth factors. *J Clin Oncol* 1995;13:1023.

Myeloid Growth Factors

6. Bregni M, Siena S, Di Nicola M, et al. Comparative effects of granulocyte-macrophage colony-stimulating factor after high-dose cyclophosphamide cancer therapy. *J Clin Oncol* 1996;14:628.
7. Bui BN, Chevallier B, Chevreau C, et al. Efficacy of lenograstim on hematologic tolerance to MAID chemotherapy in patients with advanced soft tissue sarcoma and consequences on treatment dose-intensity. *J Clin Oncol* 1995;13:2629.
8. Chi KH, Chen CH, Chan WK, et al. Effect of granulocyte-macrophage colony stimulating factor on oral mucositis in head and neck cancer patients after cisplatin, fluorouracil, and leucovorin chemotherapy. *J Clin Oncol* 1995;13:2620.
9. Dale DC, Bonilla MA, Davis MW, et al. A randomized controlled Phase

III trial of recombinant human granulocyte colony-stimulating factor (fil-grastim) for treatment of severe chronic neutropenia. *Blood* 1993;81: 2496.

10. Negrin RS, Haeuber DH, Nagler A, et al. Maintenance treatment of patients with myelodysplastic syndromes using recombinant human granulocyte colony-stimulating factor. *Blood* 1990;76:36.

11. Ribas A, Albanell J, Bellmunt J, et al. Five-day course of granulocyte colony-stimulating factor in patients with prolonged neutropenia after adjuvant chemotherapy for breast cancer is a safe and cose-effective schedule to maintain dose-intensity. *J Clin Oncol* 1996;14:1573.

12. Rowe JM, Andersen JW, Mazza JJ, et al. A randomized placebo-controlled Phase III study of granulocyte-macrophage colony-stimulating factor in adult patients (> 55 to 70 years of age) with acute myelogenous leukemia: A study of the Eastern Cooperative Oncology Group (E1490). *Blood* 1995;86:457.

13. Winter JN, Lazarus HM, Rademaker A, et al. Phase I/II Study of combined granulocyte colony-stimulating factor and granulocyte-macrophage colony-stimulating factor administration for the mobilization of hematopoietic progenitor cells. *J Clin Oncol* 1996;14:277.

Erythropoietin

14. Markham A, Bryson HM. Epoetin alfa. A review of its pharmacodynamic properties and therapeutic use in nonrenal applications. *Drugs* 1995;49:232.

15. Miller CA, Jones RJ, Piantadosi S, et al. Decreased erythropoietin response in patients with the anemia of cancer. *N Engl J Med* 1990;322: 1689.

16. Schreiber A, Howaldt S, Schnoor M, et al. Recombinant erythropoietin for the treatment of anemia in inflammatory bowel disease. *N Engl J Med* 1996;334:619.

Other Growth Factors

17. Ganser A, Lindermann A, Seipelt G, et al. Effects of recombinant human interleukin-3 in patients with normal hematopoiesis and in patients with bone marrow failure. *Blood* 1990;76:666.

18. Kaushansky K. Thrombopoietin: The primary regulator of megakaryocyte and platelet production. *Thromb Hemost* 1995;74:521.

19. Vadhan-Raj S, Broxmeyer HE, Andreef M, et al. *In vivo* biologic effects of PIXY321, a synthetic hybrid protein of recombinant human granulocyte-macrophage colony-stimulating factor and interleukin-3 in cancer patients with normal hematopoiesis: A phase I study. *Blood* 1995;86: 2098.

Toxicity

20. Brugger W, Bross KJ, Glatt M, et al. Mobilization of tumor cells and hematopoietic progenitor cells into peripheral blood of patients with solid tumors. *Blood* 1994;83:636.

21. Passos-Coehlo JL, Ross AA, Moss TJ, et al. Absence of breast cancer cells in a single-day peripheral blood progenitor cell collection after priming with cyclophosphamide and granulocyte-macrophage colony-stimulating factor. *Blood* 1996;85:1138.

CHAPTER III

Chemotherapy Regimens in Adults

Lloyd E. Damon and Alan Venook

This chapter presents commonly used chemotherapy protocols based on tumor site. The regimens selected were what we considered the standard of practice in the oncology community. However, these regimens are not an exhaustive accounting of all available therapies. After each regimen, we have provided a comment section that includes recommendations for the appropriate use and administration of the agents described.

MELANOMA

HIGH-RISK ADJUVANT

Drug	Dose	Route	Day
Interferon alfa-2b	20 MU/m^2/d	IV	1–28
Interferon alfa-2b	10 MU/m^2	subq	three times weekly

Continues for 48 weeks.

Comments:

1. This treatment conferred a survival advantage for patients with deep primary or regionally metastatic melanoma.

References:

1. Kirkwood JM, Strawderman MH, Ernstoff MS, et al: Interferon Alfa-2b Adjuvant therapy of high-risk resected cutaneous melanoma: The Eastern Cooperative Oncology Gropup Trial EST 1684. J Clin Oncol 1996: 14,7–17.

NON-SMALL CELL LUNG CANCER

ADVANCED

Drug	Dose	Route	Day
Nalvelbine	30 mg/m^2	IV	1, 8, 15, 22, 29, 36
Cisplatin	120 mg/m^2	IV	1, 29

Cycle repeated 7 days for eight cycles.

Comments:

1. This combination appears superior to others in the treatment of non-small cell lung cancer.

References:

1. LeChavalier T, Brisgand D, Douillard JY, et al: Randomized study of vinorelbine and cisplatin versus vindesine and cisplantin versus vinorelbine alone in advanced non-small cell lung cancer: results of a European multicenter trial including 612 patients. J Clin Oncol 12:360–367, 1994.

ADRENAL CORTICAL CARCINOMA

METASTATIC

Mitotane

Drug	Dose	Route	Day
Mitotane	2–10 g (in 3 or 4 divided doses)	PO	Daily

Comments:

1. The clinical response rate, particularly for hormone-related symptoms, is about 50%. Tumor regression is less common and the medication is poorly tolerated.
2. Mitotane is given in 3 or 4 divided doses (it comes in 500-mg tablets)

References:

1. Lubitz JA, Freeman L, Okun R. Mitotane use in inoperable adrenal cortical carcinoma. JAMA 1973;223:1109.

BREAST CANCER

ADJUVANT

CMF

Drug	Dose	Route	Day
Cyclophosphamide (C)	100 mg/m²/day	PO	1–14
Methotrexate (M)	40 mg/m² bolus	IV	1 and 8
5-Fluorouracil (F)	600 mg/m² bolus	IV	1 and 8

Cycle repeated every 28 days for six cycles.

Comments:

1. This study in node-positive patients set the standard for future adjuvant trials. The previous study used 12 cycles of therapy, but equal efficacy has been shown for 6 months of treatment.

References:

1. Bonadonna G, Brusamolino E, Valagussa P, et al. Combination chemotherapy as an adjuvant treatment in operable breast cancer. N Engl J Med 1976;294:405–410.

BREAST CANCER

ADJUVANT

AC

Drug	Dose	Route	Day
Doxorubicin (A)	60 mg/m² bolus	IV	1
Cyclophosphamide (C)	600 mg/m² bolus	IV	1

Cycle repeated every 21 days for four cycles.

Comments:

1. This study compared short-course AC chemotherapy to 6 months of CMF. The comparable results were achieved with much less treatment time. Higher dose AC is under investigation.

References:
1. Fisher B, Borwn AM, Dimitrov NV, et al. Two months of doxorubicin-cyclophosphamide with and without interval reinduction therapy compared with 6 months of cyclophosphamide, methotrexate and fluorouracil in positive-node breasts cancer patients with tamoxifen-non-responsive tumors: results from the National Surgical Adjuvant Breast and Bowel Project B-15. J Clin Oncol 1990;8:1483–1496.

BREAST CANCER

METASTATIC

FAC

Drug	Dose	Route	Day
5-Fluorouracil (F)	500 mg/m^2 bolus	IV	1 and 8
Doxorubicin (A)	50 mg/m^2 bolus	IV	1
Cyclophosphamide (C)	500 mg/m^2 bolus	IV	1

Cycle repeated every 21 days until disease progression occurs.

Comments:

1. This regimen first showed promise in the treatment of patients with inflammatory breast cancer.

References:
1. Buzdar AU, Montague ED, Barker JL, et al. Management of inflammatory carcinoma of breast with combined modality approach—an update. Cancer 1981;47:2537–2542.

BREAST CANCER

METASTATIC

CAF

Drug	Dose	Route	Day
Cyclophosphamide (C)	100 mg/m^2/day	PO	1–14

continued next page

CAF

Drug	Dose	Route	Day
Doxorubicin (A)	30 mg/m² bolus	IV	1 and 8
5-Fluorouracil (F)	500 mg/m² bolus	IV	1 and 8

Cycle repeated every 28 days until disease progression occurs.

Comments:

1. This regimen produced a 61% response rate in previously un-treated patients.

References:

1. Falkson G, Gelman RS, Tormey DC, et al. The Eastern Cooperative On-cology Group experience with cyclophosphamide, adriamycin, and 5-fluorouracil (CAF) in patients with metastatic breast cancer. Cancer 1985;56:219–224.

BREAST CANCER

METASTATIC

Paclitaxel

Drug	Dose	Route	Day
Paclitaxel (Taxol)	175 mg/m² infusion for 3 to 24 hours	IV	1

Cycle repeated every 21 days until disease progression occurs.

Comments:

1. Patients who have not been pre-treated with chemotherapy may tolerate higher doses. Pre-medications should include dexame-thasone and ranitidine; the 3-hour infusion schedule is well-tol-erated and is easily administered in the outpatient setting.

References:

1. Holmes FA, Walters RS, Theriault RL, et al. Phase II trial of Taxol, an active drug in the treatment of metastatic breast cancer. J Natl Cancer Inst 1991;83:1797–1805.

BREAST CANCER

METASTATIC

NFL

Drug	Dose	Route	Day
Mitoxantrone (N)	10 mg/m² bolus	IV	1
5-Fluorouracil (F)	1,000 mg/m² for 24 hours	IV	1–3
Leucovorin (L)	100 mg/m² bolus	IV	1–3

Cycle repeated every 21 days for two cycles, then assess.

Comments:

1. This regimen had activity in previously treated patients, and the toxicity was not significant.
2. Give Leucovorin during 5-fluorouracil infusion.
3. N = Novantrone®.

References:
1. Jones SE, Mennel RG, Brooks B, et al. Phase II study of mitoxantrone, leucovorin, and infusional fluorouracil for treatment of metastatic breast cancer. J Clin Oncol 1991;9:1736–1739.

BREAST CANCER

METASTATIC

MMC-VBL

Drug	Dose	Route	Day
Mitomycin-C (MMC)	10 mg/m² bolus	IV	1
Vinblastine (VBL)	5 mg/m² bolus	IV	1 and 15

Cycle repeated every 28 days until disease progression occurs.

Comments:

1. The response rate in heavily pre-treated patients is about 30% and the toxicity tolerable even with mitomycin-C dosed at 4-week intervals.

References:
1. Brambilla C, Zambetti M, Ferrari L. Mitomycin and vinblastine in advanced refractory breast cancer. Tumori 1989;75:141–144.

BREAST CANCER

METASTATIC

VATH

Drug	Dose	Route	Day
Vinblastine (V)	4.5 mg/m² bolus	IV	1
Doxorubicin (A)	45 mg/m² bolus	IV	1
Thiotepa (T)	12 mg/m² bolus	IV	1
Halotestin (H)	10 mg thrice daily	PO	Daily

Cycle repeated every 21 days for two cycles, then assess.

Comments:

1. This regimen has proven activity in patients in whom prior therapy has failed.

References:
1. Hart RD, Perloff M, Holland JF. One-day VATH (vinblastine, adriamycin, thiotepa and halotestin) therapy for advanced breast cancer refractory to chemotherapy. Cancer 1981;48:1522–1527.

BREAST CANCER

AUTOLOGOUS PERIPHERAL BLOOD STEM CELL TRANSPLANT WITH

CPB (Stamp I)

Drug	Dose	Route	Day
Cyclophosphamide (C)	1875 mg/m² over 1 hour	IV	−6 to −4
Cisplatin (P)	55 mg/m² continuous over 24 hours	IV	−6 to −4
Carmustine (BCNU) (B)	600 mg/m² over 2 hours	IV	−3

Comments:

1. Autologous peripheral blood stem cells infused IV on days -1, 0, and $+1$.
2. Autologous pelvic bone marrow infused intravenously on day $+1$.
3. Two sets of platelets transfused on day -2 to minimize the risk of hemorrhagic cardiac necrosis.
4. Drug doses based on corrected body surface area (BSA), which equals $[BSA_{Ideal} + BSA_{Actual}] \div 2$ for patients $\geq 120\%$ of their ideal body weight.
5. Continuous bladder irrigation on days -6 to -3.

References:

1. Peters WP, Ross M, Vrendenburgh JJ, et al. High-dose chemotherapy and autologous bone marrow support as consolidation after standard-dose adjuvant therapy for high-risk primary breast cancer. J Clin Oncol 1993;11:1132–43.

BREAST CANCER

AUTOLOGOUS PERIPHERAL BLOOD STEM CELL TRANSPLANT WITH

CTCb (Stamp V)

Drug	Dose	Route	Day
Cyclophosphamide (C)	1,500 mg/m^2 continuous over 24 hours (4 doses)	IV	-7 to -3
Thiotepa (T)	125 mg/m^2 continuous over 24 hours (4 doses)	IV	-7 to -3
Carboplatin (Cb)	200 mg/m^2 continuous over 24 hours (4 doses)	IV	-7 to -3

Comments:

1. Autologous hematopoietic stem cells infused IV on day zero.
2. Hemorrhagic cystitis prophylaxis suggested.
3. Autologous hemotopoietic stem cells infused IV on day zero.

References:

1. Antman K, Ayash L, Elias A, et al. A phase II study of high-dose cyclophosphamide, thiotepa, and carboplatin with autologous marrow support in women with measurable advanced breast cancer responding to standard-dose therapy. J Clin Oncol 1992;10:102–110.

BREAST CANCER

AUTOLOGOUS PERIPHERAL BLOOD STEM CELL TRANSPLANT WITH

CTM

Drug	Dose	Route	Day
Cyclophosphamide (C)	1,500 mg/m^2 over 1 hour	IV	−6 to −3
Thiotepa (T)	150 mg/m^2 over 2 hours	IV	−6 to −3
Mitoxantrone (M)	10–15 mg/m^2 over 1 hour	IV	−6 to −3

Comments:

1. Doses based on body surface area (BSA) calculated from corrected weight, which equals $[kg_{Ideal} + (0.25)(kg_{Actual} - kg_{Ideal})]$
2. Mitoxantrone dose:
   A. 10 mg/m^2/dose for Stage II–IIIA patients.
   B. 10, 12.5, or 15 mg/m^2/dose (whichever is larger) for Stage IIIB–IV patients; the dose is chosen to keep lifetime doxorubicin equivalent dose $\leq$ 400 mg/m^2 (doxorubicin equivalent dose in mg/m^2 = Σ doxorubicin dose + (2.6) (Σ mitoxantrone dose) [see Reference 2].
3. Autologous hematopoietic stem cells infused IV on day zero.

References:

1. Damon LE, Rugo HS, Ries CA, et al. Mitoxantrone, thiotepa and cyclophosphamide as preparation for autologous bone marrow transplant for

high-risk adjuvant and advanced breast cancer. J Cellular Biochem 1994;(Suppl 18B):95.

2. Henderson IC, Allegra JC, Woodcock J, et al. Randomized clinical trial comparing mitoxantrone with doxorubicin in previously untreated patients with metastatic breast cancer. J Clin Oncol 1989;7:560–571.

BREAST CANCER

RELAPSE AFTER ANTHRACYCLINE THERAPY

Docetaxel

Drug	Dose	Route	Day
Docetaxel (Taxotere)	60–100 mg/m^2	IV for 1 to 24 hours	1

Repeat cycle every 21 days for two cycles, then reevaluate.

Comments:

1. Premedication to prevent hypersensitivity reactions is dexamethsone 8 mg IV or PO bid for 5 days starting one day prior to taxotere.

References:

1. Hudis, CA, Seidman AD, Crown JP, et al. Phase II and pharmacology study of docetaxel as initial chemotherapy for metastatic breast cancer. J Clin Oncol 1996;14:58–65.

COLORECTAL CANCER

ADJUVANT

FU-Levamisole

Drug	Dose	Route	Day
5-Fluorouracil	450 mg/m^2/day bolus	IV	1–5
5-Fluorouracil	450 mg/m^2 bolus	IV	29
Levamisole	50 mg three times a day	PO	Daily for 3 days every other week

5FU is repeated weekly for a total of 52 weeks after completion of the first week induction of 5-fluorouracil.

Comments:

1. Two large studies have demonstrated a survival advantage for patients with Dukes B3 or more advanced colon cancer. Unappreciated side effects include neurologic toxicity, abnormalities in liver function tests, and unexplained changes in carcinoembryonic antigen (CEA) level.

References:

1. Moertel CG, Fleming TR, MacDonald JS, et al. Levamisole and fluorouracil for adjuvant therapy of resected colon carcinoma. N Engl J Med 1990;322:352.

COLORECTAL CANCER

METASTATIC

FU-LVR (Wolmark)

Drug	Dose	Route	Day
Fluorouracil (FU)	500 mg/m^2 bolus mid-leucovorin infusion	IV	1
Leucovorin (LVR)	500 mg/m^2 over 2 hours	IV	1

Cycle repeated every 7 days for 6 weeks, followed by 2 weeks off, then repeat for six cycles.

Comments:

1. This regimen was superior to MOF (methyl-CCNU, vincristine, 5-fluorouracil) in patients with Dukes B2 or more advanced colon cancer.

References:

1. Wolmark N, Rockette H, Fisher B, et al. The benefit of leucovorin-modulated fluorouracil as post-operative adjuvant therapy for primary colon cancer: results from National Surgical Adjuvant Breast and Bowel Protocol C-03. J Clin Oncol 1993;11:1879.

COLORECTAL CANCER

METASTATIC

FU-LVR (Petrelli)

Drug	Dose	Route	Day
Fluorouracil (FU)	500 mg/m² bolus mid-leucovorin infusion	IV	1
Leucovorin (LVR)	600 mg/m² infusion over 2 hours	IV	1

Cycle repeated every 7 days for six cycles, then 2 weeks off.

Comments:

1. This regimen may be more toxic than its counterparts, although some patients will tolerate it quite well.

References:
1. Petrelli N, Douglass HO, Herrera L, et al. The modulation of fluorouracil with leocovorin in metastatic colorectal carcinoma: a prospective randomized phase III trial. J Clin Oncol 1989;7:1419.

COLORECTAL CANCER

METASTATIC

FU-IFN

Drug	Dose	Route	Day
Fluorouracil (FU)	750 mg/m² continuous infusion for 5 days	IV	1–5
Fluorouracil*	750 mg/m² bolus	IV	8
Interferon (IFN)	9 million units	SC	Three times a week

* Repeat 5FU weekly for 8 weeks then reassess.

Comments:

1. This regimen is an example of 5-FU modulation of an uncertain mechanism. The toxicity appears to be somewhat more than with 5-FU alone, and the response rate is probably no greater than in other protocols. There is an apparent benefit to adding interferon to regimens for patients who have already had other 5-FU-based treatment.

References:
1. Wadler S, Lembersky B, Atkins M, et al. Phase II trial of 5-fluorouracil and recombinant interferon alfa-2a in patients with advanced colorectal carcinoma: an Eastern Cooperative Oncology Group Study. J Clin Oncol 1991;9:1806.

COLON/RECTAL CANCER

5FU-REFRACTORY METASTATIC

Vinotecan

Drug	Dose	Route	Day
Irinotecan	125 mg/m^2	IV	1, 8, 15, 22

Cycle repeated 42 days for two cycles, then reassess.

References:
1. Rothenberg ML, Eckardt JR, Kuhn JG, et al: Phase II trial of Irinotecan in patients with progressive or rapidly recurrent colorectal cancer. J Clin Oncol 1996:14,1128–1135.

RECTAL CANCER
ADJUVANT
FU

Drug	Dose	Route	Day
Fluorouracil (FU)	500 mg/m²/day	IV bolus	1–5, 36–40
Fluorouracil	225 mg/m²/day	Continuous IV infusion during XRT	64–106
Fluorouracil	450 mg/m²/day	IV bolus	134–138, 169–173

Comments:

1. This study demonstrates the value of 5-FU both in its prevention of distant metastases and as a radiosensitizing drug in its improvement of local tumor control in patients with Dukes B2 or more advanced rectal cancer. The continuous infusion during radiation therapy leads to a markedly increased risk of significant diarrhea.

References:
1. O'Connell MJ, Martenson JA, Wieand HS, et al. Improving adjuvant therapy for rectal cancer by combining protracted infusion fluorouracil with radiation therapy after curative surgery. N Engl J Med 1994;331:502.

ANAL CANCER

LOCALIZED

FU-MMC

Drug	Dose	Route	Day
5-Fluorouracil (FU)	1,000 mg/m² continuous infusion for 24 hours	IV	1–5, 29–33
Mitomycin-C (MMC)	10 mg/m² bolus	IV	1 and 29

Comments:

1. This chemotherapy is given concomitant to 4,500 cGy pelvic radiation. The combination showed improved colostomy-free survival compared to 5-fluorouracil alone. The incidence of Grade IV toxicity, however, is greater than 20%. The results applied to both squamous and cloacogenic tumors. Human immunodeficiency virus (HIV)-positive patients with low CD4 counts should have treatment modified.

References:

1. Flam MS, John MJ, Peters T, et al: Radiation and 5-fluorouracil vs radiation, 5-FU, mitomycin-C in the treatment of anal canal carcinoma: preliminary results of a phase III randomized RTOG/ECOG intergroup trial. Proc Amer Soc Clin Oncol 1993;12:192.

Genitourinary Cancers

BLADDER CANCER

METASTATIC

CMV

Drug	Dose	Route	Day
Cisplatin (C)	100 mg/m² infusion over 1 hour	IV	2
Methotrexate (M)	30 mg/m² bolus	IV	1 and 8
Vinblastine (V)	4 mg/m² bolus	IV	1 and 8

Cycle repeated every 21 days for two cycles and assess response.

Comments:

1. This is an active regimen in advanced bladder cancer, and could be considered for adjuvant therapy trials.

References:
1. Harker WG, Meyers FJ, Freiha FS, et al. Cisplatin, methotrexate and vinblastine (CMV): an effective chemotherapy regimen for metastatic transitional cell carcinoma of the urinary tract: a Northern California Oncology Group study. J Clin Oncol 1985;3:1463–1470.

BLADDER CANCER

METASTATIC

MVAC

Drug	Dose	Route	Day
Methotrexate (M)	30 mg/m² bolus	IV	2, 15, 22
Vinblastine (V)	3 mg/m² bolus	IV	2, 15, 22
Doxorubicin (A)	30 mg/m² bolus	IV	2
Cisplatin (C)	70 mg/m² infusion over 1 hour	IV	1

Cycle repeated every 28 days for two cycles.

Comments:

1. This regimen appears to be similar to cisplatin/metho-trexate/vinblastine (CMV) in its activity.

References:
1. Sternberg CN, Yagota A, Scher HI, et al. M-VAC (Methotrexate, Vinblas-tine, Doxorubicin, Cisplatin) for advanced transitional cell carcinoma of the urothelium. J Urol 1988;139:461–469.

RENAL CELL CANCER

METASTATIC

Floxuridine

Drug	Dose	Route	Day
Floxuridine	0.075 mg/kg/day continuous infusion	IV	1–14

Cycle repeated every 28 days for two cycles and assess response.

Comments:

1. This regimen shows modest activity with substantial toxicity. Dose escalation, if well tolerated, is advisable.

References:
1. Wilkinson MJ, Frye JW, Small EJ, et al. A phase II study of constant infusion floxuridine for the treatment of metastatic renal cell carcinoma. Cancer 1993;71:3601–3604.

PROSTATE CANCER

METASTATIC, HORMONE REFRACTORY

VBL-estramustine

Drug	Dose	Route	Day
Vinblastine	4 mg/m^2 bolus	IV	q Week for 6 weeks
Estramustine	200 mg/m^2 TID (600 mg/m^2/day)	PO	Daily for 6 weeks

Cycle is 6 weeks, then 2 weeks off.

Comments:

1. Both prostate-specific antigen (PSA) and objective tumor responses were observed.

References:

1. Hudis GR, Greenberg R, Krigel RI, et al. Phase II study of estramustine and vinblastine, two microtubule inhibitors, in hormone-refractory prostate cancer. J Clin Oncol 1992;10:1754–1761.

GERM CELL CANCERS

GOOD PROGNOSIS

Pt-E

Drug	Dose	Route	Day
Cisplatin (Pt)	20 mg/m^2 infusion over 20–60 minutes	IV	1–5
Etoposide (E)	100 mg/m^2 infusion over 1 hour	IV	1–5

Cycle repeated every 21 to 28 days for four cycles.

Comments:

1. Patients with "good risk" germ-cell tumors (pure seminoma or testicular nonseminomatous tumors likely to achieve complete response) are most appropriately treated with this regimen.

References:

1. Bosl GJ, Geller NL, Bajorin D, et al. A randomized trial of etoposide + cisplatin versus vinblastine + bleomycin + cisplatin + cyclophosphamide + dactinomycin in patients with good prognosis germ cell tumors. J Clin Oncol 1988;6:1231–1238.

GERM CELL CANCERS

METASTATIC

PEB

Drug	Dose	Route	Day
Cisplatin (P)	20 mg/m^2 infusion over 20–60 minutes	IV	1–5
Etoposide (E)	100 mg/m^2 infusion over 1 hour	IV	2, 9, 16
Bleomycin (B)	30 units (mg) bolus	IV	1–5

Cycle repeated every 21 days for four cycles.

Comments:

1. This regimen is superior to cisplatin, vinblastine, and bleomycin, with less toxicity, and should be used in patients with advanced germ-cell tumors.

References:

1. Williams SD, Birch R, Einhorn LH, et al. Treatment of disseminated germ cell tumors with cisplatin, bleomycin and either vinblastine or etoposide. N Engl J Med 1987;316:1435–1440.

GERM CELL CANCERS

METASTATIC

VIP

Drug	Dose	Route	Day
Cisplatin	20 mg/m²/day infusion over 20–60 minutes	IV	1–5
Ifosfamide	1,200 mg/m²/day continuous infusion	IV	1–5
MESNA	1,200 g/m²/day continuous infusion	IV	1–6
Vinblastine* *or*	0.11 mg/kg/day bolus	IV	1–2
Etoposide	75 mg/m²/day infusion over 1 hour	IV	1–5

Cycle repeated every 21 days for four cycles.

Comments:

1. This regimen is effective salvage therapy for patients in whom a prior regimen for advanced germ-cell tumor has failed.
2. Vinblastine or etoposide is used, depending upon which agent the patient has already received). Etoposode, ifosfamide and cisplatin may also have a role in poor-prognosis patients as initial therapy.

References:

1. Loehrer PJ, Laver R, Roth BJ, et al. Salvage therapy in recurrent germ cell cancer: ifosfamide and cisplatin plus either vinblastine or etoposide. Ann Intern Med 1988;109:540–546.

GERM CELL CANCERS
AUTOLOGOUS PERIPHERAL BLOOD STEM CELL TRANSPLANT
Indiana University

Drug	Dose	Route	Day
Carboplatin	500 mg/m² over 15 minutes	IV	−7, −5, −3
Etoposide	400 mg/m² over 15 minutes	IV	−7, −5, −3

Comments:

1. Autologous hematopoietic stem cells infused intravenously on day zero.
2. Patients responding to one course are eligible to receive a second identical course.

References:
1. Nichols CR, Andersen J, Lazarus HM, et al. High-dose carboplatin and etoposide with autologous bone marrow transplantation in refractory germ cell cancer: an Eastern Cooperative Oncology Group protocol. J Clin Oncol 1992;10:558–563.
2. Broun ER, Nichols CR, Kneelbone P, et al. Long-term outcome of patients with relapsed and refractory germ call tumors treated with high-dose chemotherapy and autologous bone marrow rescue. Ann Intern Med 1992;117:124–128.

ESOPHAGEAL

METASTATIC

Pt-FU

Drug	Dose	Route	Day
Cisplatin (Pt)	75 mg/m² infusion over 1 hour	IV	1 only
5-Fluorouracil (FU)	1,000 mg/m²/day continuous infusion	IV	1–4

Cycle repeated every 28 days for four cycles.

Comments:

1. This protocol, with concomitant radiation, showed superior results to radiation alone. This same chemotherapy is being tested as neoadjuvant treatment in esophageal cancer.

References:

1. Herskovic A, Marz K, Al-Sarraf M, et al. Combined chemotherapy and radiotherapy alone in patients with cancer of the esophagus. N Engl J Med 1992;326:1593–1598.

GASTRIC CANCER

METASTATIC

ELF

Drug	Dose	Route	Day
Etoposide (E)	120 mg/m^2/day over 1 hour	IV over 1 hour	1–3
Leucovorin (L)	300 mg/m^2/day over 2 hours	IV over 2 hours	1–3
5-Fluorouracil (F)	500 mg/m^2/day over 30 min	IV midway thru LV	1–3

Cycle repeated every 21 days for two cycles, then reassess.

Comments:

1. Relatively well tolerated, even in gastrectomized patients; has moderate response rate. No proven benefit in adjuvant setting.

References:

1. Geffen JR, Venook AP, Luce J, et al. Phase II trial of VP-16, leucovorin and fluorouracil (ELF) in advanced gastric carcinoma. Proc Am Soc Clin Oncol 1992;11:195.

GASTRIC CANCER
METASTATIC

EAP

Drug	Dose	Route	Day
VP-16 (Etoposide) (E)	120 mg/m²/day infusion over 1 hour	IV	4–6
Doxorubicin (A)	20 mg/m² bolus	IV	1 and 7
Cisplatin (P)	40 mg infusion over 1 hour	IV	2 and 8

Cycle repeated every 21–28 days for two cycles, then reassess.

Comments:

1. Initial reports were very encouraging, with high response rates. However, confirmatory studies did not verify the significant activity, and the toxicity was profound.

References:
1. Preusser P, Wilke H, Achterrath W, et al. Phase II study with the combination etoposide, doxorubicin, and cisplatin in advanced measurable gastric cancer. J Clin Oncol 1989;7:1310.

GASTRIC CANCER
METASTATIC

FAMtx

Drug	Dose	Route	Day
Fluorouracil (F)	1500 mg/m² bolus 1 hour after MTX	IV	1
Doxorubicin (A)	30 mg/m² bolus	IV	15
Methotrexate (Mtx)	1,500 mg/m² infusion 30 minutes	IV	1

Cycle repeated every 28 days for two cycles, then reassess.

Comments:

1. Generally well tolerated and appears superior to EAP regimen. May also have a role in the adjuvant setting.

References:
1. Wils JA, Klein HO, Wagener DJTh, et al. Sequential high-dose methotrexate and fluorouracil combined with doxorubicin—a step ahead in the treatment of advanced gastric cancer: a trial of the European Organization for Research and Treatment of Cancer Gastrointestinal Tract Cooperative Group. J Clin Oncol 1991;89:827.

Gynecologic Cancers

OVARIAN

METASTATIC

PAC

Drug	Dose	Route	Day
Cisplatin (P)	50 mg/m^2 infusion over 1–2 hours	IV	1
Doxorubicin (A)	50 mg/m^2 bolus	IV	1
Cyclophosphamide (C)	1,000 mg/m^2 infusion over 1–2 hours	IV	1

Cycle repeated every 21 days for eight cycles.

Comments:

1. While in this study, doxorubicin did not appear to improve results, a meta-analysis suggests that it may offer some benefit compared to cyclophosphamide and cisplatin alone.

References:

1. Omura GA, Bundy BN, Berek JS, et al. Randomized trial of cyclophosphamide plus cisplatin with or without doxorubicin in ovarian carcinoma: a Gynecologic Oncology Group study. J Clin Oncol 1989;7:457–465.

OVARIAN

METASTATIC

Altretamine

Drug	Dose	Route	Day
Altretamine	260 mg/m^2/day in four divided doses	PO	1–15

Cycle repeated every 28 days for two cycles, and assess response.

Comments:

1. Newly approved, this agent has activity in heavily pretreated patients.
2. Round to the nearest 50 mg.

References:
1. Marietta A, MacNeill C, Lyter JA, et al. Hexamethylmelamine as a single second-line agent in ovarian cancer. Gynecol Oncol 1990;36:93–96.

OVARIAN
METASTATIC
Paclitaxel

Drug	Dose	Route	Day
Paclitaxel	135 mg/m^2	IV over 3 or 24 hours	1

Cycle repeated every 21 days for two cycles and assess response

Comments:

1. Patients who have not been pretreated with chemotherapy may tolerate higher doses. Premedications should include diphenhydramine 25 mg IV, and cimetidine 300 mg IV or ranitidine 150 mg PO or 50 mg IV, all given 30 minutes prior to paclitaxel. Dexamethasone 20 mg po should be given 12 hours, 6 hours, and 30 minutes before paclitaxel.

References:
1. McGuire WP, Rowinsky EK, Rosenshein NB, et al. Taxol: a unique antineoplastic agent with significant activity in advanced ovarian epithelial neoplasms. Ann Intern Med 1989;111:273–279.

OVARIAN CANCER
METASTATIC, REFRACTORY
Topotecan

Drug	Dose	Route	Day
Topotecan	1.5 mg/m^2/day over 30 min	IV	1–5

Cycle repeated every 21 days for two cycles, then reassess.

Comments:

1. This has modest activity in refractory ovarian cancer.

References:

1. Kudelka AP, Tresukosol D, Edwards CL, et al: Phase II study of intravenous topotecan as a 5-day infusion for refractory epithelial ovarian carcinoma. J Clin Oncol 1996:14,1552–1557.

TROPHOBLASTIC DISEASE
LOW-RISK
MTX-DACT

Drug	Dose	Route	Day
Methotrexate (MTX)	20 mg	IM	1–5
Dactinomycin	0.5 mg	IV bolus	1–5

Comments:

1. These agents are effective, often alone, in the treatment of low-risk patients.

References:

1. Takamizawa H, Sekiya S, Kobayoshi, et al. Chemotherapy for gestational trophoblastic tumors. Semin Surg Oncol 1987;3:36–44.

TROPHOBLASTIC DISEASE
HIGH-RISK
EMA/CO

Drug	Dose	Route	Day
Etoposide (E)	100 mg/m^2 over 1 hour	IV	1 and 2
Methotrexate (M)	100 mg/m^2 bolus then, 200 mg/m^2 continuous infusion over 12 hours	IV bolus	1
Actinomycin D (A)	0.5 mg bolus	IV	1 and 2

continued

EMA/CO

Drug	Dose	Route	Day
Folinic Acid	15 mg/m^2 every 12 hrs × 4 doses	IM or PO	2
Cyclophosphamide (C)	600 mg/m^2 over 30 to 60 min.	IV	8
Vincristine (O)	1 mg/m^2 bolus (maximum 2 mg)	IV	8

Comments:

1. Patients with persistent elevation in human chorionic gonado-tropin (hCG) levels after evacuation of a hydatiform mole, and others with poor prognostic features, are candidates for this aggressive regimen.

References:

1. Bagshawe KD. High risk metastatic trophoblastic disease. Obstet Gynecol Clin North Amer 1988;15:531–543.

HEAD AND NECK CANCERS

METASTATIC

Pt-FU

Drug	Dose	Route	Day
Cisplatin (Pt)	100 mg/m^2 infusion over 1 hour	IV	1
Fluorouracil (FU)	1,000 mg/m^2/day continuous infusion	IV	1–5

Cycle repeated every 21 days for two cycles.

Comments:

1. This regimen was used as induction therapy in patients with advanced laryngeal cancer, and allows for larynx preservation when followed by radiation. The same chemotherapy is generally applied to a variety of head and neck cancers.

References:

1. Department of Veterans Affairs Laryngeal Cancer Study Group: Induction chemotherapy plus radiation compared with surgery plus radiation in patients with advanced laryngeal cancer. N Engl J Med 1991;324:1685–1690.

HEAD AND NECK CANCERS

METASTATIC

MTX

Drug	Dose	Route	Day
Methotrexate	40 mg/m² bolus	IV, IM	1

Cycle repeated every 7 days for six cycles.

Comments:

1. Single-agent methotrexate offers palliation to some patients. The dose may be escalated in the absence of toxicity.

References:

1. Hong WK, Bromer R: Chemotherapy in head and neck cancer. N Engl J Med 1983;308:75–79.

KAPOSI'S SARCOMA

METASTATIC

Liposomal Daunorubicin

Drug	Dose	Route	Day
Liposomal daunorubicin	40 mg/m² over 30 min	IV	1 and 15

Cycle repeat every 28 days for two cycles, then reevaluate

References:

1. Gill PS, Espina BM, Muggia F, et al. Phase I/II clinical and pharmacokinetic evaluation of liposomal daunorubicin. J Clin Oncol 1995;13:996–1003.
2. Presant CA, Scolaro M, Kennedy P, et al. Liposomal daunorubicin treatment of HIV-associated Kaposi's sarcoma. Lancet 1993;341:1242–1243.

KAPOSI'S SARCOMA

METASTATIC

Liposomal Doxorubicin

Drug	Dose	Route	Day
Liposomal doxorubicin	20 mg/m^2 over 30 min	IV	1

Cycle repeat every 21 days for two cycles, then reevaluate.

References:
1. Harrison M, Tomlinson D, Stewart S. Liposomal entrapped doxorubicin: an active agent in AIDS related Kaposi's Sarcoma. J Clin Oncol 1995;13: 914–920.

Leukemias, Acute

ACUTE LYMPHOBLASTIC LEUKEMIA

ADULTS

Induction Chemotherapy (Linker Regimen)

Drug	Dose	Route	Day
Daunorubicin	50 mg/m² bolus every 24 hours *(30 mg/m² if age > 50 years)	IV	1, 2, 3
Vincristine	2 mg bolus	IV	1, 8, 15, 22
Prednisone	60 mg/m²/day divided into 3 doses	PO	1–28
L-Asparaginase	6000 U/m²	IM	17–28

Comments:

1. Give a fourth dose of daunorubicin at 50 mg/m² for persistent leukemia on day 14.
2. For persistent leukemia on day 28, give daunorubicin 50 mg/m² IV on days 29 and 30; vincristine 2 mg IV days 29 and 36; prednisone 60 mg/m²/day on days 29 to 42; L-Asparaginase 6000 U/m² IM on days 29 to 35.
3. L-Asparaginase is derived from *Escherichia coli:* - if anaphylaxis occurs, switch to L-asparaginase derived from *Erwinia* (note - investigational drug).
4. Monitor fibrinogen and anti-thrombin III (AT III) twice weekly during L-asparaginase therapy. Replace fibrinogen with cryoprecipitate if fibrinogen falls < 100 mg/dL. Consider replacement of antithrombin III if < 50%.
5. Use for lymphoblastic lymphoma with ≥30% bone marrow involvement.

References:

1. Linker CA, Levitt LJ, O'Donnell M, et al. Improved results of treatment of adult acute lymphoblastic leukemia. Blood 1987;69:1242–1248.
2. Linker CA, Levitt LJ, O'Donnell M, et al. Treatment of adult acute lymphoblastic leukemia with intensive cyclical chemotherapy: a follow-up report. Blood 1991;78:2814–2822.

ACUTE LYMPHOBLASTIC LEUKEMIA

ADULTS

Schema for Linker protocol

Consolidation Chemotherapy A (Linker Regimen)

Drug	Dose	Route	Day
Daunorubicin	50 mg/m² bolus every 24 hours	IV	1, 2
Vincristine	2 mg bolus	IV	1, 8
Prednisone	60 mg/m²/day in 3 divided doses	PO	1–14
L-Asparaginase	12000 U/m²	IM	2, 4, 7, 9, 11, 14

Repeat for four cycles

Comments:

1. Repeat as consolidation cycles 1, 3, 5, 7.
2. Central nervous system prophylaxis: 1800 cGy whole brain radiation in 10 fractions over 12 to 14 days and 6 weekly doses of 12 mg methotrexate (intrathecal).

References:

1. Linker CA, Levitt LJ, O'Donnell M, et al. Improved results of treatment of adult acute lymphoblastic leukemia. Blood 1987;69:1242–1248.
2. Linker CA, Levitt LJ, O'Donnell M, et al. Treatment of adult acute lymphoblastic leukemia with intensive cyclical chemotherapy: a follow-up report. Blood 1991;78:2814–2822.

ACUTE LYMPHOBLASTIC LEUKEMIA

ADULTS

Consolidation Chemotherapy B (Linker Regimen)

Drug	Dose	Route	Day
Ara-C	300 mg/m² over 2 hours	IV	1, 4, 8, 11
Teniposide (VM-26)	165 mg/m² over 2 hours (four cycles)	IV	1, 4, 8, 11

Consolidation Chemotherapy C (Linker Regimen)

Drug	Dose	Route	Day
Methotrexate	690 mg/m²/over 42 hours continuous infusion	IV	1–2
Leucovorin	15 mg/m² every 6 hours (one cycle)	PO	2–5

Comments:

1. Repeat Ara-C/teniposide as consolidation cycles 2, 4, 6, 8. (B)
2. Methotrexate/leucovorin once as consolidation cycle 9. (C)
3. Maintenance chemotherapy from end of consolidation treatment to 30 months of continuous complete remission: methotrexate 20 mg/m² PO per week; 6-mercaptopurine 75 mg/m² PO daily (round to nearest 50 mg dose.)

References:

1. Linker CA, Levitt LJ, O'Donnell M, et al. Improved results of treatment of adult acute lymphoblastic leukemia. Blood 1987;69:1242–1248.
2. Linker CA, Levitt LJ, O'Donnell M, et al. Treatment of adult acute lymphoblastic leukemia with intensive cyclical chemotherapy: a follow-up report. Blood 1991;78:2814–2822.

ACUTE LYMPHOBLASTIC LEUKEMIA
ADULTS

Induction Chemotherapy-I (Hoelzer Regimen)

Drug	Dose	Route	Day
Daunorubicin	25 mg/m^2	IV	1, 8, 15, 22
Vincristine	1.5 mg/m^2 (maximum 2 mg)	IV	1, 8, 15, 22
Prednisone	60 mg/m^2	PO	1–28
L-Asparaginase	5000 U/m^2	IM	1–14

Comments:

1. Phase I of induction chemotherapy.
2. L-Asparaginase is derived from *Escherichia coli:* if anaphylaxis occurs, switch to L-asparaginase derived from *Erwinia* (note - investigational drug).
3. Monitor fibrinogen and antithrombin III (AT-III) twice weekly during L-asparaginase therapy. Replace fibrinogen with cryoprecipitate if fibrinogen falls < 100 mg/dL. Consider replacement of AT-III if < 50%.
4. Reduce daunorubicin dose for elevated total bilirubin.

References:

1. Hoelzer D, Thiel E, Loffler H, et al. Intensified therapy in acute lymphoblastic and acute undifferentiated leukemia in adults. Blood 1984;64: 38–47.
2. Hoelzer D, Thiel E, Loffler H, et al. Prognostic factors in a multicenter study for treatment of acute lymphoblastic leukemia in adults. Blood 1988;71:123–131.

ACUTE LYMPHOBLASTIC LEUKEMIA

ADULTS

Induction Chemotherapy-II (Hoelzer Regimen)

Drug	Dose	Route	Day
Cyclophosphamide	650 mg/m^2 (maximum 1,000 mg)	IV	29, 43, 57
Cytarabine (Ara-C)	75 mg/m^2 over 1 hour	IV	31–34, 38–41, 45–48, 52–55
Mercaptopurine	60 mg/m^2 (round to nearest 50 mg)	PO	29–57
Methotrexate	10 mg/m^2 (maximum, 15 mg)	IT	31, 38, 45, 52

Comments:

1. Phase 2 of induction chemotherapy.
2. Central nervous system prophylaxis: 2,400 cGy whole-brain radiation therapy.

References:

1. Hoelzer D, Thiel E, Loffler H, et al. Intensified therapy in acute lymphoblastic and acute undifferentiated leukemia in adults. Blood 1984;64:38–47.
2. Hoelzer D, Thiel E, Loffler H, et al. Prognostic factors in a multicenter study for treatment of acute lymphoblastic leukemia in adults. Blood 1988;71:123–131.

ACUTE LYMPHOBLASTIC LEUKEMIA

ADULTS

Reinduction Chemotherapy-I (Hoelzer Regimen)

Drug	Dose	Route	Day
Dexamethasone	10 mg/m^2	PO	1–28
Vincristine	1.5 mg/m^2 (maximum 2 mg)	IV	1, 8, 15, 22
Doxorubicin	25 mg/m^2	IV	1, 8, 15, 22

Comments:

1. Phase I of reinduction chemotherapy.
2. Reduce doxorubicin dose for elevated total bilirubin.

References:

1. Hoelzer D, Thiel E, Loffler H, et al. Intensified therapy in acute lymphoblastic and acute undifferentiated leukemia in adults. Blood 1984;64:38–47.
2. Hoelzer D, Thiel, Loffler H, et al. Prognostic factors in a multicenter study for treatment of acute lymphoblastic leukemia in adults. Blood 1988;71:123–131.

ACUTE LYMPHOBLASTIC LEUKEMIA

ADULTS

Reinduction Chemotherapy-II (Hoelzer Regimen)

Drug	Dose	Route	Day
Cyclophosphamide	650 mg/m^2 (maximum 1,000 mg)	IV	29
Cytarabine (Ara-C)	75 mg/m^2	IV	31–34, 38–41
Thioguanine	60 mg/m^2 (round to the nearest 40 mg)	PO	29–42

Comments:

1. Phase II of reinduction chemotherapy.
2. Maintenance chemotherapy: 60 mg/m^2/day PO 6-mercaptopurine (round to nearest 50-mg dose) and 20 mg/m^2 PO weekly methotrexate (weeks 10 to 18 and 29 to 130).
3. Round 6-thioguanine to the nearest 40 mg dose.

References:

1. Hoelzer D, Thiel E, Loffler H, et al. Intensified therapy in acute lymphoblastic and acute undifferentiated leukemia in adults. Blood 1984;64: 38–47.
2. Hoelzer D, Thiel E, Loffler H, et al. Prognostic factors in a multicenter study for treatment of acute lymphoblastic leukemia in adults. Blood 1988;71:123–131.

ACUTE LYMPHOBLASTIC LEUKEMIA

ADULTS

SCHEDULE FOR UCSF REGIMEN

Induction Chemotherapy IA (UCSF Regimen)

Drug	Dose	Route	Day
Daunorubicin	60 mg/m^2 bolus	IV	1–3
Vincristine	1.4 mg/m^2 bolus (Maximum 2 mg if ≥40 years old.)	IV	1, 8, 15, 22
Prednisone	60 mg/m^2 (tid, divided doses)	PO	1–28
L-Asparaginase	6,000 U/m^2	IM	17–28
Methotrexate	12 mg	IT	1

Comments:

1. Give a fourth dose of daunorubicin (60 mg/m^2) for persistent leukemia on day 14.
2. Proceed to consolidation IB whether or not patient is in remission on day 28.

3. L-Asparaginase derived from *Escherichia coli:* If anaphylaxis occurs, switch to L-asparaginase derived from *Erwinia* (note - investigational drug).

4. Monitor fibrinogen and antithrombin III (AT-III) twice weekly during L-asparaginase therapy. Replace fibrinogen with cryoprecipitate if fibrinogen falls <100 mg/dL. Consider replacement of AT-III if it falls <50%.

5. Use for lymphoblastic lymphoma with ≥30% bone marrow involvement.

References:
1. Linker CA, Ries CA, Damon LE, Rugo HS. Pilot study of intensified and shortened cyclical chemotherapy for adult acute lymphoblastic leukemia (ALL). Blood 1984;84(Suppl 1):143a.

ACUTE LYMPHOBLASTIC LEUKEMIA

ADULTS

Consolidation Chemotherapy IB (UCSF Regimen)

Drug	Dose	Route	Day
Etoposide (VP-16)	500 mg/m² over 3 hours	IV	1–4
Cytarabine (Ara-C)	2,000 mg/m² over 2 hours	IV	1–4
Methotrexate	12 mg	Intrathecal	Weekly for 5 doses

Comments:

1. Etoposide is mixed in NS at a concentration of 0.6 mg/mL and precedes Ara-C.
2. Chemotherapy fevers are common with this regimen.
3. No cranial radiation is needed as CNS prophylaxis.
4. Dose-adjust Ara-C based on renal function to reduce the risk of CNS toxicity:
 a. Cr 1.5 to 1.9 mg/dl, or rise in Cr 0.5 to 1.1 mg/dl: AraC: 1,000 mg/m²/dose.

b. Cr $\geq$2.0 mg/dL or rise in Cr $\geq$1.2 mg/dL:
Ara-C 100 mg/m^2/day as 24 hour continuous infusion (reference 2).

References:
1. Linker CA, Ries CA, Damon LE, Rugo HS. Pilot study of intensified and shortened cyclical chemotherapy for adult acute lymphoblastic leukemia (ALL). Blood 1984;84(Suppl 1):143a.
2. Smith G, Damon LE, Rugo HS, et al. High-dose cytarabine dose modification reduces the incidence of neurotoxicity in patients with renal insufficiency. J Clin Oncol 1997;15:833–839.

ACUTE LYMPHOBLASTIC LEUKEMIA

ADULTS

Consolidation Chemotherapy IC (UCSF Regimen)

Drug	Dose	Route	Day
Sodium Bicarbonate	1950 mg every 6 hours	PO	1–3, 15–17
Methotrexate	220 mg/m^2 over 15 minutes	IV	1 and 15
Methotrexate	60 mg/m^2/hour over 36 hours (see comment 3 below)	IV	1–2, 15–16
Leucovorin	50 mg/m^2 every 6 hours for 3 doses	IV	2 and 16
Leucovorin	10 mg/m^2 every 6 hours	PO	3–5*, 17–19*
6-Mercaptopurine	90 mg/m^2/day	PO	1–28

* Continue until predicted methotrexate level <0.05 μM.

Comments:

1. Give 150 ml/hour of D5W with 88 mEq/L of sodium bicarbonate IV on days 1 to 3 and 15 to 17.

2. Avoid trimethoprim–sulfamethoxasole, nonsteroidal anti-inflammatory drugs, penicillins, and β-lactam antibiotics during course, as they compete with methotrexate for secretion at the proximal renal tubule.
3. Methotrexate dose based on renal function.

Estimate Cr clearance (mL/min)	Methotrexate Dose (mg/m^2/hour)
>120	80
101–120	70
91–100	60
81–90	55
71–80	50
61–70	45
51–60	40
45–50	30
40–44	25

4. Goal is steady-state serum methotrexate concentration of 20 μM.
5. **A full course of treatment is as follows:**

    IA, IB, IC, IIA, IIB, IIC, IIIC, then maintenance chemotherapy (methotrexate 20 mg/m^2 PO per week; 6-mercaptopurine 90 mg/m^2 PO daily [round to the nearest 50-mg dose]) out to 30 months of continuous complete remission.
6. **Cycle IIA is modified compared to IA as follows:** daunorubicin, no change except no fourth dose; vincristine, days 1, 8, 15; prednisone, day 1 to 21; L-asparaginase, 12,000 U/m^2 day 2, 4, 7, 9, 11, 14; No IT methotrexate. Cycle IIB - No IT methotrexate.
7. Continue *Pneumocystis carinii* prophylaxis until maintenance chemotherapy is completed.

References:
1. Linker CA, Ries CA, Damon LE, Rugo HS. Pilot study of intensified and shortened cyclical chemotherapy for adult acute lymphoblastic leukemia (ALL). Blood 1994;84(Suppl):143a.
2. Hotchkiss BL, Ignoffo RJ. Evaluation of a methotrexate infusion protocol which uses a pharmacokinetic model for dosage modification. Proceedings of the Western States Conference for Pharmacy Residents, Fellows, and Preceptors, February 15, 1994, Monterey, CA.

ACUTE LYMPHOBLASTIC LEUKEMIA

ADULTS (AGE <60 YEARS)

Consolidation (Allogeneic Bone Marrow Transplant)
f TBI-E

Drug	Dose	Route	Day
Total body irradiation (TBI)	120 cGy three times daily	—	−7 to −5
Total body irradiation	120 cGy twice daily	—	−4
Etoposide (E)	60 mg/kg over 4 hours	IV	−3

Comments:

1. HLA-matched related sibling bone marrow infused IV on day zero.
2. Graft-versus-host disease prophylaxis required (cyclosporine, ± corticosteroids, ± methotrexate)
3. Considered standard therapy for young adults with high-risk features and HLA-matched siblings. This treatment has not been proven superior to intensive chemotherapy and may have similar outcomes.

References:
1. Chao NJ, Forman SJ, Schmidt GM, et al. Allogeneic bone marrow transplantation for high-risk acute lymphoblastic leukemia during first complete remission. Blood 1991;78:1923–1927.
2. Chao NJ, Schmidt GM, Niland JL, et al. Cyclosporine, methotrexate, and prednisone compared with cyclosporine and prednisone for prophylaxis of acute graft-versus-host disease. N Engl J Med 1993;329: 1225–1230.

ACUTE MYELOGENOUS LEUKEMIA

ADULTS (ANY AGE)

Induction Chemotherapy (Standard-Dose Ara-C)

Drug	Dose	Route	Day
Ara-C	100–200 mg/m² continuously over 24 hours	IV	1–7
and Daunorubicin	45 mg/m² bolus daily (30 mg/m²/dose if age ≥ 60 years)	IV	1–3 or 8–10
or Mitoxantrone	12 mg/m² bolus daily	IV	1–3
or Idarubicin	13 mg/m² bolus daily	IV	1–3

Comments:

1. For persistent leukemia on day 14, give additional Ara-C for 5 to 7 days and two or three more doses of anthracycline.
2. Reduce dose of anthracycline for elevated total bilirubin.

References:

1. Dillman, RO, Davis RB, Green MR, et al. A comparative study of two different doses of cytarabine for acute myeloid leukemia: a phase III trial of cancer and leukemia group B. Blood 1991;78:2520–2526.
2. Arlin ZA, Case DC, Moore J, et al. Randomized multicenter trial of cytosine arabinoside with mitoxantrone or daunorubicin in previously untreated adult patients with acute nonlymphocytic leukemia (ANLL). Leukemia 1990;4:177–183.
3. Wiernik PH, Banks PLC, Case DC Jr, et al. Cytarabine plus idarubicin or daunorubicin as induction and consolidation therapy for previously untreated adult patients with acute myeloid leukemia. Blood 1992;79: 313–319.

ACUTE MYELOGENOUS LEUKEMIA

ADULTS UNDER AGE 60 YEARS

Induction Chemotherapy (High-Dose Ara-C)

Drug	Dose	Route	Day
Ara-C	2000 mg/m² over 2 hours every 12 hours	IV	1–6
Daunorubicin or	60 mg/m² continous infusion 24 hours	IV	4–6
Ara-C	3000 mg/m² over 1 hour every 12 hours	IV	1–6
Daunorubicin	45 mg/m² bolus every 24 hours	IV	7–9

Comments:

1. For persistent leukemia on day 14, repeat above therapy or consider other therapy.
2. This is not considered standard induction chemotherapy. High-dose Ara-C may result in longer first remissions than standard-dose Ara-C, but this is unproven.
3. Adjust dose of Ara-C based on renal function to reduce the risk of CNS toxicity:
   a. Cr 1.5 to 1.9 mg/dL, or rise in Cr 0.5 to 1.1 mg/dl: Ara-C 1,000 mg/m²/dose
   b. Cr $\geq$ 2.0 mg/dL or rise in Cr $\geq$ 1.2 mg/dL: Ara-C 100 mg/m²/day (reference 3)
4. Adjust dose of daunorubicin based on total bilirubin.

References:

1. Damon LE, Rugo HS, Ries CA, Linker CA. Post-remission cytopenias following intense induction chemotherapy for acute myeloid leukemia. Leukemia 1994;8:535–541.

2. Phillips GL, Shepherd JD, Barnett RA, et al. High-dose cytarabine and daunorubicin induction and post-remission chemotherapy for the treatment of acute myelogenous leukemia in adults. Blood 1991;77:1429–1435.
3. Smith G, Damon L, Rugo H, et al: High-dose cytarabine dose modification reduces the incidence of neurotoxicity in patients with renal insufficiency. J Clin Oncol 1997;15:833–839.

ACUTE MYELOGENOUS LEUKEMIA

ADULTS UNDER AGE 60 YEARS

Consolidation Chemotherapy

Drug	Dose	Route	Day
Ara-C	3000 mg/m² over 3 hours every 12 hours (four cycles)	IV	1, 3, 5
then Ara-C	100 mg/m² every 12 hours	SC	1–5
and Daunorubicin	45 mg/m² bolus (four cycles)	IV	1

Comments:

1. Eight total cycles of consolidation chemotherapy, each 4 to 6 weeks apart.
2. Reduce Ara-C by 20% for marrow recovery from previous cycle > 28 days; Ara-C rash; ≥ 4 loose diarrheal stools/day; a 4-fold or greater rise in serum glutamic oxaloacetic transaminase (SGOT) or alkaline phosphatase; a total bilirubin > 3 mg/dL.
3. To be used after standard-dose ara-C induction chemotherapy.

References:

1. Mayer RJ, Davis RB, Schiffer CA, et al. Intensive post remission chemotherapy in adults with acute myeloid leukemia. N Engl J Med 1994;331:896–903.

ACUTE MYELOGENOUS LEUKEMIA

ADULTS UNDER AGE 60 YEARS

Consolidation Chemotherapy (High Dose Ara-C)

Drug	Dose	Route	Day
Ara-C	3,000 mg/m^2 over 1 hour every 12 hours	IV	1–6
Daunorubicin	30–45 mg/m^2 bolus every 24 hours	IV	7–9

Comments:

1. Two cycles of consolidation chemotherapy.
2. Adjust dose of Ara-C and daunorubicin as described for high-dose induction chemotherapy.
3. High-dose Ara-C-based consolidation chemotherapy is superior to standard-dose Ara-C in this age group (reference 3).

References:

1. Phillips GL, Reese DE, Shepherd JD, et al. High-dose cytarabine and daunorubicin induction and post-remission chemotherapy for the treatment of acute myelogenous leukemia in adults. Blood 1991;77:1429–1435.
2. Wolff SN, Herzig RH, Fay JW, et al. High-dose cytarabine and daunorubicin as consolidation therapy for acute myeloid leukemia in first remission: long-term follow-up and results. J Clin Oncol 1989;7:1260–1267.
3. Mayer RJ, Davis RB, Schiffer CA, et al. Intensive post remission chemotherapy in adults with acute myeloid leukemia. N Engl J Med 1994;331:896–903.

ACUTE MYELOGENOUS LEUKEMIA

ADULTS 60 YEARS OR OLDER

Consolidation Chemotherapy

Drug	Dose	Route	Day
Ara-C	100–200 mg/m^2 continuous over 24 hours	IV	1–5
and Daunorubicin	30–45 mg/m^2 bolus every 24 hours	IV	1, 2
or Mitoxantrone	12 mg/m^2 bolus every 24 hours	IV	1, 2
or Idarubicin	13 mg/m^2 bolus every 24 hours (2 cycles)	IV	1, 2

Comments:

1. Ara-C doses > 200 mg/m^2/day have not been shown to be superior to standard doses of Ara-C in this age group (however, higher doses are more toxic).
2. Adjust anthracycline doses based on total bilirubin.
3. The optimal consolidation treatment in this age group has yet to be defined, as curability in this age group is uncertain.

References:
1. Dillman, RO, Davis RB, Green MR, et al. A comparative study of two different doses of cytarabine for acute myeloid leukemia: a phase III trial of cancer and leukemia group B. Blood 1991;78:2520–2526.
2. Arlin ZA, Case DC, Moore J, Wiernick P, Feldman E, et al. Randomized multicenter trial of cytosine arabinoside with mitoxantrone or daunorubicin in previously untreated adult patients with acute nonlymphocytic leukemia (ANLL). Leukemia 1990;4:177–183.
3. Wiernik PH, Banks PLC, Case DC Jr, Arlin ZA, et al. Cytarabine plus idarubicin or daunorubicin as induction and consolidation therapy for previously untreated adult patients with acute myeloid leukemia. Blood 1992;79:313–319.

ACUTE MYELOGENOUS LEUKEMIA

ADULTS 60 YEARS OR OLDER

Consolidation Chemotherapy

Drug	Dose	Route	Day
Ara-C	100 mg/m² continuously over 24 hours (four cycles)	IV	1–5
then Ara-C	100 mg/m² every 12 hours	SC	1–5
Daunorubicin	45 mg/m² bolus (four cycles)	IV	1

Comments:

1. Ara-C doses > 200 mg/m²/day have not been shown to be superior to standard doses of Ara-C in this age group (however, higher doses are more toxic).
2. Adjust daunorubicin doses based on total bilirubin.
3. The optimal consolidation treatment in this age group has yet to be defined, as curability in this age group is uncertain.
4. Cycles of chemotherapy repeated every 4 to 6 weeks as tolerated.
5. Reduce Ara-C by 20% for: marrow recovery of previous cycle > 28 days; Ara-C rash; ≥4 loose diarrheal stools/day; a 4-fold or greater rise in serum glutamic oxaloacetic transaminase or alkaline phosphatase; a total bilirubin > 3 mg/dL.

References:
1. Mayer RJ, Davis RB, Schiffer CA, et al. Intensive post remission chemotherapy in adults with acute myeloid leukemia. N Engl J Med 1994;331:896–903.

ACUTE MYELOGENOUS LEUKEMIA

ADULTS UNDER AGE 60 YEARS

Consolidation Chemotherapy (Autologous Bone Marrow Transplant) BuVP; BuCy

Drug	Dose	Route	Day
Busulfan	1 mg/kg every 6 hours* (16 total doses)	PO	−7 to −4
Etoposide (VP-16)	60 mg/kg over 10 hours*	IV	−3

Drug	Dose	Route	Day
or Busulfan	1 mg/kg every 6 hours**	PO	−9 to −6
Cyclophosphamide	50 mg/Kg over 1 hour**	IV	−5 to −2

* Based on ideal body weight + (0.25) (actual − ideal body weight).
** Based on ideal body weight.

Comments:

1. Pelvic remission bone marrow (previously purged with 60 to 100 µg/mL of 4-hydroperoxycyclophosphamide [4HC: investigational] for 30 minutes) thawed and infused IV on day zero.
2. This form of consolidation therapy is investigational.
3. Autologous bone marrow transplant is performed once. If the patient receives standard-dose Ara-C induction therapy, an interim high-dose Ara-C-based consolidation cycle is given before transplantation. If the patient receives high-dose Ara-C based induction therapy, proceed straight to transplant.

References:

1. Linker CA, Ries CA, Damon LE, et al. Autologous bone marrow transplantation for acute myeloid leukemia using busulfan plus etoposide as a preparative regimen. Blood 1993;81:311–318.
2. Chao N, Stein AS, Long GD, et al. Busulfan/etoposide-initial experience

with a new preparatory regimen for autologous bone marrow transplantation in patients with acute nonlymphocytic leukemia. Blood 1993;81:319–323.

3. Yeager AM, Kaizer H, Santos GW, et al. Autologous bone marrow transplantation in patients with acute nonlymphocytic leukemia using ex vivo marrow treatment with 4-hydroperoxycyclophosphamide. N Engl J Med 1986;315:141–147.

ACUTE MYELOGENOUS LEUKEMIA
ADULTS UNDER AGE 60 YEARS

Consolidation Chemotherapy (Allogeneic Bone Marrow Transplant) BuCy; CyTBI

Drug	Dose	Route	Day
Busulfan	1 mg/Kg every 6 hours* (16 total doses)	PO	−7 to −4
Cyclophosphamide	60 mg/kg over 1 hour*	IV	−3 to −2

Drug	Dose	Route	Day
or Cyclophosphamide	60 mg/kg over 1 hour*	IV	−5 to −4
Total Body Irradiation	200 cGy twice daily	—	−2 to zero

Drug	Dose	Route	Day
or Cyclophosphamide	60 mg/Kg over 1 hour*	IV	−7 to −6
Total Body Irradiation	200 cGy QD	—	−5 to zero

* Based on ideal body weight

Comments:

1. HLA-matched related sibling bone marrow infused intravenously on day zero. (Note: for total body irradiation schedules, infuse bone marrow after final radiation dose.)

2. Graft-versus-host-disease prophylaxis required (cyclosporine ± methotrexate ± corticosteroids)

3. Considered standard treatment alternative to chemotherapy for young adults with HLA-matched siblings. This treatment has not been proven to be superior to high-dose Ara-C consolidation chemotherapy.

References:

1. Tutschka PJ, Copelan EA, Klein JP. Bone marrow transplantation for leukemia following a new busulfan and cyclophosphamide regimen. Blood 1987;70:1382–1388.

2. Blaise D, Maraninchi D, Archimbaud E, et al. Allogeneic bone marrow transplantation for acute myeloid leukemia in first remission: a randomized trial of a busulfan-cytoxan versus cytoxan-total body irradiation as preparative regimen: a report from the group d'etudes de la greffe de moelle osseuse. Blood 1992;79:2578–2582.

3. Applebaum FR, Dahlberg S, Thomas ED, et al. Bone marrow transplantation or chemotherapy after remission induction for adults with acute nonlymphoblastic leukemia. Ann Int Med 1984;101:581–588.

4. Chao NJ, Schmidt GM, Niland JL, et al. Cyclosporine, methotrexate, and prednisone compared with cyclosporine and prednisone for prophylaxis of acute graft-versus-host disease. N Engl J Med 1993;329:1225–1230.

Leukemias, Chronic

CHRONIC MYELOGENOUS LEUKEMIA

CHRONIC PHASE

IFN or HU

Drug	Dose	Route	Day
α-Interferon (IFN)	9 MU	SC	Daily
or Hydroxyurea (HU)	40 mg/kg*	PO	Daily

* Titrate dose to desired blood counts (typical dose is 1.5 to 2.5 g/day in two divided doses).

Comments:

1. Interferon alfa has been shown to prolong survival in the chronic phase, as compared to hydroxyurea. (alfa-interferon-2a; reference 1)
2. A cytogenetic response (dropout of Philadelphia chromomosome metaphases) to interferon alfa predicts longer survival than lack of a cytogenetic response.
3. Titrate interferon alfa dose to maintain white blood cell count of 2,000 to 4,000/μl.
4. Alpha-interferon decreased to 3 mU TIW in patients without a cytogenetic response at 14 months of therapy, but kept the same (9 MU/m²/day) in patients demonstrating a cytogenetic response (reference 1).

References:

1. The Italian Cooperative Study Group on Chronic Myeloid Leukemia. Interferon alfa-2a as compared with conventional chemotherapy for the treatment of chronic myeloid leukemia. N Engl J Med 1994;330:820–825.
2. Hehlmann R, Heimpel H, Hasford J, et al. Randomized comparison of busulfan and hydroxyurea in chronic myelogenous leukemia: prolongation of survival by hydroxyurea. Blood 1993;82:398–407.
3. Hehlmann R, Heimpel H, Hasford J, et al. Randomized comparison of interferon-a with busulfan and hydroxyurea in chronic myelogenous leukemia. Blood 1994;84:4064–4077.

CHRONIC MYELOGENOUS LEUKEMIA
ACCELERATED PHASE (MYELOID)
HU-Mith

Drug	Dose	Route	Day
Hydroxyurea (HU)	500 mg/day or more*	PO	Daily
Mithramycin (Mith)	25 μg/kg over 2–4 hours	IV	Daily for 3 weeks, then TIW

* Titrate according to white blood cell (WBC) count (see Comment 4 below).

Comments:

1. Responses to this regimen include improvement in blood cell counts and/or reversion to chronic phase.
2. Works only in myeloid accelerated or blast phase.
3. Monitor serum calcium and renal function closely.
4. Hydroxyurea doses based on WBC: WBC $\geq$ 100,000/μl, 4 g/day; WBC 75,000 to 99,999/μl, 3 g/day; WBC 40,000 to 74,999/μl, 2 g/day; WBC 30,000–39,999/μl, 1.5 g/day; WBC 15,000 to 29,999/μl, 1 g/day; WBC 7,5000 to 14,999/μl, 0.5 g/day; WBC < 7,500//μl, none.

References:
1. Koller CA, Miller DM. Preliminary observations on the therapy of the myeloid blast phase of chronic granulocytic leukemia with plicamycin and hydroxyurea. N Engl J Med 1986;315:1433–1438.

CHRONIC MYELOGENOUS LEUKEMIA
ALLOGENEIC BONE MARROW TRANSPLANTATION
BuCy2 or Cy TBI

Drug	Dose	Route	Day
Busulfan	1 mg/kg* every 6 hours (16 total doses)	PO	-7 to -4
Cyclophosphamide	60 mg/kg* over 1 hour	IV	-3 to -2

continued

Drug	Dose	Route	Day
or			
Cyclophosphamide	60 mg/kg over 1 hour	IV	−7 to −6
Total Body Irradiation	200 cGy daily	—	−5 to zero

* Based on ideal body weight.

Comments:

1. Infuse HLA-matched sibling allogeneic bone marrow intravenously on day zero. (Note: infuse bone marrow after final dose of radiation).
2. Graft-versus-host disease prophylaxis required (cyclosporine ± methotrexate ± corticosteroids).

References:

1. Tutschka PJ, Copeland EA, Klein JP. Bone marrow transplantation for leukemia following a new busulphan and cyclophosphamide regimen. Blood 1987;70:1382–1388.
2. Biggs JC, Szer J, Crilley P, et al. Treatment of chronic myeloid leukemia with allogeneic bone marrow transplantation after preparation with BuCy2. Blood 1992;80:1352–1357.
3. Thomas ED, Clift RA, Fefer A, et al. Marrow transplantation for the treatment of chronic myelogenous leukemia. Ann Intern Med 1986;104:155–163.
4. Clift RA, Buckner CD, Appelbaum FR, et al. Allogeneic marrow transplantation in patients with chronic myeloid leukemia in the chronic phase: a randomized trial of two irradiation regimens. Blood 1991;77:1660–1665.

CHRONIC LYMPHOCYTIC LEUKEMIA

Pulse Chlorambucil

Drug	Dose	Route	Day
Chlorambucil	0.1 mg/kg/day	PO	Daily
or Chlorambucil	0.4 mg/kg every 14 days	PO	1
and Prednisone	75 mg/day	PO	1–3

continued

Drug	Dose	Route	Day
or Chlorambucil	1.0 mg/kg every 28 days	PO	1
and Prednisone	100 mg/day	PO	1–7

Comments:

1. The value of prednisone in these regimens is uncertain.

References:

1. Kimby E, Mellstedt H. Chlorambucil/prednisone versus CHOP in symptomatic chronic lymphocytic leukemia of B-cell type. Leuk Lymphoma 1991;5(Suppl):93–96.
2. The French Cooperative Group on Chronic Lymphocytic Leukemia. A randomized trial of chrlorambucil versus COP in stage B chronic lymphocytic leukemia. Blood 1990;75:1422–1425.

CHRONIC LYMPHOCYTIC LEUKEMIA

Fludarabine-CdA

Drug	Dose	Route	Day
Fludarabine	25–30 mg/m^2/day over 30 minutes*	IV	1–5
	or		
Cladribine (CdA)	0.09 mg/kg/day continuously**	IV	1–7

* Cycle repeated every 28 days for six to 12 cycles.
** Cycle repeated every 28 to 35 days for one to nine cycles (median four cycles).

Comments:

1. May initially cause thrombocytopenia. Peripheral neuropathy often complicates fludarabine therapy.
2. Tumor lysis syndrome has been reported during the first cycle of treatment.
3. Fludarabine is the first agent to reliably produce complete remissions in this disease.

References:

1. Chun HG, Leyland-Jones B, Cheson BD. Fludarabine phosphate: a syn-

thetic purine antimetabolite with significant activity against lymphoid malignancies. J Clin Oncol 1991;9:175–188.

2. Keating MJ, Kantarjian H, Talpaz M, et al. Fludarabine: a new agent with major activity against chronic lymphocytic leukemia. Blood 1989;74: 19–25.

3. Keating MJ, Kantarjian H, O'Brien S, et al. Fludarabine: a new agent with marked cytoreductive activity in untreated chronic lymphocytic leukemia. J Clin Oncol 1991;9:44–9.

4. Saven A, Lemon RH, Kosty M, et al. 2-chlorodeoxyadenosine activity in patients with untreated chronic lymphocytic leukemia. J Clin Oncol 1995;13:570–574.

CHRONIC LYMPHOCYTIC LEUKEMIA

CVP-COP

Drug	Dose	Route	Day
(CVP) Cyclophosphamide	300–400 mg/m^2	PO	1–5
Vincristine	1.4 mg/m^2 bolus (maximum 2 mg)	IV	1
Prednisone	100 mg/m^2	PO	1–5
	or		
(COP) Cyclophosphamide	300 mg/m^2	PO	1–5
Vincristine	1 mg/m^2 bolus	IV	1
Prednisone	40 mg/m^2	PO	1–5

Comments:

1. CVP is given every 21 days and COP is given every 28 days.
2. Patients should drink 1.5 to 2 L per day of fluids and void frequently to avoid cyclophosphamide-induced hemorrhagic cystitis.

References:

1. Bagley CM Jr, DeVita VT Jr, Berard CW, et al. Advanced lymphosarcoma: intensive cyclical combination chemotherapy with cyclophosphamide, vincristine, and prednisone. Ann Intern Med 1972;76:227–234.

2. The French Cooperative Group on Chronic Lymphocytic Leukemia. A randomized trial of chlorambucil versus COP in stage B chronic lymphocytic leukemia. Blood 1990;75:1422–1425.

HAIRY CELL LEUKEMIA

2-CdA

Drug	Dose	Route	Day
Cladribine (2-CdA)	0.09 mg/m²/day continuously	IV	1–7

One cycle only.

Comments:

1. One 7-day treatment will result in an 85% complete response rate.
2. Noninfectious fevers are common in the first month after infusion.

References:

1. Piro LD, Carrera CJ, Carson DA, Beutler E. Lasting remissions in hairy-cell leukemia induced by a single infusion of 2-chlorodeoxyadenosine. N Engl J Med 1990;322:1117–1121.
2. Tallman MS, Hakimian D, Variakojis D, et al. A single cycle of 2-chlorodeoxyadenosine results in complete remission in the majority of patients with hairy cell leukemia. Blood 1992;80:2203–2209.
3. Saven A, Piro LD. Treatment of hairy cell leukemia. Blood 1992;79:1111–1120.

HAIRY CELL LEUKEMIA

Interferon alfa

Drug	Dose	Route	Day
interferon alfa (− 2a)	3 μ	SC/IM	Daily (16–24 weeks)
then interferon alfa (− 2a)	3 MU	SC/IM	tiw
or			
interferon alfa (− 2b)	2 MU/m²	SC	tiw

Comments:

1. Treatment is usually for 1 to 1½ years.
2. Relapses routinely occur when interferon alfa is discontinued.

3. There are no clear efficacy differences between the interferon types

References:
1. Jacobs AD, Naiem F, Champlin RC, Golde DW. Toxicity and bone marrow response of patients with hairy cell leukemia treated with biosynthetic (recombinant) alpha-2-interferon. Blut 1985;50:33–34.
2. Ratain MJ, Golomb HM, Vardiman JW, et al. Treatment of hairy cell leukemia with recombinant alpha-2 interferon. Blood 1985;65:644–648.
3. Thompson JA, Fefer A. Interferon in the treatment of hairy cell leukemia. Cancer 1987;59(3 Suppl):605–609.
4. Golomb HM, Ratain MJ, Fefer A, et al. Randomized study of the duration of treatment with interferon alfa-2b in patients with hairy cell leukemia. J Natl Cancer Inst 1988;80:369–373.

HAIRY CELL LEUKEMIA

Pentostatin

Drug	Dose	Route	Day
Pentostatin (2′-deoxycoformycin)	4 mg/m^2 bolus or for 20 to 30 minutes	IV	1
	or		
Pentostatin	5 mg/m^2 bolus or for 2 minutes	IV	1, 2

Cycle repeated every 14 days for six cycles.

Comments:

1. High- vs low-dose prescriptions have not been compared in prospective randomized trials.

References:
1. Cassileth PA, Cheuvart B, Spiers AS, et al. Pentostatin induces durable remissions in hairy cell leukemia. J Clin Oncol 1991;9:243–246.
2. Spiers ASD, Moore D, Cassileth PA, et al. Remissions in hairy cell leukemia with pentostatin (2′-deoxycoformycin). N Engl J Med 1987;316: 825–830.
3. Saven A, Piro LD. Treatment of hairy cell leukemia. Blood 1992;79:1111–1120.

LUNG CANCER, SMALL-CELL
EXTENSIVE

CAV

Drug	Dose	Route	Day
Cyclophosphamide	1,000 mg/m^2 bolus	IV	1
Doxorubicin	40 mg/m^2 bolus	IV	1
Vincristine	1 mg/m^2 bolus (maximum 2 mg)	IV	1

Cycle repeated every 21 days for six cycles.

Comments:

1. This regimen is equivalent to EP. Alternating this chemotherapy and etoposide/cisplatin does not improve outcome.

References:

1. Roth BJ, Johnson DH, Einhorn LH, et al. Randomized study of cyclophosphamide, doxorubicin, and vincristine versus etoposide and cisplatin versus alternation of these two regimens in extensive small-cell lung cancer: a phase III trial of the Southeastern Cancer Study Group. J Clin Oncol 1992;10:282–291.

LUNG CANCER, SMALL-CELL
EXTENSIVE

Pt-E

Drug	Dose	Route	Day
Cisplatin (Pt)	20 mg/m^2/d infusion over 20–60 minutes	IV	1–5
Etoposide (E)	80 mg/m^2 infusion over 60 minutes	IV	1–5

Cycle repeated every 21 days for six cycles.

Comments

1. This regimen is equivalent to cyclophosphamide/doxorubicin/vincristine. Alternating this chemotherapy and CAV does not improve outcome.

References:
1. Roth BJ, Johnson DH, Einhorn LH, et al. Randomized study of cyclophosphamide, doxorubicin, and vincristine versus etoposide and cisplatin versus alternation of these two regimens in extensive small-cell lung cancer: a phase III trial of the Southeastern Cancer Study Group. J Clin Oncol 1992;10:282–291.

LUNG CANCER, NON-SMALL CELL
METASTATIC

CMV

Drug	Dose	Route	Day
Cisplatin (C)	100 mg/m² infusion over 1 hour	IV	1 and 22
Mitomycin C (M)	10 mg/m² bolus	IV	1
Vinblastine (V)	1.2 mg/m² bolus	IV	1 and 2, 22 and 23

Cycle repeated every 42 days for two cycles.

Comments:

1. This is one of a number of equally effective regimens for non-small-cell lung cancer.

References:
1. Weick JK, Crowley J, Natale RB, et al. A randomized trial of five cisplatin-containing treatments in patients with metastatic non-small cell lung cancer: a Southwest Oncology Group study. J Clin Oncol 1991;9:1157–1162.

LUNG CANCER, NON-SMALL-CELL
METASTATIC

Pt-Vbl

Drug	Dose	Route	Day
Cisplatin (Pt)	100 mg/m² infusion over 1 hour	IV	1 and 29
Vinblastine (Vbl)	5 mg/m² bolus	IV	1, 8, 15, 22, 29

Comments:

1. This induction chemotherapy regimen preceding radiation improved survival in patients with Stage III non-small-cell lung cancer.

References:

1. Dillman RO, Seagren SL, Propert KL, et al. A randomized trial of induction chemotherapy plus high-dose radiation versus radiation alone in stage III non-small cell lung cancer. N Engl J Med 1990;940–945.

LUNG CANCER, NON-SMALL-CELL

METASTATIC

Pt-E

Drug	Dose	Route	Day
Cisplatin (Pt)	100 mg/m^2 infusion over 1 hour	IV	1
Etoposide (E)	100 mg/m^2 infusion over 1 hour	IV	1–3

Cycle repeated every 21 to 28 days for two cycles.

Comments:

1. This is one of a number of equally effective regimens for non-small cell cancer.

References:

1. Weick JK, Crowley J, Natale RB, et al. A randomized trial of five cisplatin-containing treatments in patients with metastatic non-small cell lung cancer: a Southwest Oncology Group study. J Clin Oncol 1991;9:1157 1162.

Lymphoproliferative Disorders

HODGKIN'S LYMPHOMA

ABVD

Drug	Dose	Route	Day
Doxorubicin (A)	25 mg/m² bolus	IV	1, 15
Bleomycin (B)	10 U/m² bolus	IV	1, 15
Vinblastine (V)	6 mg/m² bolus	IV	1, 15
Dacarbazine (D)	375 mg/m² bolus	IV	1, 15

Cycle repeated every 28 days for six to eight cycles.

Comments:

1. For patients not in complete remission by five cycles, extend to complete remission plus two cycles. (maximum eight cycles.) For patients not in remission by eight cycles, seek alternate therapy.
2. This regimen generally applies to Ann Arbor Stages IIB-IV.
3. Dose-adjust doxorubicin based on total serum bilirubin.
4. Check cardiac ejection fraction and pulmonary function tests periodically.
5. ABVD is associated with less infertility and fewer secondary leukemias than MOPP, and has better disease-free survival rates.

References:

1. Bonnadonna G, Santoro A, Zucali R, Valagussa P. Improved 5-year survival in advanced Hodgkin's disease by combined modality approach. Cancer Clin Trials 1979;2:217–226.
2. Canellos GP, Anderson JR, Propert KJ, et al. Chemotherapy of advanced Hodgkin's disease with MOPP, ABVD, or MOPP alternating with ABVD. N Engl J Med 1993;327:1478–1484.

HODGKIN'S LYMPHOMA

MOPP/ABV Hybrid

Drug	Dose	Route	Day
Mechlorethamine (M)	6 mg/m^2 bolus	IV	1
Vincristine (O)	1.4 mg/m^2 bolus (no maximum)	IV	1
Procarbazine (P)	100 mg/m^2/day	PO	1–7
Prednisone (P)	40 mg/m^2/day	PO	1–14
Doxorubicin (A)	35 mg/m^2 bolus	IV	8
Bleomycin (B)	10 U/m^2	IV	8
Vinblastine (V)	6 mg/m^2 bolus	IV	8

Comments:

1. Repeat every 28 days for eight cycles.
2. It is not yet known how this regimen compares in efficacy or toxicity to MOPP, ABVD, or MOPP/ABVD.
3. Dose-adjust doxorubicin based on total serum bilirubin.
4. Check cardiac ejection fraction and pulmonary function tests periodically.

References:

1. Klimo P, Connors JM. MOPP/ABV hybrid program: combination chemotherapy based on early induction of seven effective drugs for advanced Hodgkin's disease. J Clin Oncol 1985;3:1174–1182.

HODGKIN'S LYMPHOMA

MOPP/ABVD

Drug	Dose	Route	Day
Mechlorethamine (M)	6 mg/m^2 bolus	IV	1, 8
Vincristine (O)	1.4 mg/m^2 bolus (no maximum)	IV	1, 8
Procarbazine (P)	100 mg/m^2/day	PO	1–14
Prednisone (P)	40 mg/m^2/day	PO	1–14

Comments:

1. Alternate this regimen every 28 days with **ABVD** for a total of six cycles.
2. Because of interactions with procarbazine, avoid alcohol, sympathomimetic drugs, antidepressant drugs, and tyramine-containing foods.
3. This regimen has been shown to be superior to MOPP.

References:

1. Bonnadonna G, Valagussa P, Santoro A. Alternating non-cross-resistant combination chemotherapy or MOPP in stage IV Hodgkin's disease: report of 8-years results. Ann Intern Med 1986;104:739–746.
2. Canellos GP, Anderson JR, Propert KJ, et al. Chemotherapy of advanced Hodgkin's disease with MOPP, ABVD, or MOPP alternating with ABVD. N Engl J Med 1993;327:1478–1484.

HODGKIN'S LYMPHOMA

Stanford V

Drug	Dose	Route	Day
Doxorubicin	25 mg/m^2	IV	1, 15
Vinblastine	6 mg/m^{2*}	IV	1, 15
Mechlorethamine	6 mg/m^2	IV	1
Vincristine	1.4 mg/m2** (maximum dose 2 mg)	IV	8, 22
Bleomycin	5 U/m^2	IV	8, 22
Etoposide	60 mg/m^2	IV	15, 16
Prednisone	40 mg/m^2/day	PO	Daily (weeks 1–9)

* Decrease to 4 mg/m^2 during cycle 3 if ≥50 years of age.
** Decrease to 1 mg/m^2 during cycle 3 if ≥50 years of age.
Repeat every 28 days for three total cycles.

Comments:

1. Failure-free 3-year survival is 87% (Stages II to IV); these are single-institution, unconfirmed results.
2. Prednisone tapered by 10 mg daily starting at week 10.
3. Adjust dose of doxorubicin based on serum total bilirubin.
4. Prophylxis with trimethoprim–sulfamethoxazole (one double-strength tablet daily), acyclovir (200 mg thrice daily), ketoconazole (200 mg daily) and H_2-blockers suggested to prevent *Pneumocystitis carinii, Herpes zoster,* thrush, and gastritis/peptic ulcers (respectively).
5. Radiation therapy to sites of bulky disease is recommended following chemotherapy.

References:

1. Bartlett NL, Rosenberg SA, et al. Brief chemotherapy, Stanford V, and adjuvant radiotherapy for bulky or advanced-stage Hodgkin's disease: a preliminary report. J Clin Oncol 1995;13:1080–1088.

HODGKIN'S LYMPHOMA

EVA (Salvage Regimen)

Drug	Dose	Route	Day
Etoposide (E)	100 mg/m² over 2 hours	IV	1, 2, 3
Vinblastine (V)	6 mg/m² bolus	IV	1
Doxorubicin (A)	50 mg/m² bolus	IV	1

Cycle repeated every 28 days for six cycles.

Comments:

1. Generally, this regimen is used as salvage chemotherapy.
2. Adjust dose of doxorubicin based on total serum bilirubin.
3. Check cardiac ejection fraction periodically.

References:

1. Canellos GP, Anderson JR, Peterson BA, Gottlieb AJ. EVA: etoposide, vinblastine, doxorubicin (Adriamycin) - an effective regimen for the

treatment of Hodgkin's disease in relapse following MOPP. A study of the cancer and leukemia group B. Proc Am Soc Clin Oncol 1991;10:273.

HODGKIN'S LYMPHOMA

B-CAVe (Salvage Regimen)

Drug	Dose	Route	Day
Bleomycin (B)	5 U/m² bolus	IV	1
Lomustine (CCNU)	100 mg/m²	PO	1
Doxorubicin (A)	60 mg/m² bolus	IV	1
Vinblastine (Ve)	5 mg/m² bolus	IV	1

Cycle repeated every 28 days for eight cycles.

Comments:

1. Generally, this is used as salvage chemotherapy.
2. Dose-adjust doxorubicin based on total serum bilirubin.
3. Check cardiac ejection fraction and pulmonary function tests periodically.

References:

1. Harker WG, Kushlan P, Rosenberg SA. Combination chemotherapy for advanced Hodgkin's disease after failure of MOPP: ABVD and B-CAVe. Ann Intern Med 1984;101:440–446.

HODGKIN'S LYMPHOMA

AUTOLOGOUS STEM CELL TRANSPLANTATION

CBV

Drug	Dose	Route	Day
Cyclophosphamide (C)	1.8 g/m²/day over 2 hours	IV	−7, −6, −5, −4
Carmustine (BCNU) (B)	600 mg/m²/day over 2–6 hours	0IV	−3
Etoposide (V)	400 mg/m²/day over 1 hour every 12 hours	IV	−7, −6, −5

Comments:

1. Autologous hematopoietic stem cells infused intravenously on day zero.
2. Chemotherapy doses based on the lesser of ideal or actual body weight.
3. Hyperhydration, mesna, and/or bladder irrigation should be considered to reduce the risk of cyclophosphamide-induced hemorrhagic cystitis.
4. Some investigators have reduced the carmustine dose to 450 mg/m² to decrease the incidence of interstitial pneumonitis.
5. Consider post-transplant radiation therapy to sites of bulky disease.

References:
1. Reece DE, Barnett MJ, Connors JM, et al. Intensive chemotherapy with cyclophosphamide, carmustine, and etoposide followed by autologous bone marrow transplantation for relapsed Hodgkin's disease. J Clin Oncol 1991;9:1871–1879.

NON-HODGKIN'S LYMPHOMA, LOW GRADE

Pulse Chlorambucil

Drug	Dose	Route	Day
Chlorambucil	0.4 mg/kg every 14 days	PO	1
Prednisone	75 mg/day	PO	1–3
or Chlorambucil	1 mg/kg every 28 days	PO	1
± Prednisone	100 mg/day	PO	1–7
or			
Chlorambucil	16 mg/m²/day every 28 days	PO	1–5

Comments:
1. The value of prednisone in this regimen is uncertain.

References:

1. Kimby E, Mellstedt H. Chlorambucil/prednisone versus CHOP in symptomatic chronic lymphocytic leukemia of B-cell type. Leuk Lymphoma 1991;5(suppl):93–96.
2. The French Cooperative Group on Chronic Lymphocytic Leukemia. A randomized trial of chlorambucil versus COP in stage B chronic lymphocytic leukemia. Blood 1990;75:1422–1425.
3. Portlock CS, Fischer DS, Cadman E, et al. High-dose pulse chlorambucil in advanced, low-grade Non-Hodgkin's lymphoma. Cancer Treat Rep 1987;71:1029–1031.

NON-HODGKIN'S LYMPHOMA

LOW GRADE

CVP

Drug	Dose	Route	Day
Cyclophosphamide (C)	300–400 mg/m^2/day	PO	1–5
Vincristine (V)	1.4 mg/m^2 bolus (maximum 2 mg)	IV	1
Prednisone (P)	100 mg/m^2/day	PO	1–5

Cycle repeated every 21 days to maximum response.

Comments:

1. For New Working Formulation classes A–C.

References:

1. Bagley CM Jr, DeVita VT Jr, Berard CW, Canellos GP. Advanced lymphosarcoma: intensive cyclical combination chemotherapy with cyclophosphamide, vincristine, and prednisone. Ann Intern Med 1972;76:227–234.
2. Portlock CS, Rosenberg SA, Glatstein E, Kaplan HS. Treatment of advanced Non-Hodgkin's lymphomas with favorable histologies: preliminary results of a prospective trial. Blood 1976;47:747–756.

NON-HODGKIN'S LYMPHOMA

LOW-GRADE

I-COPA

Drug	Dose	Route	Day
Interferon alfa (-2a) (I)	6 MU/m^2	IM	22–26
Cyclophosphamide (C)	600 mg/m^2	IV	1
Vincristine (O)	1.2 mg/m^2 push (maximum 2 mg)	IV	1
Prednisone (P)	100 mg/m^2/day	PO	1–5
Doxorubicin (A)	50 mg/m^2 bolus	IV	1

Repeat cycles every 28 days for eight to ten cycles.

Comments:

1. Premedicate prior to interferon alfa ($-$2a) with 650 mg acetaminophen PO and then every 4 h for four doses.
2. I-COPA is associated with longer complete responses and possibly improved survival compared to COPA.
3. To be used in New Working Formulation histologic classes B and C.
4. Adjust doxorubicin dose based on serum total bilirubin.

References:

1. Smalley RV, Andersen JW, Hawkins MJ, et al. Interferon alfa combined with cytotoxic chemotherapy per patients with non-Hodgkins lymphoma. N Engl J Med 1992;327:1336–1341.

NON-HODGKIN'S LYMPHOMA

LOW-GRADE

Fludarabine-CdA

Drug	Dose	Route	Day
Fludarabine	25 mg/m²/day over 30 minutes	IV	1–5
or Fludarabine	20 mg/m²/day	IV	1–5
and Cyclophosphamide	600–1,000 mg/m²	IV	1
or Cladribine (2'-chlorode-oxyadenosine)	0.1 mg/m²/day continuously	IV	1–7

Fludarabine cycles: every 28 days;
2'-Chlorodeoxyadenosine cycles: every 35 days.

Comments:

1. Fludarabine may cause thrombocytopenia. Peripheral neuropathy often complicates fludarabine treatment.
2. Due to a high incidence of *Pneumocystis carinii* pneumonia and *Herpes zoster* infections, prophylaxis is recommended against these organisms in the fludarabine/cyclophosphamide combination.
3. Noninfectious fevers are common in the first month after 2-CDA infusion.
4. For use in New Working Formulation Classes A–C.

References:
1. Solol-Celigny P, Brice P, Brousse N, et al. Phase II trial of fludarabine monophosphate (FAMP) as first line treatment in patients (pts) with advanced follicular lymphoma (FL). Blood 1994;84(Supp 1):383a.
2. Hochster H, Oken M, Bennett J, et al. Efficacy of cyclophosphamide (CYC) and fludarabine (FAMP) as first line therapy of low-grade non-Hodgkins lymphoma (NHL) - ECOG 1491. Blood 1994;84(Suppl 1):383a.
3. Kay AC, Saven A, Carrera CJ, et al. 2-chlorodeoxyadenosine treatment of low-grade lymphomas. J Clin Oncol 1992;10:371–377.

NON-HODGKIN'S LYMPHOMA

INTERMEDIATE GRADE

CHOP or CNOP

Drug	Dose	Route	Day
Cyclophosphamide (C)	750 mg/m^2 bolus	IV	1
Doxorubicin (H)	50 mg/m^2 bolus	IV	1
Vincristine (O)	1.4 mg/m^2 bolus (maximum 2 mg)	IV	1
Prednisone (P)	100 mg/day (single daily dose)	PO	1–5
or (CNOP) Mitoxantrone (N) (replaces doxorubicin)	*or* 12 mg/m^2 bolus	IV	1

Cycle repeated every 21 days for six to eight cycles

Comments:

1. Patients in complete remission after four cycles should receive six total cycles of CHOP; patients in complete remission after six cycles should receive eight total cycles of CHOP; patients not in complete remission after six cycles need salvage therapy.
2. Adjust dose of doxorubicin for total serum bilirubin.
3. Check cardiac ejection fraction periodically
4. For use in Working Formulation classes D–H
5. Mitoxantrone can be used to replace doxorubicin in patients >60 years old to reduce cardiac complications.

References:

1. McKelvey EM, Gottlieb JA, Wilson MD, et al. Hydroxyldaunomycin (Adriamycin) combination chemotherapy in malignant lymphoma. Cancer 1976;38:1484–1493.
2. Armitage JO, Fyfe MA, Lewis J. Long-term remission durability and functional status of patients treated for diffuse histiocytic lymphoma with the CHOP regimen. J Clin Oncol 1984;2:898–902.
3. Paulovsky S, Santarelli MT, Erazo A, et al. Results of a randomized study of previously untreated intermediate and high grade lymphoma using CHOP versus CNOP. Ann Oncol 1992;3:205–209.

NON-HODGKIN'S LYMPHOMA
INTERMEDIATE GRADE
MACOP-B

Drug	Dose	Route	Day
Methotrexate (M)	100 mg/m² bolus then 300 mg/m² over 4 hours	IV	8, 36, 64
Leucovorin	15 mg every 6 hours × 6 hours	PO	9, 37, 65
Doxorubicin (A)	50 mg/m² bolus	IV	1, 15, 29, 43, 57, 71
Cyclophosphamide (C)	350 mg/m² bolus	IV	1, 15, 29, 43, 57, 71
Vincristine (O)	1.4 mg/m² bolus (maximum 2 mg)	IV	8, 22, 36, 50, 64, 78
Prednisone (P)	75 mg/day	PO	Daily (12 weeks)
Bleomycin (B)	10 U/m² bolus	IV	22, 50, 78

One 12-week cycle.

Comments:

1. Patients should receive H$_2$-blockers and *Pneumocystis carinii* prophylaxis (trimethoprim–sulfamethoxazole one DS tablet twice daily for 12 weeks)
2. Give CNS prophylaxis if bone marrow, testicles, paranasal sinus, or Waldeyer's ring is involved.
   - Methotrexate 12 mg intrathecal twice weekly (weeks 6 to 8).
   - Ara-C 30 mg intrathecally twice weekly (weeks 6 to 8)
   - Methotrexate + AraC may be given in same syringe.
3. Mucositis is common with this regimen.
4. Periodic check of cardiac ejection fraction and pulmonary function tests are necessary.
5. For use in Working Formulation classes G–H.

References:
1. Klimo P, Connors JM. MACOP-B chemotherapy for the treatment of diffuse large cell lymphoma. Ann Intern Med 1985;102:596–602.

2. Cooper IA, Wolf MM, Robertson TI, et al. Randomized comparison of MACOP-B with CHOP in patients with intermediate-grade non-Hodgkins lymphoma. J Clin Oncol 1994;12:769–778.

NON-HODGKIN'S LYMPHOMA
INTERMEDIATE GRADE
VACOP-B

Drug	Dose	Route	Day
Etoposide (V)	50 mg/m^2	IV	15, 43, 71
Etoposide	100 mg/m^2	PO	16, 17, 44, 45, 72, 73
Doxorubicin (A)	50 mg/m^2 bolus	IV	1, 15, 29, 43, 57, 71
Cyclophosphamide (C)	350 mg/m^2 bolus	IV	1, 29, 57
Vincristine (O)	1.2 mg/m^2 bolus	IV	8, 22, 36, 50, 64, 78
Prednisone (P)	45 mg/m^2/day (round to nearest 25 mg)	PO	Daily × 1 week qod × 11 weeks
Bleomycin (B)	10 U/m^2 bolus	IV	8, 22, 36, 50, 64, 78

Comments:

1. Patients should receive H$_2$-blockers and *Pneumocystis carinii* prophylaxis (trimethoprim–sulfamethoxazole one DS tablet twice daily for 14 weeks) and ketoconazole 200 mg PO daily.
2. Give CNS prophylaxis if bone marrow, testicles, paranasal sinus, or Waldeyer's ring is involved.
   • Methotrexate 12 mg intrathecally twice weekly (weeks 6 to 8).
   or
   • Ara-C 30 mg intrathecal twice weekly (weeks 6 to 8).
3. Periodic check of cardiac ejection fraction and pulmonary function tests are necessary.
4. For use in Working Formulation classes F–H.

References:
1. Connors JM, Hoskins P, Klasa R, et al. VACOP-B: 12 week chemotherapy for advanced stage diffuse large cell lymphoma. Efficacy is sustained and toxicity reduced compared to MACOP-B. Proc Am Soc Clin Oncol 1990;9:254.

NON-HODGKIN'S LYMPHOMA

INTERMEDIATE GRADE

m-BACOD/M-BACOD

Drug	Dose	Route	Day
Methotrexate (m) (M)	200 mg/m² over 4 hours (m) *or* 3000 mg/m² over 4 hours (M)	IV IV	8, 15 *or* 15
Leucovorin	10 mg/m² every 6 hours × 6 doses	PO	9, 16 *or* 16
Bleomycin (B)	4 U/m² bolus	IV	1
Doxorubicin (A)	45 mg/m² bolus	IV	1
Cyclophosphamide (C)	600 mg/m² bolus	IV	1
Vincristine (O)	1 mg/m² bolus	IV	1
Dexamethasone (D)	6 mg/m²/day	PO	1–5

Cycle repeated every 21 days for ten cycles.

Comments:

1. Check cardiac ejection fraction and pulmonary function tests periodically.
2. For use in Working Formulation classes E–H.

References:
1. Shipp MA, Harrington DP, Klatt MM, et al. Identification of major prognostic subgroups of patients with large-cell lymphoma treated with m-BACOD or M-BACOD. Ann Int Med 1986;140:757–765.
2. Skarin AT, Canellos GP, Rosenthal DS, et al. Improved prognosis of diffuse histiocytic and undifferentiated lymphoma by use of high-dose

methotrexate alternating with the standard agent (M-BACOD). J Clin Oncol 1983;1:91–98.

NON-HODGKIN'S LYMPHOMA

INTERMEDIATE GRADE

ProMACE/CytaBOM

Drug	Dose	Route	Day
Cyclophosphamide	650 mg/m^2 over 30 minutes	IV	1
Doxorubicin	25 mg/m^2 bolus	IV	1
Etoposide (VP-16)	120 mg/m^2 over 1 hour	IV	1
Prednisone	60 mg/day	PO	1–14
Cytarabine	300 mg/m^2 bolus	IV	8
Bleomycin	5 U/m^2 bolus	IV	8
Vincristine	1.4 mg/m^2 bolus	IV	8
Methotrexate	120 mg/m^2 bolus	IV	8
Leucovorin	25 mg/m^2 every 6 hours × 4 doses	PO	9

Repeat cycle every 14 days for six to eight cycles.

Comments:

1. For use in Working Formulation classes D–H
2. *Pneumocystis carinii* prophylaxis is suggested.

References:

1. Longo DL, DeVita VT Jr., Duffey PL, et al. Superiority of ProMACE-CytaBOM over ProMACE-MOPP in the treatment of advanced diffuse aggressive lymphoma: results of a prospective randomized trial. J Clin Oncol 1991;9:25–38.

NON-HODGKIN'S LYMPHOMA
LOW AND INTERMEDIATE GRADE

ESHAP (Salvage Regimen)

Drug	Dose	Route	Day
Etoposide (E)	40 mg/m² over 2 hours	IV	1–4
Methylprednisolone (S)	500 mg/day for 15 minutes	IV	1–4
Cytarabine (HA)	2000 mg/m² over 3 hours	IV	5
Cisplatin (P)	25 mg/m²/day continuous over 24 hours	IV	1–4

Repeat Cycle every 28 days for six cycles.

Comments:

1. Primarily used as a salvage regimen for first relapse or primary treatment failures.
2. Monitor electrolytes frequently (K^+, Mg^{++}).
3. Because of high-dose corticosteroids consider *Pneumocystis carinii* prophylaxis.
4. For use in Working Formulation classes A–H.

References:

1. Velasquez WS, McLaughlin P, Tucker S, et al. ESHAP - an effective combination chemotherapy regimen in refractory and relapsing lymphoma: a 4-year follow-up study. J Clin Oncol 1994;12:1169–1176.

NON-HODGKIN'S LYMPHOMA
INTERMEDIATE GRADE

MINE (Salvage Regimen)

Drug	Dose	Route	Day
Ifosfamide (I)	1,330 mg/m² for 1 hour	IV	1–3

continued

MINE (Salvage Regimen)

Drug	Dose	Route	Day
MESNA (M)	1,330 mg/m² over 1 hour in ifosfamide bag, then 266 mg/m² bolus 4 and 8 hours after each ifosfamide dose	IV	1–3
Mitoxantrone (N)	8 mg/m² over 15 minutes	IV	1
Etoposide (E)	65 mg/m²/day over 1 hour	IV	1–3

Repeat cycle every 21 days.

Comments:

1. Primarily used as salvage therapy for first relapse or primary treatment failures.
2. For use in Working Formulation classes E–H.
3. Modify mitoxantrone doses for serum total bilirubin.

References:

1. Cabanillas F, Rodriguez MA, Swan F, Jr. Recent trends in the management of lymphomas at M.D. Anderson Cancer Center. Semin Oncol 1990;17(Suppl 10):28–33.

NON-HODGKIN'S LYMPHOMA

HIV-ASSOCIATED

m-BACOD

Drug	Dose	Route	Day
Methotrexate (m)	200 mg/m² over 2 hours	IV	15
Leucovorin	25 mg every 6 hours × 6	IV/PO	16, 17
Bleomycin (B)	4 mg/m² bolus	IV	1

continued

m-BACOD

Drug	Dose	Route	Day
Doxorubicin (A)	25 mg/m² bolus	IV	1
Cyclophosphamide (C)	300 mg/m² over 30 minutes	IV	1
Vincristine (O)	1.4 mg/m² bolus (2 mg maximum)	IV	1
Dexamethasone (D)	3 mg/m²/day	PO/IV	1–5

Repeat every 21 to 28 days for six to eight cycles.

Comments:

1. Do not use in patients with pleural effusions, ascites, or renal failure.
2. Due to better bone marrow tolerance, this regimen is felt to be superior to standard-dose m-BACOD (cyclophosphamide dose = 600 mg/m² and doxorubicin dose = 45 mg/m²).
3. *Pneumocystis carinii* prophylaxis, fungal prophylaxis, and antiviral therapy should be concurrently administered.
4. Adjust dose of doxorubicin based on serum total bilirubin.
5. Check cardiac ejection fraction and pulmonary function tests periodically.
6. For use in New Working Formulation classes G,H,J.
7. Intrathecal cytarabine 50 mg on days 1, 8, 15, 22 of first cycle.

References:

1. Kaplan L, Straus D, Testa M, et al for the NIAID AIDS Clinical Trials Group. Low-dose compared with standard-dose m-BACOD chemotherapy non-Hodgkins lymphoma associated with human immunodeficiency virus infection. NEJM 1997; 336;1641–8.

NON-HODGKIN'S LYMPHOMA
BURKITT'S/SMALL-CELL NON-CLEAVED/LYMPHOBLASTIC

Magrath Regimen (Cycle 1)

Drug	Dose	Route	Day
Cytarabine	30 mg/m²	IT	1, 2, 3, 7
Cyclophosphamide	1200 mg/m² bolus	IV	1

continued

Magrath Regimen (Cycle 1)

Drug	Dose	Route	Day
Methotrexate	12.5 mg/m^2 (maximum 12.5 mg)	IT	10
Methotrexate	300 mg/m^2/day over 1 hour then 60 mg/m^2/h for 41 hours	IV	10–11
Leucovorin	15 mg/m^2 bolus every 6 hours × 8	IV	Beginning hour 42 of methotrexate

Comments:

1. For use in Working Formulation classes I–J.
2. Determine baseline ejection fraction and reassess periodically.
3. Monitor methotrexate levels at hours 24, 48, and 72 (continue leucovorin until methotrexate level is ≤0.05 μM).

References:

1. Magrath IT, Janus C, Edwards BK, et al. An effective therapy for both undifferentiated (including Burkitt's) lymphomas and lymphoblastic lymphoma in children and young adults. Blood 1984;63:1102–1111.

NON-HODGKIN'S LYMPHOMA

BURKITT'S/SMALL-CELL NON-CLEAVED/LYMPHOBLASTIC

Magrath Regimen (Cycles 2–15)

Drug	Dose	Route	Day
Cytarabine	45 mg/m^2	IT	1, 2 (cycles 2, 3); 1 (cycles 4–6)
Cyclophosphamide	1,200 mg/m^2 bolus	IV	1

continued

Magrath Regimen (Cycles 2–15)

Drug	Dose	Route	Day
Doxorubicin	40 mg/m² bolus	IV	1
Vincristine	1.4 mg/m² bolus (maximum 2 mg)	IV	1
Methotrexate	12.5 mg/m² (maximum 12.5 mg)	IT	3, 10 (cycles 2, 3); 10 (cycles 4–6)
Methotrexate	300 mg/m² over 1 hour then 60 mg/m²/hour over 41 hours	IV	10, 11 (cycles 2–6); 14, 15 (cycles 7–15)
Leucovorin	15 mg/m² bolus every 6 hours × 8	IV	Begin hour 42 of methotrexate
Prednisone	40 mg/m²/day	IV/PO	1–5

Cycles repeated every 28 days for fourteen cycles.

Comments:

1. Begin cycles as soon as granulocytes are > 1500/µl.
2. Adjust dose of doxorubicin based on total serum bilirubin.
3. Monitor methotrexate levels at hours 24, 48, and 72 (continue leucovorin until methotrexate level is ≤ 0.05 µM).

References:

1. Magrath IT, Janus C, Edwards BK, et al. An effective therapy for both undifferentiated (including Burkitt's) lymphomas and lymphoblastic lymphoma in children and young adults. Blood 1984;63:1102–1111.

NON-HODGKIN'S LYMPHOMA

BURKITT'S/SMALL-CELL NON-CLEAVED

Stanford Induction Regimen

Drug	Dose	Route	Day
Cyclophosphamide	1,200 mg/m²	IV	1
Doxorubicin	40 mg/m² bolus	IV	1
Vincristine	1.4 mg/m² bolus (maximum 2 mg)	IV	1
Prednisone	40 mg/m²/day	PO	1–5
Methotrexate	3,000 mg/m² for 6 hours	IV	10 (cycles 1–5)
Leucovorin	25 mg/m² every 6 hours × 12 doses	PO/IV	11–13 (cycles 1–5)
Methotrexate	12 mg/m²	Intra-thecally	1, 10 (cycles 1–5)

Cycle repeated every 28 days for six cycles (Stages A, AR, B) or for eight cycles (Stage C, D).

Comments:

1. Used for Working Formulation classes I–K.
2. Radiation added (125 cGy twice daily for 6 to 9 days) for un-resected abdominal mass ≥ 10 cm (omit cycle 1 doxorubicin if radiation is given during cycle).

References:

1. Bernstein JI, Coleman CN, Strickler JG, et al. Combined modality therapy for adults with small noncleaved cell lymphoma (Burkitt's or non-Burkitt's types). J Clin Oncol 1986;4:847–858.

NON-HODGKIN'S LYMPHOMA

ADULTS AND CHILDREN

BURKITT'S/SMALL-CELL NON-CLEAVED/LYMPHOBLASTIC

Cytoreductive Phase (LMB-86)

Drug	Dose	Route	Day
Cyclophosphamide	300 mg/m²	IV	1
Vincristine	2 mg bolus	IV	1
Prednisone	60 mg/m²/day	PO	1–7
Methotrexate	8 mg, 10 mg, or 12 mg*	IT	1, 3, 5
Cytarabine (Ara-C)	30 mg, 50 mg, or 70 mg*	IT	1, 3, 5
Hydrocortisone	20 mg, 30 mg, or 50 mg*	IT	1, 3, 5

One cycle.

* Based on ages <2 years, 2 to 3 years, or >3 years (respectively).

Comments:

1. Used to reduce tumor bulk and allow metabolic disturbances to flare and correct before beginning intense chemotherapy.
2. Used for New Working Formulation Classes I-J and Burkitt's leukemia (FAB L₃).

References:

1. Soussain C, Patte C, Ostronoff M, et al. Small non-cleaved cell lymphoma and leukemia in adults. A retrospective study of 65 adults treated with the LMB pediatric protocols. Blood 1995;85:664–674.
2. Finlay JL, Trigg ME, Link MP, Frierdich S. Poor-risk non-lymphoblastic lymphoma of childhood: results of an intensive pilot study. Med Pediatr Oncol 1989;17:29–38.

NON-HODGKIN'S LYMPHOMA

ADULTS AND CHILDREN

BURKITT'S/SMALL-CELL NON-CLEAVED/LYMPHOBLASTIC

Induction Regimen I (LMB-86)

Drug	Dose	Route	Day
Cyclophosphamide	500 mg/m^2/day	IV	2–4
Vincristine	2 mg	IV	1
Methotrexate	8,000 mg/m^2 over 4 hours	IV	1
Leucovorin	**		2
Doxorubicin	60 mg/m^2 bolus	IV	2
Prednisone	60 mg/m^2/day	PO	1–7
Methotrexate	8 mg, 10 mg, or 12 mg*	IT	2, 4, 6
Cytarabine (AraC)	30 mg, 50 mg, or 70 mg*	IT	2, 4, 6
Hydrocortisone	20 mg, 30 mg, or 50 mg*	IT	2, 4, 6

* Based on ages <2 years, 2 to 3 years, or >3 years (respectively).
** Leucovorin dose not stated in references 1, 2.

Comments:

1. One cycle only
2. Adjust doxorubicin dose based on serum total bilirubin.

References:

1. Soussain C, Patte C, Ostronoff M, et al. Small-non-cleaved-cell lymphoma and leukemia in adults. A retrospective study of 65 adults treated with the LMB pediatric protocols. Blood 1995;85:664–674.
2. Finlay JL, Trigg ME, Link MP, Frierdich S. Poor-risk non-lymphoblastic lymphoma of childhood: results of an intensive pilot study. Med Pediatr Oncol 1989;17:29–38.

NON-HODGKIN'S LYMPHOMA

ADULTS AND CHILDREN

BURKITT'S/SMALL-CELL NON-CLEAVED/LYMPHOBLASTIC

Induction Regimen II (LMB-86)

Drug	Dose	Route	Day
Cyclophosphamide	1,000 mg/m²	IV	2–4
Vincristine	2 mg bolus	IV	1, 6
Methotrexate	8,000 mg/m² over 4 hours	IV	1
Leucovorin	**		2
Doxorubicin	60 mg/m² bolus	IV	2
Prednisone	60 mg/m²/day	PO	1–7
Methotrexate	8 mg, 10 mg, or 12 mg*	IT	2, 4, 6
Cytarabine (Ara-C)	30 mg, 50 mg, or 70 mg*	IT	2, 4, 6
Hydrocortisone	20 mg, 30 mg, or 50 mg*	IT	2, 4, 6

One cycle.

* Based on ages <2 years, 2 to 3 years, or >3 years (respectively).
** Leucovorin dose not stated in references 1, 2.

Comments:

1. Begin as soon as blood counts recover from induction regimen I.
2. Adjust doxorubicin dose based on serum total bilirubin.

References:

1. Soussain C, Patte C, Ostronoff M, et al. Small non-cleaved cell lymphoma and leukemia in adults. A retrospective study of 65 adults treated with the LMB pediatric protocols. Blood 1995;85:664–674.
2. Finlay JL, Trigg ME, Link MP, Frierdich S. Poor-risk non-lymphoblastic lymphoma of childhood: results of an intensive pilot study. Med Pediatr Oncol 1989;17:29–38.

NON-HODGKIN'S LYMPHOMA

ADULTS AND CHILDREN

BURKITT'S/SMALL-CELL NON-CLEAVED/LYMPHOBLASTIC

Consolidation Regimen (LMB-86)

Drug	Dose	Route	Day
Etoposide (VP-16)	200 mg/m² daily	IV	2–5
Cytarabine (Ara-C)	50 mg/m² over 12 hours (given prior to each high-dose Ara-C)	IV	1–4
Cytarabine (Ara-C)	3000 mg/m² daily	IV	2–5

Two cycles.

Comments:

1. Infusion times for etoposide and high-dose Ara-C not specified in reference 1.

References:
1. Soussain C, Patte C, Ostronoff M, et al. Small non-cleaved cell lymphoma and leukemia in adults. A retrospective study of 65 adults treated with the LMB pediatric protocols. Blood 1995;85:664–674.
2. Finlay JL, Trigg ME, Link MP, Frierdich S. Poor-risk non-lymphoblastic lymphoma of childhood: results of an intensive pilot study. Med Pediatr Oncol 1989;17:29–38.

NON-HODGKIN'S LYMPHOMA

ADULTS AND CHILDREN

BURKITT'S/SMALL-CELL NON-CLEAVED/LYMPHOBLASTIC

Maintenance Regimen (LMB-86)

Drug	Dose	Route	Day
SEQUENCE 1 Vincristine	2 mg bolus	IV	2
Cyclophosphamide	500 mg/m^2	IV	2, 3
Doxorubicin	60 mg/m^2 bolus	IV	3
Methotrexate	8,000 mg/m^2 for 4 hours	IV	1
Leucovorin	*		2
Prednisone	60 mg/m^2/day	PO	1–5
SEQUENCE 2 Etoposide (VP-16)	150 mg/m^2	IV	1–3
Cytarabine (Ara-C)	100 mg/m^2	SC	1–5
SEQUENCE 3 Same as sequence 1 without methotrexate and leucovorin			
SEQUENCE 4 Same as sequence 2.			

Sequences 1 through 4 done once.

* Leucovorin dose not stated in references 1, 2.

Comments:

1. Intrathecal methotrexate/Ara-C/hydrocortisone given on day 2 of sequence 1.
2. CNS radiation given therapeutically for positive spinal fluid or brain/cranial nerve involvement.
3. Prophylaxis for *Pneumocystis carinii* recommended.
4. Adjust doxorubicin dose for serum total bilirubin.

References:

1. Soussain C, Patte C, Ostronoff M, et al. Small non-cleaved cell lymphoma and leukemia in adults. A retrospective study of 65 adults treated with the LMB pediatric protocols. Blood 1995;85:664–674.
2. Finlay JL, Trigg ME, Link MP, Frierdich S. Poor-risk non-lymphoblastic lymphoma of childhood: results of an intensive pilot study. Med Pediatr Oncol 1989;17:29–38.

NON-HODGKIN'S LYMPHOMA

LYMPHOBLASTIC

Induction (Stanford Regimen)

Drug	Dose	Route	Day
Cyclophosphamide	400 mg/m²	PO	1–3, 22–24
Doxorubicin	50 mg/m² bolus	IV	1, 22
Vincristine	2 mg bolus	IV	1, 8, 15, 22, 29, 36
Prednisone	40 mg/m²	PO	1–28, then taper
L-Asparaginase	6,000 U/m²	IM	1, 8, 15, 22, 29
Methotrexate	12 mg	IT	29, 36, 43, 50, 57

Comments:

1. Cranial radiation therapy (2400 cGy in 12 fractions) to begin in fifth week of induction as CNS prophylaxis.
2. L-Asparaginase is derived from *Escherichia coli.* If anaphylaxis occurs, switch to L-asparaginase derived from *Erwinia* (note - investigational drug).
3. Adjust doxorubicin dose based on serum total bilirubin.
4. For lymphoblastic lymphoma Stages I-II, this regimen is appropriate; for Stage III-IV or low stage with adverse features, use acute lymphoblastic leukemia treatment.

References:

1. Coleman CN, Picozzi VJ Jr, Cox RS, et al. Treatment of lymphoblastic lymphoma in adults. J Clin Oncol 1986;4:1628–1637.

NON-HODGKIN'S LYMPHOMA
LYMPHOBLASTIC

Consolidation (Stanford Regimen)

Drug	Dose	Route	Day
Cyclophosphamide	400 mg/m²/day	PO	1–3
Doxorubicin	50 mg/m² bolus	IV	1
Vincristine	2 mg bolus	IV	1
Prednisone	40 mg/m²/day	PO	1–5

Repeat every 21 days for four cycles.

Comments:

1. Adjust doxorubicin dose based on serum total bilirubin.
2. Maintenance chemotherapy given after completing consolidation chemotherapy and ending at 1 year from initiation of induction chemotherapy: methotrexate (30 mg/m² PO weekly) and 6-mercaptopurine (75 mg/m² PO daily; round to nearest 50 mg).

References:
1. Coleman CN, Picozzi VJ Jr, Cox RS, et al. Treatment of lymphoblastic lymphoma in adults. J Clin Oncol 1986;4:1628–1637.

NON-HODGKIN'S LYMPHOMA

INTERMEDIATE - HIGH GRADE

TVC (Autologous Stem Cell Transplant)

Drug	Dose	Route	Day
Thiotepa (T)	325 mg/m²/day over 2 hours	IV	−7, −6
Etoposide (VP-16)	200 mg/m²/day over 2 hours every 12 hours	IV	−7 to −3
Cyclophosphamide (C)	1000 mg/m² day over 1 hour	IV	−7 to −3

Comments:

1. Autologous hematopoietic stem cells infused IV on day zero.
2. Twice-daily showers days -7 to -3 to reduce cutaneous toxicity (high sweat levels of thiotepa and cyclophosphamide)
3. Continuous bladder irrigation (500 mL/hour normal saline) days -7 to -2 or mesna (1,200 mg/m^2 continuous over 24 hours days -7 to -3) with 250 mL/hour NS IV as cyclophosphamide-induced hemorrhagic cystitis prophylaxis.
4. Doses based on body surface area calculated on corrected weight = [kg$_{Ideal}$ + (0.25)(kg$_{Actual}$ $-$ kg$_{Ideal}$)]
5. The optimal conditioning regimen for NHL ABMT is not determined and other alternatives are available.

References:

1. Damon L, Wolf J, Rugo H, et al. Autologous bone marrow transplant (ABMT) for non-Hodgkin's (NHL) and Hodgkin's (HD) lymphoma using a thiotepa-based preparative regimen. Blood 1994;84(Suppl I):706a.

WALDENSTROM'S MACROGLOBULINEMIA

CVP

Drug	Dose	Route	Day
Cyclophosphamide (C)	300–400 mg/m^2/day	PO	1–5
Vincristine (V)	1.4 mg/m^2 bolus (maximum 2 mg)	IV	1
Prednisone (P)	100 mg/m^2/day	PO	1–5

Cycle repeated every 21 days indefinitely.

Comments:

1. Patients should drink 1.5–2 liters per day of fluid and void frequently to avoid cyclophosphamide-induced hemorrhagic cystitis.

References:

1. Dimopoulos MA, Alexanian R. Waldenstrom's macroglobulinemia. Blood 1994;83:1452–9.
2. Portlock CS, Rosenberg SA, Glatstein E, Kaplan HS. Treatment of ad-

vanced Non-Hodgkin's lymphomas with favorable histologies: preliminary results of a prospective trial. Blood 1976;47:747–56.

WALDENSTROM'S MACROGLOBULINEMIA
Chlorambucil - Prednisone

Drug	Dose	Route	Day
Chlorambucil*	8 mg/m²	PO	1
Prednisone*	40 mg/m²/day	PO	1–10

*Cycles repeated every 6 weeks

Comments:

1. Treatment continued (chorambucil/prednisone) until IgM monoclonal protein plateau is established.
2. Adjust chlorambucil dose based on nadir blood counts.

References:
1. Dimopoulos MA, Alexanian R. Waldenstrom's macroglobulinemia. Blood 1994;83:1452–1459.
2. MacKenzie MR, Fudenberg HH. Macroglobulinemia: An analysis for forty patients. Blood 1972;39:874–889.

WALDENSTROM'S MACROGLOBULINEMIA
Fludarabine-CdA

Drug	Dose	Route	Day
Fludarabine	25–30 mg/m² for 30 minutes	IV	1–5
or			
Cladribine (CdA)	0.09 mg/kg/day continuous infusion	IV	1–7

Cycle repeated every 28 days for six to twelve cycles (fludarabine) and every 28 days for two cycles (2-CdA)

Comments:

1. Fluderabine may initially cause thrombocytopenia. Peripheral neuropathy often complicates fludarabine therapy.
2. Not effective agents for multiple myeloma.

References:
1. Kantarjian HM, Alexanian R, Koller CA, et al. Fludarabine therapy in macroglobulinemic lymphoma. Blood 1990;75:1928–1931.
2. Dimopoulos MA, Kantarjian H, Estey E, et al. Treatment of Waldenstrom macroglobulinemia with 2-chlorodeoxyadenosine. Ann Intern Med 1993;118:195–198.

MELANOMA

METASTATIC

DTIC/TAM

Drug	Dose	Route	Day
Dacarbazine (DTIC)	250 mg/m²/day infusion over 15–30 minutes if given centrally or 30 minutes if given peripherally and diluted in 250 mL solution	IV	1–5
Tamoxifen (TAM)	20 mg/m²/day	PO	1–5

Cycle repeated every 21 days for four cycles.

Comments:

1. As in other series, the addition of other agents appears to increase the activity of dacarbazine.
2. Round tamoxifen dose to nearest 10 mg.

References:
1. Cocconi G, Bella M, Calabresi F, et al. Treatment of metastatic malignant melanoma with dacarbazine plus tamoxifen. N Engl J Med 1992;327: 516.

MELANOMA
METASTATIC
Interleukin-2

Drug	Dose	Route	Day
Interleukin-2	100,000 Cetus U/Kg/day	IV	1–5 15–19

Cycle repeated every 28 days for two cycles.

Comments:

1. Although IL-2 is quite toxic and may be given in a variety of schedules, this approach yielded a few durable complete responses.

References:

1. Parkinson DR, Abrams JS, Wiernik PH, et al. Interleukin-2 therapy in patients with metastatic malignant melanoma: a phase II study. J Clin Oncol 1990;8:1650.

MELANOMA
METASTATIC
Pt-DTIC-BCNU-TAM (DARTMOUTH)

Drug	Dose	Route	Day
Cisplatin	25 mg/m^2 infusion over 1 hour	IV	1–3
Dacarbazine	220 mg/m^2/day infusion over 15–30 minutes. Infusion over 15 minutes if given centrally; 30 minutes diluted in 250 mL if given peripherally.	IV	1–3
BCNU	150 mg/m^2 infusion over 1 hour	IV	1
Tamoxifen	10 mg bid	PO	Twice daily

Cycle repeated every 21 days, except BCNU repeated every 42 days.

Comments:

1. This regimen appears to be the most active chemotherapy combination for metastatic melanoma. Deletion of any of the agents, including tamoxifen, seems to reduce response rates.

References:

1. Del Prete SA, Maurer LH, O'Donnell J, et al. Combination chemotherapy with cisplatin, carmustine, dacarbazine, and tamoxifen in metastatic melanoma. Canc Treat Rep 1984;68:1403.

MELANOMA

Adjuvant

IFN

Drug	Dose	Route	Day
Interferon Alfa-2b	20 MIU/m^2	IV	1–5, 8–12, 15–19, 22–26
Interferon Alfa-2b	10 MIU/m^2	SC	TIW × 48 weeks

Comments:

1. This study demonstrated an increased median overall survival (3.8 vs 2.8 years) compared to observation.

Reference:

1. Kirkwood JM, Strawderman MH, Ernstaff MS, Smith TJ, Borden EC, and Blum RH. Interferon Alfa-2b adjuvant therapy of high-risk resected cutaneous melanoma: the Eastern Cooperative Oncology Group Trial EST 1684. J Clin Oncol 1996; 14:7–17.

MELANOMA

METASTATIC

IFN-DTIC

Drug	Dose	Route	Day
Interferon alfa-2B induction	15 MU/m^2/day	IV	1–5, 8–12, 15–19

continued

IFN-DTIC

Drug	Dose	Route	Day
Interferon alfa-2B	10 MU/m²	SC	Starting after induction interferon
Dacarbazine	200 mg/m²/day	IV	22–26

[Cycle repeated q 28 days] for 2 cycles
Interferon given three times weekly, dacarbazine repeated every 28 days for two cycles, then reassess.

Comments:

1. This study demonstrated the superiority of the combination of these two agents compared to dacarbazine alone.

References:
1. Falkson CI, Falkson G, Falkson HC. Improved results with the addition of Interferon alfa-2B to Dacarbazine in the treatment of patients with metastatic malignant melanoma. J Clin Oncol 1991;9:1403–1408.

MULTIPLE MYELOMA

M-P

Drug	Dose	Route	Day
Melphalan (M)	0.25 mg/kg/day	PO	1–4
Prednisone (P)	100 mg/day	PO	1–4
or Melphalan	9 mg/m²/day	PO	1–4
Prednisone	100 mg/day	PO	1–4

Cycle repeated every 4 to 6 weeks for at least twelve cycles.

Comments:

1. Titrate melphalan dose based on nadir blood counts.
2. Some oncologists advocate α-interferon maintenance (3 MU/m² SC thrice weekly) following the plateau response to melphalan and prednisone. This prolongs chemotherapy-free remission time and overall survival in patients responsive to M and P (reference 3).
3. Some oncologists give prednisone at a dose of 2 mg/kg/day (days 1 through 4); see reference 1.

References:

1. Alexanian R, Hart A, Khan A. Treatment for multiple myeloma. Combination chemotherapy with different melphalan dose regimens. JAMA 1969;208:1680–1685.
2. Belch A, Shelley W, Bergsagel D, et al. A randomized trial of maintenance versus no maintenance melphalan and prednisone in responding multiple myeloma patients. Br J Cancer 1988;57:94–9.
3. Mandelli F, Avvisati G, Amadari S, et al. Maintenance treatment with recombinant interferon alfa-2b in patients with multiple myeloma responding to conventional induction chemotherapy. N Engl J Med 1990;322:1430–1434.

MULTIPLE MYELOMA

VAD

Drug	Dose	Route	Day
Vincristine	0.4 mg/day continuously over 24 hours	IV	1–4
Doxorubicin	9 mg/m²/day continuously over 24 hours	IV	1–4
Dexamethasone	40 mg/day	PO	1–4, 9–12, 17–20

Cycle repeated every 28 days for an indefinite number of cycles.

Comments:

1. Most commonly used salvage regimen.
2. Produces a rapid catabolism of the monoclonal protein.
3. Because of the intense corticosteroid usage, patients should receive H$_2$-blockers and *Pneumocystis carinii* prophylaxis.
4. Infusional vincristine and doxorubicin must be administered through a central venous line due to their vesicant properties.

References:

1. Barlogie B, Smith L, Alexanian R. Effective treatment of advanced multiple myeloma refractory to alkylating agents. N Engl J Med 1984;310:1353–1356.

MULTIPLE MYELOMA

MP - alpha-interferon

Drug	Dose	Route	Day
Melphalan (M)	0.25 mg/kg/day	PO	1–4
Prednisone (P)	2 mg/kg/day	PO	1–4
Interferon-alfa	7 MU/m^2/day	SC	1–5 and 22–26

Cycle repeated every 42 days indefinitely.

Comments:

1. Interferon alfa used in this study was natural (leukocyte-derived).
2. When patients reached response criteria, melphalan and prednisone were continued as above, and the interferon-alfa dose was dropped to 3 MU thrice weekly.

References:

1. Osterborg A, Bjorkholm M, Bjoreman M, et al. Natural interferon-α in combination with melphalan/prednisone versus melphalan/prednisone in the treatment of multiple myeloma stages II and III: a randomized study from the Myeloma Group of Central Sweden. Blood 1993;81:1428–1434.

MULTIPLE MYELOMA

VCAP or VBAP

Drug	Dose	Route	Day
Vincristine (V)	1 mg/m^2 bolus (maximum 1.5 mg)	IV	1
Doxorubicin (A)	30 mg/m^2 bolus	IV	1
Prednisone (P)	60 mg/m^2/day	PO	1–4
Cyclophosphamide (C) [VCAP]	125 mg/m^2/day	PO	1–4
or Carmustine (BCNU) [VBAP]	30 mg/m^2 for 1 hour	IV	1

Comments:

1. Adjust dose of doxorubicin based on total serum bilirubin.

References:
1. Salmon SE, Haut A, Bonnet JD, et al. Alternating combination chemotherapy and levamisole improves survival in multiple myeloma: a Southwest Oncology Group study. J Clin Oncol 1983;1:453–461.

MULTIPLE MYELOMA

VMCP

Drug	Dose	Route	Day
Vincristine (V)	1 mg/m^2/day bolus (maximum 1.5 mg)	IV	1
Melphalan (M)	6 mg/m^2/day	PO	1–4
Cyclophosphamide (C)	125 mg/m^2/day	PO	1–4
Prednisone (P)	60 mg/m^2/day	PO	1–4

Cycle repeated every 21 days.

Comments:

1. This regimen (VMCP) is alternated every 21 days with VCAP for 6 to 12 months; or repeated every 21 days for three total cycles, followed by three cycles of VBAP, then VMCP-VBAP is repeated again.

References:
1. Salmon SE, Haut A, Bonnet JD, et al. Alternating combination chemotherapy and levamisole improves survival in multiple myeloma: a Southwest Oncology Group study. J Clin Oncol 1983;1:453–461.

NEUROENDOCRINE TUMOR

METASTATIC

Pt-E

Drug	Dose	Route	Day
Etoposide (E)	130 mg/m²/day infusion over 1 hour	IV	1–3
Cisplatin (Pt)	45 mg/m²/day infusion over 1 hour	IV	2 and 3

Cycle repeated every 28 days for two cycles and assess response.

Comments:

1. This regimen is active in patients with anaplastic neuroendocrine tumors. Patients with well-differentiated neuroendocrine (islet cell) tumors should be treated with streptozocin–doxorubicin.

References:

1. Moertel CG, Kvols LK, O'Connell MJ, et al: Treatment of neuroendocrine carcinomas with combined etoposide and cisplatin. Cancer 1991;68:227.

PANCREATIC ADENOCARCINOMA

ADVANCED

Drug	Dose	Route	Day
Gemcitabine	1,000 mg/m^2 over 30 minutes	IV	1,8,15,22, 29,36,43, then start again on 57, three weeks on, 1 week off

Comments:

1. When compared to 5-fluorouracil, gemcitabine conferred an improvement in quality of life and survival.

References:
1. Moore M, Anderson J, Burris H, et al. A randomized trial of gemcitabine versus 5-fluorouracil as first-line therapy in advanced pancreatic cancer. Proc Am Soc Clin Oncol 1995;14:473.

PANCREATIC ISLET CELL CARCINOMA

METASTATIC

Streptozocin/Doxorubicin

Drug	Dose	Route	Day
Streptozocin	500 mg/m^2/day infusion over 30–60 minutes	IV	1–5
Doxorubicin	50 mg/m^2 bolus	IV	1 and 22

Cycle repeated every 42 days for two cycles.

Comments:

1. This appears to be the most effective regimen for differentiated islet-cell carcinoma. Its emetogenicity is minimized with current antiemetics.

References:
1. Moertel CG, Lefkopoulo M, Lipsitz S, et al: Streptozocin-doxorubicin, streptozocin-fluorouracil, or chlorozotocin in the treatment of advanced islet-cell carcinoma. N Engl J Med 1992;326:519.

SARCOMAS SOFT TISSUE
METASTATIC
MAID

Drug	Dose	Route	Day
Mesna (M)	2,500 mg/m²/day continuous infusion	IV	1–4
Doxorubicin (A)	20 mg/m²/day continuous infusion	IV	1–3
Ifosfamide (I)	2,500 mg/m²/day continuous infusion	IV	1–3
Dacarbazine (D)	300 mg/m²/day continuous infusion	IV	1–3

Cycle repeated every 21 days for two cycles, then reassess.

Comments:

1. While this is the most popular sarcoma regimen, it is quite toxic and the deletion of darcarbazine probably does not diminish its efficacy. Mesna may be given on a bolus schedule rather than by the infusional route.
2. Mesna may be admixed with ifosfamide. Doxorubicin may be admixed with dacarbazine.

References:
1. Elias A, Ryan L, Sulkes A, et al. Response to mesna, doxorubicin, ifosfamide and dacarbazine in 108 patients with metastatic or unresectable sarcoma and no prior chemotherapy. J Clin Oncol 1989;7:1208.

SARCOMAS, SOFT TISSUE

METASTATIC

CYVADIC

Drug	Dose	Route	Day
Cyclophosphamide (CY)	500 mg/m² bolus	IV	1
Vincristine (V)	1.5 mg/m² bolus	IV	1
Doxorubicin (A)	50 mg/m² bolus	IV	1
Dacarbazine (DIC)	250 mg/m²/day infusion over 15–30 minutes	IV	1–5

Cycle repeated every 28 days for two cycles, then reassess and stop if it isn't working.

Comments:

1. This regimen leads to some complete responses but, as with other sarcoma protocols, no survival advantage has been clearly demonstrated.

References:
1. Pinedo HM, Bramwell VHC, Morridsen HT, et al. CYVADIC in advanced soft tissue sarcoma: a randomized study comparing two schedules. Cancer 1984;53:1825.

CHAPTER IV

Chemotherapy Regimens in Pediatric Tumors

Bruce Shiramizu

Ken DeSantes

PEDIATRIC MALIGNANCIES

General Comments

The majority of children diagnosed with malignancies are treated at Institutions participating in cooperative-group regimens. Therefore, chemotherapy dosages and schedules will vary. The following tables are not inclusive, but include guidelines for the common drugs used in most standardized regimens.

PEDIATRIC EWING'S SARCOMA/PRIMITIVE
NEUROECTODERMAL TUMOR (PNET)

VCR-Doxo-CY-Ifos-Mesna-E

Drug	Dose	Route	Day
Vincristine	2 mg/m^2 bolus (maximum dose = 2mg)	IV	1,8,15,43
Doxorubicin	30 mg/m^2/day over 24 hours	IV	1–3,43–45
Cyclophosphamide	2.2 g/m^2 over 30 minutes	IV	1,43
Ifosfamide	1,800 mg/m^2/day over 1 hour	IV	22–26,63–67
Mesna	360 mg/m^2 over 15 minutes for 5 doses every 3 hours	IV	Given with cyclophosphamide and ifosfamide
Etoposide	100 mg/m^2 over 1 hour	IV	22–26,63–67

6–10 cycles, depending on stage and response.

Comments:

1. Following completion of chemotherapy, evaluation of the tumor site(s) is made to determine the extent of local control (radiation therapy, surgery), followed by additional chemotherapy

References:
1. Meyer WH, Kun L, Marina N, et al. Ifosfamide plus etoposide in newly diagnosed Ewing's sarcoma of bone. J Clin Oncol 1992;10:1737–42.
2. Bergert EO, Nesbit ME, Garnsey LA, et al. Multimodal therapy for the management of nonpelvic, localized Ewing's sarcoma of bone: intergroup study IESS-II. J Clin Oncol 1990;8:1514–24.

EWING'S SARCOMA AND PRIMITIVE NEUROECTODERMAL TUMOR (PNET)

PEDIATRIC AUTOLOGOUS BONE MARROW TRANSPLANTATION

TBI-Melph-VP-16

Drug	Dose	Route	Day
Total Body Irradiation	150 cGy twice daily	—	$-7, -6, -5, -4$
Melphalan	45 mg/m^2/day for 30 minutes	IV	$-7, -6, -5, -4$
Etoposide	60 mg/kg for 4 hours	IV	-3

General Comments:

1. The role of high-dose chemoradiotherapy with hematopoietic stem-cell rescue to treat Ewing's sarcoma/PNET has not been clearly defined. Patients presenting with multifocal disease or distant bone marrow metastases, or those who relapse within 2 years of diagnosis may benefit from this approach.
2. The optimal conditioning regimen for Ewing's sarcoma/PNET has not been determined. Most patients have been treated on protocols that include melphalan and/or TBI, but other drugs have also been utilized (e.g., carboplatin, busulfan).
3. Autologous stem cells are infused on day zero.

Drug Information:

1. It is essential to maintain adequate urine output prior to and for 24 hours after melphalan infusion to reduce bladder irritation. This may be accomplished with hyperhydration and use of furosemide.
2. Etoposide is administered undiluted and piggybacked in free-flowing normal saline over a period of 4 hours. Children should be bathed frequently to minimize cutaneous toxicity. Some patients experience intense pruritus during the etoposide infusion which often responds to diphenhydramine (or ranitidine) and intravenous hydrocortisone.

Reference:
Burdach S, Jurgens H, Peters C, et al. Myeloablative radiochemotherapy and hematopoietic stem-cell rescue in poor-prognosis Ewing's sarcoma. J Clin Oncol 1993;11(8):1482–1488.

PEDIATRIC ACUTE LYMPHOBLASTIC LEUKEMIA (ALL)

Induction Chemotherapy (Days 1-30)

Drug	Dose	Route	Day
Vincristine	1.5 mg/m² bolus (maximum dose = 2 mg)	IV	1,8,15,22
L-Asparaginase	6,000 IU/m²	IM	3 times per week (9 doses)
Prednisone	60 mg/m² (divided doses thrice daily)	PO	1–28, then taper
Daunorubicin	25 mg/m² over 15 minutes	IV	1,8,15,22
Methotrexate	See comments	IT	15,28
Cytarabine	See comments	IT	1

Comments:

1. Doses of intrathecal (IT) medications are based on age: Methotrexate 6 mg (≤1 year); 8 mg (1 to 2 years); 10 mg (2 to 3 years); 12 mg (≥3 years). Patients with CNS disease at diagnosis received additional IT methotrexate on D8,22. Cytarabine 20 mg (0 to 1 year); 30 mg (1 to 2 years); 50 mg (2 to 3 years); 70 mg (≥3 years).

2. If the bone marrow on day 28 shows remission, patients continue on with the next phase of chemotherapy. If the day-28 bone marrow shows residual disease, consider other therapy.

References:

1. Gaynon, P.S., Steinherz, P.G., Bleyer, W.A., et al. Chappell R.J., Sather H.N., Hammond D.G. Improved therapy for children with acute lymphoblastic leukemia and unfavourable presenting features: A follow-up report of the Children's Cancer Group Study CCG-106. J Clin Oncol 1993;11:2234–2242.

2. Pullen J, Boyett J, Shuster J, et al. Extended triple intrathecal chemotherapy trial for prevention of CNS relapse in good-risk and poor-risk patients with B-progenitor acute lymphoblastic leukemia, Pediatric Oncology Group study. J Clin Oncol 1993;11:839–849.

3. Land, V.J., Shuster, J.J., Crist, W.M., et al. Comparison of two schedules of intermediate-dose methotrexate and cytarabine consolidation therapy for childhood B-precursor cell acute lymphoblastic leukemia: a Pediatric Oncology Group study. J Clin Oncol 1994;12:1939–1945.

PEDIATRIC ACUTE LYMPHOBLASTIC LEUKEMIA

Consolidation/Maintenance Chemotherapy

Drug	Dose	Route	Day
Cyclophosphamide	1,000 mg/m^2 for 30 minutes	IV	1,15,122
L-Asparaginase	6,000 U/m^2	IM	Three times/week from day 97–122
Cytarabine	75 mg/m^2/day for 15 minutes	IV/SC	Four consecutive days starting day 2,9,16,23, 123,130
Doxorubicin	25 mg/m^2 over 15 minutes	IV	94,101,108

continued

Consolidation/Maintenance Chemotherapy

Drug	Dose	Route	Day
Mercaptopurine	60 mg/m²/day	PO	1–93, 143 to end of therapy
Methotrexate	20 mg/m²	PO	Weekly day 36–72, 143 to end of therapy
Prednisone	40 mg/m²/day in divided doses thrice daily	PO	Five consecutive days per month starting day 143 to end of therapy
Thioguanine	60 mg/m²/day	PO	122–135
Vincristine	1.5 mg/m² bolus (maximum dose = 2mg)	IV	94,101,108, then monthly starting day 143 to end of therapy
Methotrexate	See comments	IT	1,8,15,22, 123,130, then every 3 months starting day 143

Comments:

1. Doses of intrathecal (IT) medications are based on age: Methotrexate 6 mg (≤1 year); 8 mg (1 to 2 years); 10 mg (2 to 3 years); 12 mg (≥3 year).
2. End of therapy is 2 years from day 36.
3. Craniospinal irradiation may be indicated for patients with persistent CNS disease.

References:

1. Gaynon, P.S., Steinherz, P.G., Bleyer, W.A., et al. Chappell R.J., Sather H.N., Hammond D.G. Improved therapy for children with acute lymphoblastic leukemia and unfavourable presenting features: A follow-up report of the Children's Cancer Group Study CCG-106. J Clin Oncol 1993;11:2234–2242.

2. Pullen J, Boyett J, Shuster J, et al. Extended triple intrathecal chemotherapy trial for prevention of CNS relapse in good-risk and poor-risk patients with B-progenitor acute lymphoblastic leukemia, Pediatric Oncology Group study. J Clin Oncol 1993;11:839–849.

3. Land, V.J., Shuster, J.J., Crist, W.M., et al. Comparison of two schedules of intermediate-dose methotrexate and cytarabine consolidation therapy for childhood B-precursor cell acute lymphoblastic leukemia: a Pediatric Oncology Group study. J Clin Oncol 1994;12:1939–1945.

PEDIATRIC ACUTE LYMPHOBLASTIC LEUKEMIA (ALL)

ALLOGENEIC BONE MARROW TRANSPLANTATION

TB1-CY-VP-16

Drug	Dose	Route	Day
Cyclophosphamide (CY)	60 mg/kg/day for 1 hour	IV	$-8, -7$
Etoposide (VP-16)	900 mg/m²/day for 24 hours	IVCI	$-6, -5$
Total Body Irradiation (TBI)	200 cGy twice daily	-	$-3, -2, -1$
GVHD Prophylaxis			
Cyclosporine	1.5 mg/kg every 12 hours	IV	-1 to $+50$
Methotrexate	15 mg/m²	IV	$+1$
Methotrexate	10 mg/m²/day	IV	$+3, +6, +11$

General Comments:

1. Children with ALL are usually considered candidates for allogeneic bone marrow transplantation (BMT) if they experience a

bone marrow relapse during or shortly after discontinuing chemotherapy (i.e., within 6 to 12 months).

2. Certain patients with high risk ALL are considered for BMT in first complete remission (e.g., patients with t(9;22), infants with t(4;11)).

3. The optimal conditioning regimen for children with ALL has not been determined. Most centers utilize TBI with cyclophosphamide, etoposide, and Ara-C either alone or in various combinations. Busulfan has been used by some institutions in lieu of TBI.

4. Allogeneic bone marrow is infused on day zero.

Drug Information

1. Hyperhydration and/or mesna is utilized to minimize the risk of hemorrhagic cystitis associated with cyclophosphamide use. Furosemide or mannitol may also be administered to maintain a brisk diuresis.

2. Etoposide is generally administered as a continuous infusion over 4 to 48 hours. The concentration should *not* exceed 0.4 mg/ml for prolonged infusions. Children should be bathed frequently to minimize cutaneous toxicity. Some patients experience intense pruritus during the etoposide infusion, which often responds to diphenhydramine (or ranitidine) and IV hydrocortisone.

3. Cyclosporine may be changed to an oral dose of 6 mg/kg twice daily as tolerated. After day +50 the drug is tapered by 5% per week. Adjust dose for renal insufficiency.

References:

1. Cole CH, Pritchard S, Rogers PCJ, et al. Intensive conditioning regimen for bone marrow transplantation in children with high-risk haematological malignancies. Med Pediatr Oncol 1994;23:464–469.

2. Dopfer R, Henze G, Bender-Gotze C, et al. Allogeneic bone marrow transplantation for childhood acute lymphoblastic leukemia in second remission after intensive primary and relapse therapy according to the BFM- and CoALL-protocols: Results of the German Cooperative Group. Blood 1991;78:2780–2784.

3. Bordigoni P, Vernant JP, Souillet G, et al. Allogeneic bone marrow transplantation for children with acute lymphoblastic leukemia in first remis-

sion: A cooperative study of the Group d'Etude de la Greffe de Moelle Osseuse. J Clin Oncol 1989;7:747–753.

PEDIATRIC ACUTE MYELOID LEUKEMIA

Induction Chemotherapy

Drug	Dose	Route	Day
Daunorubicin	20 mg/m²/day over 24 hours	IV	1–4, 10–13
Cytarabine	200 mg/m²/day over 24 hours	IV	1–4, 10–13
Thioguanine	100 mg/m²/day over in divided doses twice daily	PO	1–4, 10–13
Etoposide	100 mg/m² for 24 hours	IV	1–4, 10–13
Dexamethasone	6 mg/m² divided doses thrice daily	IV/PO	1–4, 10–13
Cytarabine	See comments	IT	1

Comments:

1. Doses of intrathecal (IT) medications are based on age: Cytarabine 20 mg (0 to 1 year); 30 mg (1 to 2 years); 50 mg (2 to 3 years); 70 mg (≥3 years).
2. Cycle is repeated on day 28.

References:

1. Nesbit, M.E., Buckley, J.D., Feig, S.A., et al. Chemotherapy for induction of remission of childhood acute myeloid leukemia followed by marrow transplantation or multiagent chemotherapy: a report from the Children's Cancer Group. J Clin Oncol 1994;12:127–135.
2. Wells, R.J., Woods, W.G., Buckley, J.D., et al. Treatment of newly diagnosed children and adolescents with acute myeloid leukemia: a Children's Cancer Group study. J Clin Oncol 1994;12:2367–2377.
3. Ravindranath Y, Steuber P, Krischer J, et al. High-dose cytarabine for intensification of early therapy of childhood acute myeloid leukemias: A Pediatric Oncology Group study. J Clin Oncol 1991;9:572–580.

PEDIATRIC ACUTE MYELOID LEUKEMIA

Consolidation/Maintenance Chemotherapy

Drug	Dose	Route	Day
Cytarabine	3,000 mg/m² over 3 hours every 12 hours	IV	Every 12 hours, days 1–2, 8–9
L-Asparaginase	6,000 IU/m²; 3 hours after cytarabine	IM	2,9
Vincristine	1.5 mg/m² bolus (maximum dose = 2 mg)	IV	28, 56
Thioguanine	75 mg/m²/day	PO	28–84
Cytarabine	75 mg/m²/day over 15 minutes	IV	28–31, 56–59
Cyclophosphamide	75 mg/m²/day over 30 minutes	IV	28–31, 56–59
Cytarabine	25 mg/m²/day bolus	SC/IV	89–93
Thioguanine	50 mg/m²/day	PO	89–93
Etoposide	100 mg/m² for 1 hour	IV	89, 92
Dexamethasone	2 mg/m²/day	PO	89–92
Daunorubicin	30 mg/m² over 15 minutes	IV	89
Cytarabine	See comments	IT	1, 28, 56

Comments:

1. During high-dose cytarabine administration, dexamethasone eye drops 0.1% are administered in each eye every 2 hours until 6 hours after infusion of cytarabine.
2. Doses of intrathecal (IT) medications are based on age: Cytarabine 20 mg (0 to 1 year); 30 mg (1 to 2 years); 50 mg (2 to 3 years); 70 mg (≥3 years).

References:

1. Nesbit, M.E., Buckley, J.D., Feig, S.A., et al. Chemotherapy for induction of remission of childhood acute myeloid leukemia followed by marrow transplantation or multiagent chemotherapy: a report from the Children's Cancer Group. J Clin Oncol 1994;12:127–135.
2. Wells, R.J., Woods, W.G., Buckley, J.D., et al. Treatment of newly diagnosed children and adolescents with acute myeloid leukemia: a Children's Cancer Group study. J Clin Oncol 1994;12:2367–2377.
3. Ravindranath Y, Steuber P, Krischer J, et al. High-dose cytarabine for intensification of early therapy of childhood acute myeloid leukemias: A Pediatric Oncology Group study. J Clin Oncol 1991;9:572–580.

PEDIATRIC ACUTE MYELOGENOUS LEUKEMIA (AML)

ALLOGENEIC OR AUTOLOGOUS BONE MARROW TRANSPLANTATION

BU-CY

Drug	Dose	Route	Day
Busulfan	1 mg/kg every 6 hours (16 total doses)	PO/nasogastric	−9, −8, −7, −6
Cyclophosphamide	50 mg/kg/day for 1 hour	IV	−5, −4, −3, −2
GVHD Prophylaxis			
Cyclosporine	1.5 mg/kg every 12 hours	IV	−1 to +50
Methotrexate	15 mg/m²	IV	+1
Methotrexate	10 mg/m²/day	IV	+3, +6, +11

General Comments:

1. Allogeneic marrow transplantation is recommended for patients in first complete remission if an HLA-identical family donor is available.
2. Unrelated donor or autologous transplantation (if remission marrow has been stored) should be considered for relapsed patients.

3. Some centers utilize total body irradiation and Ara-C or cyclo-phosphamide $+/-$ etoposide as the conditioning regimen for AML.

4. Bone marrow is infused on day zero.

Drug Information:

1. Phenytoin prophylaxis is often utilized to prevent busulfan-induced seizures. Phenytoin may be discontinued 24 hours after the last busulfan dose.

2. Busulfan tablets may be crushed, resuspended in sterile water and simple syrup, and administered through a nasogastric tube for children unable to swallow tablets or capsules.

3. Hyperhydration and/or mesna is utilized to minimize risk of hemorrhagic cystitis associated with cyclophosphamide use. Furosemide or mannitol may also be administered to maintain a brisk diuresis.

4. Cyclosporine may be changed to an oral dose of 6 mg/kg twice daily as tolerated. After day $+50$ the drug is tapered by 5% per week. Adjust dose for renal insufficiency.

References:

1. Michel G, Gluckman E, Esperou-Bourdeau H, et al. Allogeneic bone marrow transplantation for children with acute myeloblastic leukemia in first remission: Impact of conditioning regimen without total-body irradiation -a report from the Societe Francaise de Greffe de Moelle. J Clin Oncol 1994;12:1217–1222.

2. Chopra R, Goldstone AH, McMillan AK, et al. Successful treatment of acute myeloid leukemia beyond first remission with autologous bone marrow transplantation using busulfan/cyclophosphamide and unpurged marrow: The British autograft group experience. J Clin Oncol 1991;9:1840–1847.

3. Santos GW, Tutschka PJ, Brookmeyer R, et al. Marrow transplantation for acute nonlymphocytic leukemia after treatment with busulfan and cyclophosphamide. N Engl J Med 1983;309:1347–1353.

JUVENILE CHRONIC MYELOGENOUS LEUKEMIA (JCML)

ALLOGENEIC BONE MARROW TRANSPLANTATION

BU-CY-Melph

Drug	Dose	Route	Day
Busulfan	1 mg/kg every 6 hours (16 total doses)	PO/naso-gastric	-7, -6, -5, -4
Cyclophosphamide	60 mg/kg/day for 1 hour	IV	-3, -2
Melphalan	140 mg/m^2 for 30 min	IV	-1
GVHD Prophylaxis			
Cyclosporine	1.5 mg/kg every 12 hours	IV	-1 to $+50$
Methotrexate	15 mg/m^2	IV	$+1$
Methotrexate	10 mg/m^2/day	IV	$+3$, $+6$, $+11$

General Comments:

1. Currently, allogeneic marrow transplantation is thought to be the only curative therapy for children with JCML.
2. The optimal conditioning regimen for JCML has not been determined. Many centers have utilized cyclophosphamide and TBI with or without other agents. Etoposide and Ara-C have also been used in conjunction with TBI or busulfan/cyclophosphamide.
3. Allogeneic bone marrow is infused on day zero.

Drug Information:

1. Phenytoin prophylaxis is often utilized to prevent busulfan induced seizures. Phenytoin may be discontinued 24 hours after the last busulfan dose.
2. Busulfan tablets may be crushed, resuspended in sterile water and simple syrup, and administered through a nasogastric tube for children unable to swallow tablets or capsules.

3. Hyperhydration and/or mesna is utilized to minimize risk of hemorrhagic cystitis associated with cyclophosphamide use. Furosemide (Lasix) or mannitol may also be administered to maintain a brisk diuresis.
4. It is essential to maintain adequate urine output prior to and for 24 hours after melphalan infusion to reduce bladder irritation. This may be accomplished with hyperhydration and use of furosemide.
5. Cyclosporine may be changed to an oral dose of 6 mg/kg twice daily as tolerated. After day +50 the drug is tapered by 5% per week. Dosing may have to be adjusted for renal insufficiency.

References:

1. Locatelli F, Pession A, Bonetti F, et al. Busulfan, cyclophosphamide and melphalan as conditioning regimen for bone marrow transplantation in children with myelodysplastic syndromes. Leukemia 1994;8:844–849.
2. Donadieu J, Stephan J, Blanche S, et al. Treatment of juvenile chronic myelomonocytic leukemia by allogeneic bone marrow transplantation. Bone Marrow Transpl 1994;13:777–782.
3. Bunin N, Casper J, Lawton C, et al. Allogeneic marrow transplantation using T cell depletion for patients juvenile chronic myelogenous leukemia without HLA-identical siblings. Bone Marrow Transpl 1992;9:119–122.

PEDIATRIC HISTIOCYTOSIS

Pred-VBL

Drug	Dose	Route	Day
Prednisone	40 mg/m^2/day in divided doses thrice daily	PO	Daily
Vinblastine	6 mg/m^2 bolus	IV	Once a week

Comments:

1. Treatment continues for 6 months or until signs or symptoms disappear.

References:

1. Ladisch S, Gadner H. Treatment of Langerhans cell histiocytosis—evolution and current approaches. Br J Cancer. 1994;(Suppl) 23:S41–6.
2. Ceci A, de Terlizzi M, Colella R, Loiacono G, Balducci D, Castello M, Testi AM, De Bernard B, Indolfi P. Langerhans cell histiocytosis in childhood: results from the Cooperative AIEOP-CNR-HX '83 study. Med Pediatr Oncol 1993;21:259–64.
3. Ishii E, Matsuzaki A, Okamura J, et al. Matsumoto T. Treatment of Langerhans cell histiocytosis in children. Am J Clin Oncol 1992;15:515–517.

PEDIATRIC HODGKIN'S LYMPHOMA

MOPP-ABVD

Drug	Dose	Route	Day
Mechlorethamine (M)	6 mg/m² bolus	IV	1, 8
Vincristine (O)	1.5 mg/m² bolus (maximum, 2 mg)	IV	1, 8
Procarbazine (P)	100 mg/m²/day	PO	1–14
Prednisone (P)	40 mg/m²/day in divided doses thrice daily	PO	1–14
Doxorubicin (A)	25 mg/m² for 15 minutes	IV	29, 43
Bleomycin (B)	10 U/m² for 15 minutes	IV	29, 43
Vinblastine (V)	6 mg/m² bolus	IV	29, 43
Dacarbazine (D)	375 mg/m² for 15 minutes	IV	29, 43

Comments:

1. Cycles are every 8 weeks for six cycles.
2. If residual disease is present after six cycles of chemotherapy, radiation therapy may be indicated.

References:

1. Gehan EA, Sullivan MP, Fuller LM, et al. The Intergroup Hodgkin's disease in children: A study of stages I and II. Cancer 1990;65:1429–1437.

2. Hunger SP, Link MP, Donaldson SS. ABVD/MOPP and low-dose involved-field radiotherapy in pediatric Hodgkin's disease: the Stanford
experience. J Clin Oncol 1994;12:2160–2166.

3. Hudson MM, Greenwald C, Thompson E, et al. Efficacy and toxicity of
multiagent chemotherapy and low-dose involved-field radiotherapy in
children and adolescents with Hodgkin's disease. J Clin Oncol
1993;11:100–108.

PEDIATRIC HODGKIN'S DISEASE
AUTOLOGOUS BONE MARROW TRANSPLANTATION
CBV

Drug	Dose	Route	Day
Cyclophosphamide (C)	900 mg/m²/day over 1 hour every 12 hrs	IV	−7, −6, −5, −4
Carmustine (BCNU) (B)	112 mg/m²/day over 30 minutes	IV	−7, −6, −5, −4
Etoposide (V)	250 mg/m²/day over 1 hour every 12 hours	IV	−7, −6, −5, −4

General Comments:

1. The use of high-dose chemotherapy with hematopoietic stem-
cell rescue for Hodgkin's disease is generally limited to patients
who have failed one or more standard chemotherapy protocols.

2. The optimal conditioning regimen for Hodgkin's disease has not
been determined. Varying doses of cyclophosphamide, carmustine, and etoposide have been used by different investigators.
Other regimens have also been utilized including: BCNU + etoposide + Ara-C + melphalan (BEAM), cyclophosphamide +
TBI, and busulfan + cyclophosphamide.

3. Autologous stem cells are infused on day zero.

Drug Information:

1. Hyperhydration and/or mesna is utilized to minimize risk of
hemorrhagic cystitis associated with cyclophosphamide use. Furosemide or mannitol may also be administered to maintain a
brisk diuresis.

2. Some patients experience intense pruritis during the etoposide infusion, which often responds to diphenhydramine (or ranitidine) and IV hydrocortisone. Children should be bathed frequently to minimize cutaneous toxicity.

References:

1. Chopra R, McMillan A, Linch D, et al. The place of high-dose BEAM therapy and autologous bone marrow transplantation in poor-risk Hodgkin's disease. A single-center eight-year study of 155 patients. Blood 1993;81:1137–1145.
2. Wheeler C, Antin J, Churchill W, et al. Cyclophosphamide, Carmustine, and Etoposide with autologous bone marrow transplantation in refractory Hodgkin's disease and non-Hodgkin's lymphoma: A dose-finding study. J Clin Oncol 1990;8:648–656.
3. Jones R, Piantadosi S, Mann R, et al. High-dose cytotoxic therapy and bone marrow transplantation for relapsed Hodgkin's disease. J Clin Oncol 1990;8:527–537.

CHILDHOOD LYMPHOBLASTIC LYMPHOMA

Induction Chemotherapy

Drug	Dose	Route	Day
Cyclophosphamide	1,200 mg/m^2 for 30 minutes	IV	1
Cytarabine	See comments	IT	1
Vincristine	1.5 mg/m^2 bolus (maximum dose = 2 mg)	IV	3, 10, 17, 24
Prednisone	60 mg/m^2/day divided doses thrice daily	PO	3–28, then taper
Daunorubicin	60 mg/m^2 over 15 minutes	IV	17
L-Asparaginase	6,000 U/m^2/day	IM	17–35 (three times per week)
Methotrexate	See comments	IT	17, 31

Comments:

1. Doses of intrathecal (IT) medications are based on age: Methotrexate 6 mg ($\leq$1 year); 8 mg (1 to 2 year); 10 mg (2 to 3 years); 12 mg ($\geq$3 years). Cytarabine 20 mg (0 to 1 year); 30 mg (1 to 2 years); 50 mg (2 to 3 years); 70 mg ($\geq$3 years).

References:

1. Patte C, Kalifa C, Flamant F, et al. Results of the LMT81 protocol, a modified LSA2L2 protocol with high dose methotrexate, on 84 children with non-B-cell (lymphoblastic) lymphoma. Med Ped Oncol 1992;20: 105–113.
2. Reiter A, Schrappe M, Parwaresch R, et al. Non-Hodgkin's lymphomas of childhood and adolescence: results of a treatment stratified for biologic subtypes and stage—a report of the Berlin-Frankfurt-Munster Group. J Clin Oncol 1995;13:359–72.
3. Meadows AT, Sposto R, Jenkin RD, et al. Similar efficacy of 6 and 18 months of therapy with four drugs (COMP) for localized non-Hodgkin's lymphoma of children: a report from the Children's Cancer Study Group. J Clin Oncol 1989;7:92–99.

CHILDHOOD LYMPHOBLASTIC LYMPHOMA

Maintenance Chemotherapy

Drug	Dose	Route	Day
Cyclophosphamide	1000 mg/m² for 30 minutes	IV	1
Vincristine	1.5 mg/m² bolus (maximum dose = 2mg)	IV	1,15
Prednisone	60 mg/m²/day in divided doses thrice daily	PO	1–5 (courses 2–10)
Methotrexate	300 mg/m² (60% for 15 minutes then 40% for 4 hours)	IV	15
Leucovorin	10 mg/m² every 6 hours for 6 doses	PO	16

continued

Maintenance Chemotherapy

Drug	Dose	Route	Day
Daunorubicin	30 mg/m^2 over 30 min.	IV	29
Methotrexate	See comments	IT	1,8,15 (course 1) 1 monthly (courses 2–10)

Comments:

1. Dose of intrathecal (IT) medications are based on age: Methotrexate 6 mg ($\leq$1 year); 8 mg (1 to 2 years); 10 mg (2 to 3 years); 12 mg ($\geq$3 years).
2. Total of 10 courses are administered.
3. At the beginning of Course 1, prednisone is tapered over 10 days from the Induction course.

FAMILIAL ERYTHROPHAGOCYTIC LYMPHOHISTIOCYTOSIS (FEL) ALLOGENEIC BONE MARROW TRANSPLANTATION

BU-CY-VP-16

Drug	Dose	Route	Day
Etoposide (VP-16)	300 mg/m^2/day for 4 hours	IV	-12, -11, -10
Busulfan (BU)	1 mg/kg every 6 hours (16 total doses)	PO/naso-gastric	-9, -8, -7, -6
Cyclophosphamide (CY)	50 mg/kg/day for 1 hour	IV	-5, -4, -3, -2
GVHD Prophylaxis			
Cyclosporine	1.5 mg/kg every 12 hours	IV	-1 to $+50$
Methotrexate	15 mg/m^2	IV	$+1$
Methotrexate	10 mg/m^2/day	IV	$+3$, $+6$, $+11$

General Comments:

1. It is important to differentiate FEL from a virus-associated hemophagocytic syndrome, since the latter may resolve spontaneously or after withdrawal of immunosuppressive therapy.
2. Some transplant centers have also incorporated Ara-C into the preparative regimen.
3. Allogeneic bone marrow is infused on day zero.

Drug Information

1. Phenytoin prophylaxis is often utilized to prevent busulfan-induced seizures. Phenytoin may be discontinued 24 hours after the last busulfan dose.
2. Busulfan tablets may be crushed, resuspended in sterile water and simple syrup, and administered through a nasogastric tube for children unable to swallow tablets or capsules.
3. Hyperhydration and/or mesna is utilized to minimize risk of hemorrhagic cystitis associated with cyclophosphamide use. Furosemide or mannitol may also be administered to maintain a brisk diuresis.
4. Cyclosporine may be changed to an oral dose of 6 mg/kg twice daily as tolerated. After day +50 the drug is tapered by 5% per week. Dosing may have to be adjusted for renal insufficiency.

References:

1. Blanche S, Caniglia, M Girault D, et al. Treatment of hemophagocytic lymphohistiocytosis with chemotherapy and bone marrow transplantation: A single center study of 22 cases. Blood 1991;78:51–54.
2. Fischer A, Cerf-Benussan N, Blanche S, et al. Allogeneic bone marrow transplantation for erythrophagocytic lymphohistiocytosis. J Pediatr 1986;108:267–270.

PEDIATRIC NEUROBLASTOMA

Doxo-E-CY-Pt

Drug	Dose	Route	Day
Doxorubicin (Doxo)	25 mg/m^2 over 15 minutes	IV	2,30,58
Etoposide (E)	100 mg/m^2 over 1 hour	IV	2,5,30,33, 58,61
Cyclophosphamide (CY)	1000 mg/m^2 over 30 minutes	IV	3,4,31,32, 59,60
Cisplatin (Pt)	60 mg/m^2 over 6 hours	IV	1,28,56

Comments:

1. Evaluation for therapeutic response is performed after 9 weeks to decide on additional therapy (surgical resection, radiation therapy or further chemotherapy).

References:

1. Castleberry RP, Shuster JJ, Altshuler G, et al. Infants with neuroblastoma and regional lymph node metastases have a favorable outlook after limited postoperative chemotherapy: a Pediatric Oncology Group study. J Clin Oncol 1992;10:1299–1304.
2. Garaventa A, de Bernardi B, Pianca C, et al. Localized but unresectable neuroblastoma: treatment and outcome of 145 cases. J Clin Oncol 1993;11:1770–1779.
3. West DC, Shamberger RC, Macklis RM, et al. Stage III neuroblastoma over 1 year of age at diagnosis: improved survival with intensive multimodality therapy including multiple alkylating agents. J Clin Oncol 1992;11:84–90.

PEDIATRIC NEUROBLASTOMA

AUTOLOGOUS BONE MARROW TRANSPLANTATION

TBI-Carbo-E-Melph

Drug	Dose	Route	Day
Carboplatin (Carbo)	250 mg/m^2/day	IVCI	$-8, -7, -6, -5$
Etoposide (E)	160 mg/m^2/day	IVCI	$-8, -7, -6, -5$
Melphalan (Melph)	140 mg/m^2 over 30 minutes	IV	-7
Melphalan	70 mg/m^2 over 30 minutes	IV	-6
Total Body Irradiation	333 cGy/day	—	$-3, -2, -1$

General Comments:

1. The role of bone marrow transplantation (BMT) in the treatment of neuroblastoma has not been clearly defined. Children with advanced-stage disease may be candidates for BMT once tumor cytoreduction has been achieved with conventional therapy (usually chemotherapy, surgery and radiotherapy)

2. The optimal conditioning regimen for children with neuroblastoma has not been determined. Most centers utilize TBI (or local radiotherapy) and melphalan either alone or in combination with other agents (e.g., carboplatin, BCNU, thiotepa, etoposide).

3. Most transplants are performed with autologous marrow that has been purged of tumor cells utilizing immunomagnetic beads or chemotherapy.

4. Autologous purged bone marrow is infused on day zero.

Drug Information

1. The creatinine clearance (Cr Cl) should be measured prior to carboplatin administration and the dose adjusted for renal insufficiency (Cr Cl $<$ 100 ml/min/1.73 m^2) to achieve an AUC of

3.4/day. If the CrCl is <65 ml/min/1.73 m^2, alternative therapy should be considered. The carboplatin dose may be calculated by utilizing a modified Calvert formula:

$$\text{Total dose (mg) per day} = \left[\frac{(\text{Corrected Cr Cl} \times \text{surface area})}{1.73} + (15 \times \text{surface area}) \right] \times 3.4$$

2. It is essential to maintain adequate urine output prior to and for 24 hours after melphalan infusion to reduce bladder irritation. This may be accomplished with hyperhydration and use of furosemide.

3. Etoposide is generally administered as a continuous infusion in a concentration *not* to exceed 0.4 mg/mL.

References:

1. Matthay KK, Seeger RC, Reynolds CP, et al. Allogeneic versus autologous purged bone marrow transplantation for neuroblastoma: A report from the Children's Cancer Group. J Clin Oncol 1994;12:2382–2389.

2. Pole JG, Casper J, Elfenbein G, et al. High-dose chemoradiotherapy supported by marrow infusions for advanced neuroblastoma: A Pediatric Oncology Group study. J Clin Oncol 1991;9:152–158.

3. Kushner BH, O'Reilly, Mandell LR, et al. Myeloablative combination chemotherapy without total body irradiation for neuroblastoma. J Clin Oncol 1991;9:274–279.

PEDIATRIC OSTEOSARCOMA

Doxo-Pt-MTX-Lcv

Drug	Dose	Route	Day
Doxorubicin (Doxo)	25 mg/m^2/day over 24 hours	IV	1–3
Cisplatin (Pt)	120 mg/m^2/day over 6 hours	IV	1
Methotrexate (MTX)	12 gm/m^2 over 1 hour	IV	21,28
Leucovorin (Lcv)	10 mg/m^2 every 6 hours	PO	22,29

Comments:

1. Leucovorin is continued after methotrexate administration until serum methotrexate levels are less than 0.1 μM.
2. Two cycles of chemotherapy are administered, followed by surgery for local control. Chemotherapy is then resumed for ten cycles.

References:

1. Meyers PA, Heller G, Healey J, et al. Chemotherapy for nonmetastatic osteogenic sarcoma: The Memorial Sloan-Kettering experience. J Clin Oncol 1992;10:5–15.
2. Bramwell VHC, Burgers M, Sneath R, et al. A comparison of two short intensive adjuvant chemotherapy regimens in operable osteosarcoma of limbs in children and young adults: The first study of the European osteosarcoma intergroup. J Clin Oncol 1992;10:1579–1591.
3. Hudson M, Jaffe MR, Jaffe N, et al. Pediatric osteosarcoma: Therapeutic strategies, results and prognostic factors derived from a 10 year experience. J Clin Oncol 1990;8:1988–1997.

PEDIATRIC RHABDOMYOSARCOMA

Vcr-Dact-CY-MESNA

Drug	Dose	Route	Day
Vincristine (Vcr)	1.5 mg/m² bolus (maximum dose = 2 mg)	IV	1,8,15,22, 29,36,43, 50,57
Dactinomycin (Dact)	0.015 mg/kg bolus (Total maximum daily dose 0.5 mg)	IV	1–5, 22–27, 43–47
Cyclophosphamide (CY)	2.2 g/m² over 1 hour	IV	1, 22, 43
MESNA	360 mg/m² over 15 minutes every 3 hours times 5 doses	IV	1, 22, 43

Comments:

1. After 9 weeks of therapy, response to therapy is evaluated for local control (surgery, radiation therapy, continuation of chemotherapy).

References:
1. Maurer H, Gehen E, Beltangady M, et al. The Intergroup Rhabdomyosarcoma Study-II. Cancer 1993;71:1904–1922.
2. Mandell LR. Ongoing progress in the treatment of childhood rhabdomyosarcoma. Oncology 1993;7:71–83.

PEDIATRIC WILMS' TUMOR

Vcr-Dact

Drug	Dose	Route	Day
Vincristine (Vcr)	2 mg/m^2 bolus (maximum dose = 2 mg)	IV	7, then weekly
Dactinomycin (Dact)	0.045 mg/kg bolus (≤30 kg) 1.35 mg/m^2 (>30 kg); (maximum dose = 3 mg)	IV	1, then every 3 weeks

Comments:

1. Surgical resection and staging are initially performed.
2. Radiation therapy is used depending on the stage of disease.

References:
1. D'Angio GJ, Breslow N, Beckwith JB, et al. Treatment of Wilms' tumor: Results of the Third National Wilms' Tumor Study. Cancer 1989;64:349–360.
2. Green DM, Breslow NE, Beckwitch JB, et al. Treatment outcomes in patients less than 2 years of age with small, stage I, favorable-histology Wilms' tumors: a report from the National Wilms' Tumor Study. J Clin Oncol 1993;11:91–95.

AUTOLOGOUS BONE MARROW TRANSPLANTATION

PEDIATRIC WILMS' TUMOR

E-Thio-CY

Drug	Dose	Route	Day
Etoposide (E)	1800 mg/m^2	IVCI	-8
Thiotepa (Thio)	300 mg/m^2/day for 2 hours	IV	-7, -6, -5
Cyclophosphamide (CY)	50 mg/kg/day for 1 hour	IV	-4, -3, -2, -1

General Comments:

1. The role of high-dose chemotherapy with hematopoietic stem-cell rescue for the treatment of Wilms' tumor has not been defined. Children with primary refractory Wilms' tumor or those who relapse during or within 6 months after completing chemotherapy may be candidates for this approach.
2. The optimal conditioning regimen for Wilms' tumor has not been determined. Other agents have been utilized including TBI, melphalan, cisplatin, carboplatin, BCNU, vincristine, and busulfan.
3. Autologous stem cells are infused on day zero.

Drug Information:

1. Etoposide is administered as a continuous infusion over 24 hours in a concentration *not* to exceed 0.4 mg/ml. Children should be bathed frequently to minimize cutaneous toxicity. Some patients experience intense pruritus during the etoposide infusion, which often responds to diphenhydramine (or ranitidine) and intravenous hydrocortisone.
2. Thiotepa concentration should not exceed 10 mg/mL.
3. Hyperhydration and/or mesna is utilized to minimize risk of hemorrhagic cystitis associated with cyclophosphamide use. Furosemide or mannitol may also be administered to maintain a brisk diuresis.

References:
1. Garaventa A, Hartman O, Bernard JL, et al. Autologous bone marrow transplantation for pediatric Wilms' tumor: The experience of the European Bone Marrow Transplant Registry. Med Pediatr Oncol 1994;22: 11–14.
2. Warkentin PI, Brochstein JA, Strandjord SE, et al. High dose therapy followed by autologous stem cell rescue for recurrent Wilms' tumor. Proc Am Soc Clin Oncol 1993;12:414 (Abstr).

CHAPTER V

Antiemetic Therapy in the Cancer Patient

Robert J. Ignoffo

A survey performed in the early 1980s reported that nausea and vomiting were the most feared complications associated with cytotoxic chemotherapy. Recent advances in the development and selection of new antiemetic drugs has improved the control of both nausea and vomiting from conventional-dose chemotherapy. However, the impact has been less dramatic in high-dose chemotherapy programs and in delayed emesis. Since emesis is related to the dose of agent administered, it is likely that nausea and vomiting will continue to substantially affect the quality of life of cancer patients given chemotherapy. This chapter will discuss some of the risk factors and strategies that may be utilized in the management of chemotherapy-induced nausea and vomiting.

In designing prophylactic strategies, the clinician should consider those major risk factors associated with chemotherapy-induced emesis (CIE) (Table 5-1). One of the most important risk factors is the emetogenic potential of the individual agents (Table 5-2). From Table 5-2 it can be seen that some agents, such as vincristine and bleomycin, produce such mild nausea and vomiting that a less aggressive approach in prevention of emesis may be employed. In contrast, highly emetogenic drugs require the most aggressive and appropriate schedule to prevent emesis. Unfortunately, even the most effective antiemetic regimens may be insufficient to prevent acute emesis and, even if controlled acutely, delayed emesis may ensue several days after chemotherapy, and is often poorly controlled with standard antiemetics.

General guidelines for the use of antiemetics are shown in Table 5-3. Specific recommendations for certain antiemetic agents are preferred, depending on patient risk factors and other drug factors (Table

Table 5-1. RISK FACTORS ASSOCIATED WITH POOR CONTROL OF CIE

Patient Factor	Comment
Age	Younger age is associated a higher incidence of nausea and vomiting
Gender	Women have a higher incidence of nausea and vomiting
Alcohol intake	More than 10 drinks per week is associated with a lower incidence of emesis
Drug Factor	**Comment**
Emetogenicity of chemotherapy	Cisplatin, dacarbazine, mechlorethamine
Dose of chemotherapy	Higher doses greater than lower doses
Schedule of chemotherapy	Bolus greater than infusion

5-4). The newer 5-HT$_3$ antagonists, ondansetron, and dolasetron granisetron, should be reserved for highly emetogenic chemotherapy. For moderately emetogenic chemotherapy, the use of dexamethasone alone or in combination with a lower dose of a 5-HT$_3$ antagonist is effective. Furthermore, lower-dose regimens of 5-HT$_3$ antagonists have been shown to be cost effective.

Delayed emesis is a more difficult problem to manage than acute emesis in the cancer patient. Only a few studies of this problem have been performed, which have demonstrated that conventional antiemetics are as efficacious as the 5-HT$_3$ antagonists. However, the effectiveness of phenothiazines, butyrophenones, and cannabinoids is limited by their higher toxicity profile compared to the 5-HT$_3$ antagonists. The recent release of oral formulations of the 5-HT$_3$ antagonists

Table 5-2. EMETOGENIC POTENTIAL OF CYTOTOXIC DRUGS

Class III HIGH (60–100%)	Class II MODERATE (10–60%)	Class I LOW (⊂10%)
Busulfan (>40 mg)	Asparaginase	Bleomycin
Carmustine	Azacitidine	Busulfan < 10 mg
Cisplatin >50 mg/m^2	Busulfan (10–40 mg)	Chlorambucil
Cyclophosphamide (≥400 mg/m^2)	Carboplatin	Cladribine (2-CdA)
Cytarabine (>400 mg/m2)	Cisplatin < 50 mg/m^2	Cytarabine < 20 mg IV or < 50 mg/m^2 Intrathecally
Dacarbazine (≥500 mg)	Cyclophosphamide (<400 mg/m^2)	Docetaxel Doxorubicin < 20 mg
Dactinomycin	Cytarabine 100–400 mg/m^2	Floxuridine
Etoposide, high-dose (≥400 mg/m^2)	Dacarbazine (<500 mg)	Fluorouracil < 1000 mg
Ifosfamide > 2,500 mg/m^2	Daunorubicin	Melphalan < 10 mg
Lomustine (>60 mg)	Doxorubicin > 20 mg	Mercaptopurine
Mechlorethamine	Estramustine phosphate	Methotrexate < 100 mg
Melphalan (>100 mg)	Etoposide 200–400 mg/m^2	Paclitaxel
Methotrexate, high-dose (>3,000 mg)	Floxuridine IV	Tamoxifen

continued

Table 5-2. EMETOGENIC POTENTIAL OF CYTOTOXIC DRUGS *(continued)*

Class III HIGH (60–100%)	Class II MODERATE (10–60%)	Class I LOW (⊂10%)
Pentostatin	Fludarabine	Thioguanine
Plicamycin	Fluorouracil > 1,000 mg	Vinblastine
Streptozocin	Gemcitabine	Vincristine
Thiotepa, high-dose (≥200 mg)	Hydroxyurea	Vinorelbine
	Idarubicin Ifosfamide < 2.5 g/m^2	
	Lomustine < 60 mg	
	Melphalan 10–100 mg	
	Methotrexate 100–3,000 mg	
	Mitomycin	
	Mitoxantrone	
	Procarbazine	
	Teniposide	
	Thiotepa 30–200 mg	

Antiemetic Therapy in the Cancer Patient **379**

Table 5-3. GUIDELINES FOR THE GENERAL USE OF ANTIEMETICS IN THE PREVENTION OF EMESIS

1. Give antiemetics in advance of chemotherapy (at least 30 minutes prior to treatment). If oral agents are given, give one or two doses at least 2 hours prior to treatment.
2. For chemotherapy that is severely emetogenic, use 5-HT$_3$ antagonists on each day of chemotherapy. If not contraindicated, include dexamethasone in combination with 5-HT$_3$ antagonists.
3. For highly emetogenic agents, such as cisplatin, give antiemetics that will inhibit emetic stimulus for 24 hours.
4. Give anxiolytic agents to patients receiving their first cycle of chemotherapy to prevent anticipatory nausea and vomiting. Lorazepam is the anxiolytic of choice and may be given parenterally or sublingually.
5. For cisplatin or chemotherapy that may cause delayed emesis, give oral antiemetics (phenothiazines or metoclopramide) with or without dexamethasone for 2 or three days starting 16 hours after chemotherapy.

Table 5-4. GUIDELINES FOR THE USE OF 5-HT$_3$ ANTAGONISTS IN THE MANAGEMENT OF CIE

5-HT$_3$3 antagonists are indicated in the following situations:

1. Patients receiving one or more highly emetogenic chemotherapeutic agents (Class III).
2. Patients receiving combinations of two or more Class II emetogenic chemotherapy drugs.
3. Patients receiving single agent moderate (Class II) or low (Class I) emetogenic cancer chemotherapy regimens not responding to ***prior*** antiemetic therapy with dexamethasone, prochlorperazine, dronabinol, thiethylperazine or metoclopramide, or chlorpromazine.

continued

Table 5-4. GUIDELINES FOR THE USE OF 5-HT₃ ANTAGONISTS IN THE MANAGEMENT OF CIE *(continued)*

The dosage of 5-HT$_3$ antagonist should be based on the emetogenicity of the chemotherapeutic agent in adults

Class III—Granisetron 10 μg/kg (**round to nearest 50 μg**) IV over a period of 5 to 15 minutes every 24 hrs or granisetron 1 mg po bid (*on each day of chemotherapy*) **plus** dexamethasone 10 to 20 mg IV 30 minutes prior to chemotherapy for 1 to 5 days (if not contra-indicated)

OR

Ondansetron 10 mg IV every 8 hours or Ondansetron 24–32 mg IV × 1 for 15 minutes (*on each day of chemotherapy*) **plus** dexamethasone 10 to 20 mg IV 30 minutes prior to chemotherapy for 1 to 5 days (if not contraindicated)

Class II—Ondansetron 10 to 20 mg IV over a period of 15 to 30 minutes × 1 (*for each day of chemotherapy*) **plus** dexamethasone 10 to 20 mg IV 30 minutes prior to chemotherapy for 1 to 5 days (if not contraindicated)

OR

Ondansetron 8 mg PO thrice daily (*for each day of chemotherapy*) or granisetron 1 mg PO twice daily (*for each day of chemotherapy*) **plus** dexamethasone as above.

The selection and dose of 5-HT$_3$ antagonist in pediatric patients

Ondansetron 0.15 mg/kg every 4 hours for 3 doses or every 8 hours.

or

Granisetron 10 μg/kg (**use exact dosage**) IV for 15 minutes every 24 hours.

plus

Dexamethasone 0.8 mg/kg given in three divided doses IV 30 minutes prior to chemotherapy every 8 hours for 1 to 5 days (if not contraindicated).

Table 5-5. GUIDELINES FOR THE MANAGEMENT OF DELAYED EMESIS FROM CYTOTOXIC CHEMOTHERAPY

Day	Agent	Dose
2–5	Metoclopramide *plus*	0.5–1 mg/kg IV/PO every 4 hours × 3 doses
	Dexamethasone *or*	8 mg po bid
	Ondansetron *plus*	8 mg po bid
	Dexamethasone *or*	8 mg po bid
	Prochlorperazine Spansules *plus*	15 mg po bid
	Dexamethasone	8 mg po bid

may demonstrate cost effectiveness, but further studies are needed Our current recommendations for the management of delayed emesis are shown in Table 5-5. Notice that the use of a 5-HT$_3$ antagonist is reserved for patients with refractory emesis or those experiencing severe side effects from conventional antiemetics.

References

1. Coates A, Abraham S, Kaye SB, et al. On the receiving end—patient perception of side effectas of cancer chemotherapy. Eur J Cancer Clin Oncol 1983;19:203–208.
2. Pisters KM and Kris MG. Management of nausea and vomiting caused by anticancer drugs: State of the Art. Oncology (Suppl) 1992;99–104.
3. Borison HL, Mc Carthy LE. Neuropharmacology of chemotherapy-induced emesis. Drugs 1983;25:8–17.
4. Merrifield KR, Chafee BJ. Recent advances in the management of nausea and vomiting caused by antineoplastic agents. Clin Pharm 1991;8:187–99.
5. Triozzi PL and Laszlo J. Optimum management of nausea and vomiting in cancer chemotherapy. Drugs 1987;34:136–149.
6. Gralla RJ. Antiemetic Therapy. In: DeVita V, Hellman S, Rosenberg S. (eds) Cancer: Principles and Practice of Oncology. 4th Ed. J.B. Lippincott, Philadelphia. 1993,pp. 2338–2348.

7. Kris M. Rationale for combination antiemetic therapy and strategies for the use of ondansetron in combinations. Semin Oncol 1992;19 (Suppl 10); 61–66.

8. Sridhar KS, Donnelly E. Combination antiemetics for cisplatin chemotherapy. Cancer 1988;61:1508–1517.

9. Schmoll HJ. The role of ondansetron in the treatment of emesis induced by noncisplatin-containing chemotherapy regimens. Eur J Cancer Clin Oncol 1989;(Suppl 1); 25:S35–S39.

10. Fraschini G. Antiemetic activity of ondansetron in cancer patients receiving non cisplatin chemotherapy. Semin Oncol 1992;(Suppl 10); 19: 41–47.

11. Hainsworth J, Harvey W, Pendergrass K, Kasimis B, Oblon D, Monaghan G, Gandara D, Hesketh P, Khojastch A, Harker G, York M, and Finn A. A single-blind comparison of intravenous ondansetron with intravenous metoclopramide in the prevention of nausea and vomiting associated with high-dose cisplatin chemotherapy. J Clin Oncol 1991;9:721–728.

12. Beck TM, Heketh PJ, Madajewicz S, Navari RM, Pendergrass K, Lester EP, Kish JA, Murphy WK, Hainsworth JD, Gandura DR, Bricker LJ, Keller AM, Mortimer J, Galvin DV, House KW, and Bryson JC. Stratified, randomized, double-blind comparison of intravenous ondansetron administered as a multiple-dose regimen versus two single-dose regimens in the prevention of cisplatin-induced nausea and vomiting. J Clin Oncol 1992;10:1969–1975.

13. Finn A. Toxicity and side effects of ondansetron. Semin Oncol 1992;19 (Suppl 10); 53–60.

14. Kris MG. Phase II trials of ondansetron with high dose cisplatin. Semin Oncol 1992;19 (Suppl 10); 22–27.

15. Roila F, et al. Prevention of cisplatin-induced emesis: A double-blind multicenter randomized crossover study comparing ondansetron and ondansetron plus dexamethasone. J Clin Oncol 1991;9:675–678.

16. Hesketh PJ, Gandara DR. Serotonin antagonists: a new class of antiemetic agents. J Natl Cancer Inst 1991;83:613–20.

17. Kamanasbrou D. Intravenous granisetron—establishing the optimal dose. Eur J Cancer 1992; (Suppl 1); 28A:S6–11.

18. Kris M, Gralla R, Tyson LB, et al. Controlling delayed vomiting: double-blind randomized, trial comparing placebo, dexamethasone alone, and metoclopramide and dexamethasone in patients receiving cisplatin. J Clin Oncol 1989;7:108–114.

19. Hesketh PJ, Beck T, Uhlenhopp M, et al. Adjusting the dose of intravenous ondansetron plus dexamethasone to the emetogenic potential of the chemotherapy regimen. J Clin Oncol 1995;13:2117–2122.

20. Navari R, Gandara d, Hesketh P, et al. Comparative clinical trial of granisetron and ondansetron in the prophylaxis of cisplatin-induced emesis. The Granisetron Study Group. J Clin Oncol 1995;13:1242–1248.

21. Perez EA. Review of the preclinical pharmacology and comparative efficacy of 5-hydroxytryptamine-3 receptor antagonists for chemotherapy-induced emesis. J Clin Oncol 1995;13:1036–1043.

22. Yarker YE, McTavish D. Granisetron: An update of its therapeutic use in nausea and vomiting induced by antineoplastic therapy. Drugs 1994;48:761–793.

23. Heron JF, GoedhalsL, Jordaan JP, Cunningham J, and Cedar E. Oral granisetron alone and in combination with dexamethasone: a double-blind randomized comparison against high dose metoclopramide plus dexamethasone in prevention of cisplatin-induced emesis. The Granisetron Study Group. Ann Oncol 1994;5:579–584.

24. The Italian Group for Antiemetic Research. Dexamethasone, granisetron, or both for the prevention of nausea and vomiting during chemotherapy for cancer. N Engl J Med 1995;332:1–5.

25. Gebbia V, Cannata G, Testa A, et al. Ondansetron versus granisetron in the prevention of chemotherapy-induced nausea and vomiting. Results of a prospective randomized trial. Cancer 1994;74:1945–1952.

26. Hesketh P, Beck T, Uhlenhopp M, et al. Adjusting the dose of intravenous ondansetron plus dexamethasone to the emetogenic potential of the chemotherapy regimen J Clin Oncol 1995;13:2117–2122.

27. Hesketh PJ, Kris MG, Grunberg SM, Beck T, Hainsworth JD, Harket G, Apro MS, Gandara D, and Lindley CM. Proposal for classifying the acute emetogenicity of cancer chemotherapy. J Clin Oncol 1997;15:103–109.

28. Italian Group for Antiemetic Research. Ondansetron vs metoclopramide, both combined with dexamethasone, in the prevention of cisplatin-induced delayed emesis. J Clin Oncol 1997;15:124–130.

CHAPTER VI

Pain Management of the Cancer Patient

Elaine Harney
Donald W. Northfelt

This chapter provides an overview for clinicians treating pain in the cancer patient. It is designed as a guide to understanding pain, its etiologies, and different treatment modalities for it. The following topics will be discussed:

Pain Assessment, including assessment tools commonly used to document pain intensity, with a comparison of the characteristics of acute and chronic pain.

Pain Management: to help develop a strategy for treating pain; contains the WHO three-step analgesic ladder. For specific drugs and doses, refer to Tables 6-8 through 6-14.

Guidelines for pain management in substance abusers with cancer.

Side effects of analgesics and their management, including symptoms of withdrawal.

Analgesics, adjuvant drugs, and doses.

ASSESSMENT OF PAIN

Pain is underrecognized in cancer patients: underreported by patients, and undertreated by physicians.

1. Types of pain in cancer patients
   a. Directly related to tumor
      Bone metastases
      Infiltration of brachial/lumbar plexus
      Infiltration of viscera
   b. Associated with therapy of cancer
      Postsurgical

Postchemotherapy
Postradiation
  c. Pain unrelated to cancer or treatment
  2. Evaluation of pain
  a. History and physical
Patient report is primary source of data.
Vital signs and other physiologic criteria are not useful in evaluation.
  b. Neurologic and psychiatric evaluation is critical, and can usually be adequately obtained by a well-trained internist.
  c. Frequent reassessment is critical.
  d. Use brief, easy-to-use assessment tools that reliably document pain intensity and pain relief (10-cm baselines recommended for each) (Table 6-1).
  3. Characteristics of pain (Table 6-2)
  a. Elements of both acute and chronic pain

Table 6-1. PAIN INTENSITY ASSESSMENT TOOLS

Simple descriptive pain intensity scale					
No pain	Mild pain	Moderate pain	Severe pain	Very severe	Worst possible pain

0–10 Numeric pain intensity scale										
No pain					Moderate pain				Worst possible pain	
0	1	2	3	4	5	6	7	8	9	10

Visual analog scale		
None	Moderate	Worst possible pain
0————————————————————————————————10		

Table 6-2. CHARACTERISTICS OF ACUTE AND CHRONIC PAIN

Acute	Chronic
Recent onset, short duration	Persistence of pain for 1 month or more beyond usual for acute injury.
Expectation of resolution	Association with chronic pathologic process.
Serving as warning signal; adaptive	Less well-defined temporal onset; no adaptive function.
Tissue damage, objective physical signs	Lack of objective signs.
Anxiety as the primary effect	Depression as the primary effect, often masked by pain preoccupation.

      b. Anxiety and depression
      c. Life-threatening nature of illness
   4. Four aspects of cancer pain that require ongoing evaluation:
      a. Pain intensity
      b. Pain relief
      c. Mood state or psychological distress
      d. Narcotic-drug effects such as side effects and abuse

CANCER PAIN MANAGEMENT

General principles

Treat acute pain with rapidly acting medication, anticipate need for frequent dosing (Tables 6-3 and 6-4).

Treat chronic pain with long-acting medication, try to achieve infrequent dosing (Table 6-3).

Anticipate narcotic side effects and treat expectantly (see Tables 6-5 through 6-7).

Table 6-3. STRATEGIES FOR THE MANAGEMENT OF ACTUE PAIN AND CANCER PAIN

Strategy	Acute Pain	Cancer Pain
Aim	Pain relief	Pain relief
Sedation	Useful	Undesirable
Desired duration of effect	2–4 hours	As long as possible
Timing	On demand	Regular anticipation
Dose	Standard	Determined by patient
Route	Parenteral	Oral
Adjuvant medication	Rare	Frequent

Table 6-4. RECOMMENDED CLINICAL APPROACH TO CANCER PAIN— ABCDE

A	Ask about pain regularly; assess pain systematically.
B	Believe the patient and family in their reports of pain and what relieves it.
C	Choose pain-control options appropriate for the patient, family, and setting.
D	Deliver interventions in a timely, logical, coordinated fashion.
E	Empower patients and their families; enable patients to control their course to the greatest extent possible.

Table 6-5. INCIDENCE AND MANAGEMENT OF ADVERSE EFFECTS WITH NARCOTICS

Adverse Effect	Incidence	Management
Gastrointestinal—nausea	Common	See Table 5
Gastrointestinal—constipation	Common	See Table 6
Sedation	Infrequent	Psychostimulants
CNS—twitching	Rare, occurs at high doses (meperidine, morphine > hydromorphone > methadone > levor	Change drug
Respiratory depression	infrequent, occur at high doses	Decrease dose and/or use naloxone 0.4 mg IV

Use non-narcotics for additive effects and specific actions (e.g. NSAIDs for bone pain, amitriptyline for neurologic cancer pain) (see Tables 6-8, 6-11, and 6-12).

The WHO three-step analgesic ladder (Figure 6-1) encompasses five important concepts for cancer pain: by the mouth, by the clock, by the ladder, for the individual, and with attention to detail.

For patients with mild to moderate pain attempt pain relief with the use of oral opioids with or without adjuvants (see Tables 6-6, 6-9, 6-11 and 6-12).

Once patient has reached third-step opioid requirements for severe pain, prescribe narcotics freely (see Table 6-10).

Specific recommendations

1. Use oral medications whenever possible.
2. Never prescribe meperidine (Demerol®) when continued opioid use is anticipated.

Table 6-6. MECHANISMS OF OPIOID-INDUCED NAUSEA AND VOMITING, AND THEIR MANAGEMENT

Mechanism	Suggestive clinical features	Anti-emetic drugs
Stimulation of medullary chemoreceptor trigger zone	Nausea/vomiting shortly after opioid administrat	Metoclopramide, lorazepam, prochlorperazine, haloperidol, chlorpromazine, or corticosteroid
Enhanced vestibular sensitivity	Prominent movement-induced nausea/vomiting or vertigo	Scopolamine, meclizine, or lorazepam
Increased gastric antral tone	Early satiety, postprandial bloating, vomiting	Metoclopramide

   3. Avoid prescribing medications for chronic pain on an as needed basis.

   4. There is no ceiling effect with narcotics: "The dose that works is the dose that works."

   5. When initiating narcotic therapy

      a. For inpatients use a morphine infusion or a PCA device (see Table 6-14).

      b. For outpatients use oral liquid morphine.

      c. Allow the nursing staff/patient to vary the dose rate liberally.

   6. Use equianalgesic doses when changing from one narcotic to another.

ADDICTION, DEPENDENCE, TOLERANCE IN SUBSTANCE ABUSERS WITH CANCER

Opioid tolerance and physical dependence are expected with long-term opioid treatment, and should not be confused with addiction.

Table 6-7. TREATMENT LADDER FOR CONSTIPATION

Step I: Recommended to start patients with 1 senna (Senokot)
tablet per 30 mg morphine

or

Docusate 100 mg twice daily + senna (Senokot) or
bisacodyl (Dulcolax) 5 mg daily

Step II: Senna or bisacodyl 5 mg twice daily→ 10 mg twice
daily→15 mg twice daily

Step III: Senna 20 mg twice daily + lactulose 15cc twice
daily→senna 20 mg twice daily + sorbitol 30 mL twice
daily

Step IV: Senna 20 mg PO twice daily + lactulose 30 mL twice or
thrice daily

If a patient has not had a bowel movement in 3 days, the nurse
will use one of the following treatments once or twice daily until
results are obtained:

a) Digital disimpaction followed by 2 bisacodyl suppositories

OR

b) Sodium phosphate 30 mL PO repeated in 2 hours if needed

OR

c) Mineral oil or Fleet's enema.

After successful treatment, the patient will resume the escalated
maintenance regimen.

Addiction—a pattern of compulsive drug use characterized by a continued craving for an opioid and the need to use the opioid for
effects other than pain relief.

Dependence—chronic opioid use that results in the development of
the abstinence syndrome when the medication is discontinued or
an opioid antagonist is administered.

Tolerance—the tendency for the effect of a drug to wane over time at
a given dose, requiring that an increased dose be given to produce the same effect; this occurs principally with the nonanalgesic
effects of narcotics, and tends not to occur with the analgesic
effect.

Table 6-8. 1ST STEP—FOR MILD TO MODERATE PAIN: NONOPIOID ANALGESTIC

Generic	Trade Name	Usual adult dose (⊃50kg)	Comments
Acetaminophen	Tylenol	650 mg every 4 hours	Hepatic toxicity w/high doses (>4 Gm/day)
Aspirin	Various	650 mg every 4 hours	Standard for comparison among nonopioid analgesics
Choline magnesium trisalicylate	Disalcid, Trilisate	1,000–1,500 mg thrice daily	Less GI toxicity; no effect on platelet function at usual doses
Ibuprofen	Motrin, Advil, etc.	400–600 mg every 6 hours	Available over-the-counter (OTC) Can inhibit platelet function
Naproxen	Naprosyn	250–500 mg twice daily	Tablet or suspension; available OTC
Naproxen sodium	Anaprox, Aleve	275–550 mg twice daily	Available OTC
Ketoprofen	Orudis	25–60 mg every 6–8 hours	Sustained-release product (Oruvail) available: 100, 150, 200 mg
Indomethacin	Indocin	50 mg thrice daily	Sustained release: SR (75 mg twice daily), PR (50 mg), and suspension available
Sulindac	Clinoril	200 mg twice daily	Less renal toxicity
Diclofenac	Voltaren	50 mg thrice daily	
Ketorolac	Toradol	10 mg po every 4–6 hours; maximum dose = 40 mg/day Do not exceed 5 days of IM Toradol.	Parenteral: 60 mg IM initially, then 30 mg IM every 6 hours. Caution with renal dysfunction.

[1] SR = sustained release; PR = per rectum

Table 6-9. 2ND STEP—FOR MODERATE PAIN: OPIOIDS ADMINISTERED ORALLY

Generic Name	Trade Name	Average adult dose	Ratio of Opioid/ APAP or ASA	Comments
Codeine	Various	1–2 tablets every 6 hours	15, 30, or 60 mg/300 or 325 mg	Nausea common
Oxycodone	Oxycontin	1–3 tablets every 4 hours	10, 20, 40 mg	No APAP or ASA
Oxycodone ± ASA	Roxicodone Percodan (ASA)	1 tablet every 6 hours	5 mg/650 mg (ASA)	Roxicodone available as single agent
Oxycodone + APAP	Percocet	1 tablet every 6 hours	5 mg/500 mg (APAP)	Do not exceed 4 g
Hydrocodone	Vicodin, Lortab	1–2 every 4–6 hours, up to 8 tablets/day	5 or 7.5 mg/500 mg (APAP)	APAP per day.[1]
Propoxyphene (w/APAP)	Darvocet-N Darvocet-N-100	2 tablets every 4 hours 1 tablet every 4 hours	50 mg/325 mg 100 mg/650 mg	Toxic metabolite norpropoxyphene accumulates with repeated dosing
Propoxyphene (ASA + caffeine)	Darvon	1–2 capsules every 4 hours	65 mg/389 mg/32.4 mg caff.	
Meperidine	Demerol	1 tablet every 4–6 hours	50 mg/25 mg prometh	Not recommended[2]

[1] Preparations with >500 capsules mg acetaminophen per tablet are not recommended; excessive doses of acetaminophen (>4 g) may lead to hepatic toxicity.

[2] Accumulation of metabolite normeperidine increases risk of seizure.

Table 6-10. 3RD STEP—FOR SEVERE PAIN: OPIOIDS[1]

Drug: generic (Trade)	Equianalgesic Doses		Duration of Action	Comments
Morphine	10 mg IM/IV/SC	30 mg PO	Short acting MS 4 hours *SR* (i.e., MS Contin) 8–12 hours	PO: wide range of formulations: long-acting (SR) tablets (MS Contin, Roxanol SR); short-acting solution and tablets
Hydromorphone (Dilaudid)	2 mg IM	8 mg PO	4 hours	
Meperidine (Demerol)	75 mg IM	300 mg PO	3 hours	Not recommended for cancer pain[2]
Levorphanol (Levo-Dromoran)	2 mg IM	4 mg PO	6 hours	Delayed toxicity due to plasma accumulation
Methadone (Dolophine)	10 mg IM	20 mg PO	6 hours	Delayed toxicity due to accumulation; half-life = 15–150 hours
Fentanyl (Sublimaze)	See Table 14		1 hour	See Table 14

[1] Patients who are opioid-naive should begin with a dose equivalent to 4 to 8 mg morphine IV every 3–4 hours. For patients with good pain control but unacceptable side effects, the starting dose of the new drug should be reduced to 50 to 75% equianalgesic dose to account for incomplete cross-tolerance.

[2] Accumulation of metabolite normeperidine increases risk of seizure.

Table 6-11. ADJUVANT ANALGESICS

Class	Indication	Preferred Drug	Schedule	Daily Dose	Comment
Tricyclic antidepressants	Neuropathic pain, depression, insomnia	Amitriptyline Doxepin Imipramine	qhs	50–150 mg (for pain), to 300 mg for depression	Use nortriptyline for excess sedation
Anticonvulsants	Lancinating neuropathic pain	Clonazepam Carbamazepine	every 12 hours every 6–8 hours	2–7 mg 600–1,600 mg	Serum concentration of carbamazepine 4–10 mg/L
Oral local anesthetics	Neuropathic pain	Mexilitene	every 8 hours	150 mg/d × 3 d, 3 days, then 300 mg/days then 10 mg/kg/day	
Neuroleptics	Refractory neuropathic pain and delirium	Haloperidol Fluphenazine	every 6–12 hours every 8 hours	2–10 mg 3–6 mg	Not used as first-line agents
Antihistamines	Anxiety, nausea	Hydroxyzine[1] Diphenhydramine	every 6–8 hours every 6–8 hours	200 mg 100–200 mg	No evidence of analgesia
Corticosteroids	Bone pain, infiltration of neural structures	Dexamethasone	every 6–8 hours	2–24 mg	Less mineralocorticoid effect than prednisone
Psychostimulant	Reverse opioid-induced sedation	Methylphenidate Dexedrine	twice daily twice daily	10–40 mg 10–40 mg	CII substances: need triplicate prescriptions

[1] Do not administer hydroxyzine by vein (IV) as it can cause phlebitis.

Table 6-12. TRADE AND GENERIC NAMES, AVAILABLE ROUTES OF ADMINISTRATION—ADJUVANT ANALGESICS

Generic Name	Trade Name	Available Routes
Amitriptyline	Elavil	PO,IM,PR
Nortriptyline	Pamelor, Aventyl	PO
Imipramine	Tofrenil	PO,IM
Doxepin	Sinequan	PO,IM
Clonazepam	Klonopin	PO
Carbamazepine	Tegretol	PO
Mexilitene	Mexitil	PO
Haloperidol	Haldol	PO,IM,IV
Fluphenazine	Prolixin	PO,IM
Hydroxizine	Vistaril, Atarax	PO,IM
Diphenhydramine	Benadryl	PO,IM,IV
Dexamethasone	Decadron	PO,IV
Methylphenidate	Ritalin	PO
Dextroamphetamine	Dexedrine	PO

Table 6-13. FENTANYL TRANSDERMAL SYSTEM (Dose Based on Daily Morphine Equivalence)

Oral 24 hour morphine (mg/day)—6 : 1 ratio[1]	Oral 24 hour morphine (mg/day)—3 : 1 ratio[2]	IM 24 hr morphine (mg/day)	Fentanyl transdermal (μg/hour)
45–134	24–66	8–22	25
135–224	67–101	23–37	50
225–314	102–156	38–52	75
315–404	157–201	53–67	100
405–494	202–226	68–82	125
495–584	227–291	83–97	150
585–674	292–336	98–112	175
675–764	337–381	113–127	200
765–854	382–426	128–142	225
855–944	427–471	143–157	250
945–1034	472–516	158–172	275
1035–1124	517–561	173–187	300

[1] The package insert suggests that 60 mg PO or 10 mg IM of morphine (6:1 ratio) every 4 hours × 24 hours (360 mg/day oral or 60 mg/day IM) is approximately equivalent to 100 μg/hour of transdermal fentanyl. That is, fentanyl is supposedly 150 and 25 times more potent than oral and IM morphine.

[2] The literature shows fentanyl is closer to 100 times more potent than injectable morphine. Most sources and clinical experience suggest the use of a PO:IV or IM ratio for morphine of 2 to 4:1. A ratio of 3:1 is shown.

[3] Available in cartons of 5 patches: 25, 50,75 and 100 μg/hour; multiple patches may be applied simultaneously.

Table 6-14. PATIENT CONTROLLED ANALGESIA (PCA)[1]

Drug	Conc.	Delay	Basal Rate	1 hr. Limit[2]	Bolus
Morphine	1 mg/mL	6–10 minutes	1 mg/hour	25 mg/hour	1 mg
Hydromorphone	0.2 mg/mL	6–10 minutes	0.2 mg/hour	2.2 mg/hour	0.2 mg
Meperidine	10 mg/mL	6–10 minutes	10 mg/hour	70 mg/hour	10 mg
Fentanyl	10 mcg/mL	6–10 minutes	10 mcg/hour	110 mcg/hour	10 μg

[1] These are guidelines with which a patient might be started on PCA; the values contained within this table are very general; ranges may vary greatly: "the dose that works is the dose that works."

[2] One-hour limits will vary depending on clinician's judgement and patient's pain.

GUIDELINES FOR PAIN MANAGEMENT IN SUBSTANCE ABUSERS WITH CANCER

1. Accept and respect the report of acute pain in spite of the possibility of being "duped."
2. Prevent or minimize withdrawal symptoms.
3. Define the pain syndrome and provide treatment for both the underlying disorder and the pain complaint.
4. Utilize WHO analgesic ladder schema to select appropriate pharmacologic approach.
5. Apply appropriate pharmacologic principles when using opioids.
6. Provide nonopioid and nonpharmacologic therapies as indicated.
7. Recognize specific drug-abuse behaviors.
8. Set realistic goals for pain therapy.
9. The care of the substance-abusing cancer patient with pain requires a team effort.
10. Evaluate and treat other distressing physical and psychological symptoms that may contribute to pain and suffering.

11. Constant assessment and re-evaluation of the effects of pain interventions must take place in order to optimize care.

MANAGEMENT OF NARCOTIC SIDE EFFECTS

Constipation is a common problem associated with long-term opioid administration, and should be anticipated, treated prophylactically, and monitored constantly. The "ladder" of increasing potency that can be used for treating constipation is found in Table 6-7.

Symptoms of withdrawal:

1. Early: Yawning; lacrimation; rhinorrhea; sweating.
2. Intermediate: Mydriasis; piloerection; flushing; tachycardia; twitching; tremor; restlessness; irritability; anxiety; anorexia.
3. Late: Muscle spasm; fever; nausea; diarrhea; vomiting; severe backache; abdominal and leg pains; abdominal and muscle cramps; hot and cold flashes; insomnia; intestinal spasm; coryza and repetitive sneezing; increase in body temperature, blood pressure, respiratory rate and heart rate; spontaneous orgasm; chills.

DRUGS AND DOSES

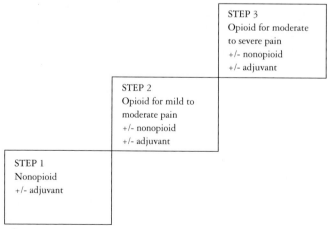

Figure 1. WHO three-step analgesic ladder.

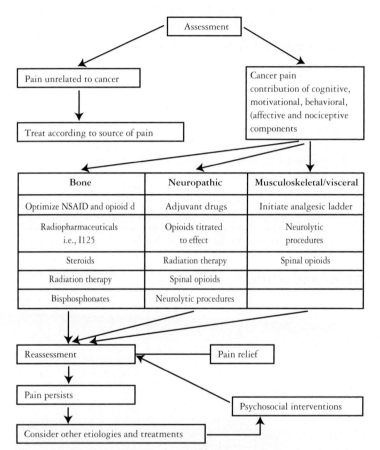

Figure 2. Continuing pain management for cancer patients.

References

1. Agency for Health Care Policy and Research. Management of cancer pain: Adults. Am J Pharm 1994;51:1643–1656.
2. American Pain Society. Principles of analgesic use in the treatment of acute pain and chronic cancer pain, 2nd Ed. Clin Pharm 1990;9:601–611.
3. Breitbart W, & Lefkowitz M. Pain in AIDS. Bulletin of Experimental Treatments for AIDS. 1995 March 16–29.
4. Calis KA, Kohler DR, Corso DM. Transdermally administered fentanyl for pain management. Clin Pharm 1992;11:22–36.
5. Cherny NI, Foley KM. Current approaches to the management of cancer pain: A review. Ann Acad Med 1994;23:139–159.
6. Jacox A, Carr DB, Payne R, et al. Management of Cancer Pain. Clinical Practice Guideline No. 9. AHCPR Publication No. 94-0592. Rockville, MD. Agency for Health Care Policy and Research, U.S. Department of Health and Human Services, Public Health Service, March 1994.
7. Levy MH. Pharmacologic management of cancer pain. Seminars in Oncology. 1994;21:718–739.
8. Kastrup EK (ed): Drug Facts and Comparisons: Facts and Comparisons, Inc., St. Louis, MO. 1997, pp. 242–252f.

CHAPTER VII

Management of Tumor Lysis Syndrome and Hypercalcemia

Reginald S. King

The maintenance of normal serum calcium is dependent on three systemic hormones: vitamin D (as calcitriol), parathyroid hormone (PTH), and calcitonin. Calcitriol increases intestinal calcium absorption and PTH directly stimulates bone resorption and renal calcium reabsorption and indirectly stimulates production of vitamin D by the kidneys. Calcitonin inhibits bone resorption, thereby serving as a counterregulator to PTH. It is the free ionized, or active calcium, that determines the actions of these hormones. Protein-bound and free ionized calcium each comprises approximately 50% of total serum calcium.

Hypercalcemia is defined as an elevation of total serum calcium above a normal range of approximately 8.5 to 10.5 mg/dL. Caution needs to be taken when interpreting a total serum calcium level, depending on the patient's clinical condition. For example, it should be ascertained whether the patient has received hydration or not. Additionally, if a patient is hypoalbuminemic, regardless of the etiology, his/her total serum calcium level needs to be corrected as follows:

Corrected calcium (mg/dL) = measured calcium + 0.8 (4.0 − albumin)

As calcium levels approach 12 mg/dL, symptoms of hypercalcemia become more common. When calcium levels exceed 14 mg/dL or symptoms are severe, immediate treatment is indicated to avoid life-threatening complications. On the other hand, if a patient is in the end-stage of disease and chemotherapy is not indicated to treat the underlying process, less aggressive or even no management of hypercalcemia may be appropriate. Signs and symptoms of hypercalcemia are patient-specific and may depend on age, concurrent conditions, duration of hypercalcemia, and rate of increase of calcium (see Table 7-1).

403

Table 7-1. SIGNS AND SYMPTOMS OF HYPERCALCEMIA

Body System	Patient Presentation
Central Nervous System	Altered mental status (personality changes, impaired concentration, mild confusion, lethargy) Weakness Decreased deep tendon reflexes Stupor Coma
Renal	Interference with renal mechanisms for sodium/water reabsorption in proximal tubule resulting in: Loss of urine-concentrating ability (polyuria→polydipsia) Dehydration/hypovolemia Decreased glomerular filtration rate Renal insufficiency→increased serum calcium
Cardiovascular	Electrocardiographic changes consistent with slowed conduction or bradyarrhythmias Complete heart block Cardiac arrest

There are two types of malignant hypercalcemia. Humoral hypercalcemia of malignancy involves the systemic secretion of PTH-related protein or other bone-resorbing substances by the tumor, resulting in osteoclast activation and accelerated bone resorption. PTH-related protein stimulation of renal tubular reabsorption of calcium further impairs the kidney's ability to excrete the increased filtered load of calcium. Metastatic hypercalcemia, also referred to as the "local osteolytic" type, is a result of bone destruction caused by factors secreted at the site of bone metastases. Regardless of the etiology, the homeostatic mechanisms of serum calcium maintenance are overwhelmed.

Malignancies associated with hypercalcemia include carcinoma of the breast and lung, multiple myeloma, and lymphomas. Breast cancer is commonly associated with osteolytic metastases, and multiple my-eloma is believed to produce cytotoxins that mediates extensive os-teolytic bone destruction. Non-small-cell lung cancer also commonly leads to lytic bone metastases. Lymphomas are postulated to produce one or more bone-resorbing cytokines.

There are several goals to consider in the management of hyper-calcemia of malignancy. The first of these is to initiate treatment for the underlying disorder if possible or if the disorder is known. Next, dehydration needs to be corrected. Renal calcium clearance can be increased by improving the glomerular filtration rate through the res-toration of intravascular volume, preferably with normal saline (NS). Depending on the severity of dehydration and tolerability of the pa-tient's cardiovascular system, fluid should be administered at a rate of 100 to 250 mL/hour, or approximately 3 L/m^2. Serum calcium may be expected to decrease by 1 to 2 mg/dL but will rarely return to normal with hydration alone. Loop diuretics should also be employed to fa-cilitate the renal excretion of calcium as well as aid in the prevention of fluid overload. Of note, thiazide diuretics may exacerbate existing hypercalcemia by enhancing distal tubular reabsorption of calcium.

Pharmacologic intervention for hypercalcemia of malignancy comprises several classes of agents:

CALCITONIN

Most widely used as a salmon derived preparation, calcitonin acts on bone to inhibit osteoclast resorption and on the kidney to promote urinary calcium excretion. Of the agents that can be used, calcitonin has the most rapid onset of action. Hypocalcemic effects may be ob-served in as soon as 2 to 4 hours. The duration of effect of calcitonin is typically only 2 to 3 days secondary to the development of tachy-phylaxis, otherwise known as the escape phenomenon. The usual dose of calcitonin is 4 units/kg administered IM/SC every 12 hours. Doses up to 8 units/kg every 6 hours have been used. Adverse effects are generally mild and include nausea, vomiting, and flushing. Calci-tonin acutely lowers the serum calcium concentration by 2 to 3 mg/dL.

PLICAMYCIN

Previously investigated as an antitumor agent, plicamycin is believed to inhibit RNA synthesis in osteoclasts. It may also act as a direct toxin on the osteoclasts, therefore serving as a potent inhibitor of bone resorption. Plicamycin's onset of action is at 12 to 24 hours, with its maximum hypocalcemic effects occurring in 48 to 72 hours. The duration of its action ranges from a few days to several weeks. Usual dosing of plicamycin is 25 μg/kg, with the drug administered IV by slow infusion over a period of 4 to 6 hours. Repeat administration of plicamycin may be considered in several days; however, a single dose can produce normocalcemia. The potential for certain adverse effects may limit the usefulness of plicamycin. These include nausea and vomiting, hepatotoxicity manifested by elevation in serum aminotransferases, nephrotoxicity, and thrombocytopenia. Plicamycin is considered to be relatively safe at doses used for hypercalcemia in comparison to those studied in connection with its use as a cytotoxic agent.

GALLIUM NITRATE

Another agent initially investigated for its antineoplastic effects, gallium nitrate appears to inhibit bone resorption by adsorbing to and reducing the solubility of hydroxyapatite crystals. Its onset of action is within 24 to 48 hours, with maximal hypocalcemic effects achieved at approximately 7 days. Gallium nitrate is administered at a dose of 100 to 200 mg/m²/day in 1 L of NS by continuous IV infusion over a period of 5 days. The major adverse effect associated with gallium nitrate is nephrotoxicity. The drug should be avoided in patients whose serum creatinine is greater than 2.5 mg/dL or who are receiving other nephrotoxins. Hypophosphatemia may also be seen.

BISPHOSPHONATES

The bisphosphonates are the newest group of agents to become available for the management of hypercalcemia of malignancy. These compounds are analogs of the natural substrate, pyrophosphate, and are distinguished by a P-C-P bond instead of a P-O-P bond. They have a high affinity for hydroxyapatite, which is a potent inhibitor of bone-crystal dissolution.

Etidronate

Etidronate (Didronel®) is a first-generation bisphosphonate that inhibits osteoclast-mediated bone resorption. It is 50% bound to bone and

Table 7-2. GUIDELINES FOR PAMIDRONATE DOSING

Corrected Serum Calcium	Dose Regimen
12 to 14 mg/dL	45–60 mg in 1 L 0.9% NaCl over 2–4 hours*
>14 mg/dL	60–90 mg in 1 L 0.9% NaCl over 2–4 hours*

exhibits a half-life of greater than 90 days. The onset of etidronate's hypocalcemic effects is approximately 24 to 48 hours, and may be as long as 72 hours. Peak effects are realized in about 7 days. The usual dose of etidronate is 7.5 mg/kg administered as a slow IV infusion over 2 hours daily for 3 days. Patients may need to be retreated after 7 days if optimal effects are not achieved. Adverse effects include nausea, a metallic taste, and transient increases in serum creatinine and phosphorous.

Pamidronate

Pamidronate (Aredia®) is a second-generation bisphosphonate. Like etidronate, it is 50% bound to bone and inhibits osteoclast-mediated bone resorption. Additionally, pamidronate appears to possess a direct cytotoxic effect on osteoclast viability. The onset of its hypocalcemic effects occurs within 24 to 48 hours, with peak effects occurring in 7 days and a duration of effect of about 2 weeks. Pamidronate's adverse effects include: mild, transient fever; phlebitis; asymptomatic hypophosphatemia; nausea; and a transient increase in serum creatinine and leukopenia. Because there appears to be a significant dose–response relationship between pamidronate dose and hypocalcemia, guidelines have been recommended to optimally tailor the pamidronate dose to the severity of hypercalcemia (see Table 7-2).

References

1. Bilezikian JP. Management of acute hypercalcemia. N Engl J Med 1992;326:1196–1203.
2. Galpin AJ, Irvin RJ, Kuhn JG. Hypercalcemia of malignancy. In: Dorr

RT, Von Hoff DD (eds): Cancer Chemotherapy Handbook, 2nd Ed. Appleton & Lange, Norwalk, CT; 1994, pp. 35–53.

3. Hall TG and Schaiff RAB. Update on the medical treatment of hypercalcemia of malignancy. Clin Pharm 1993;12:117–125.

4. Kinirons MT. Newer agents for the treatment of malignant hypercalcemia. Am J Med Sci 1993;305:403–406.

5. Nussbaum SR. Pathophysiology and management of severe hypercalcemia. Endocrine and Metab Clin North Am 1993;22:343–362.

6. Ritch PS. Treatment of cancer-related hypercalcemia. Semin Oncol 1990;17:26–33.

7. Dodwell, Howell A, Morton AR, Daley-Yates PT, and Hoggarth CR. Infusion rate and pharmacokinetics of intravenous pamidronate in the treatment of tumour-induced hypercalcemia. Postgrad Med J 1992;68:434–439.

CHAPTER VIII

Management of Malignant Effusions

Robert Robles

Malignant effusions are a frequent complication of advanced cancers. The development of malignant effusions produces significant morbidity in patients who are typically near the end of their lives because of their advanced cancers. Prompt treatment can provide significant palliation. The clinically significant malignant effusions are those of the pleura, peritoneum, and pericardium. Malignant effusions represent an inappropriate accumulation of protein-rich fluid in a potential space of the body. Because ascites and pleural and pericardial effusions may also occur as a result of pathologic processes other than malignancies, an appropriate and timely evaluation is required in order to direct therapy.

Table 8-1. CANCERS ASSOCIATED WITH MALIGNANT EFFUSIONS

Ascites	Pleural effusion	Pericardial effusion
Ovarian, colorectal, gastric, endometrial	Lung, breast, mesothelioma, lymphoma, ovary, melanoma	Lung, breast, leukemia, lymphoma, melanoma, gastrointestinal, sarcomas

SIGNS AND SYMPTOMS OF MALIGNANT EFFUSIONS

Table 8-2. SIGNS AND SYMPTOMS OF MALIGNANT ASCITES

Symptoms:	Signs:
Anorexia Early satiety Abdominal distention Abdominal discomfort Respiratory compromise Lower extremity edema	Abdominal distention Fluid wave Shifting dullness Bulging flanks

Table 8-3. SIGNS AND SYMPTOMS OF MALIGNANT PLEURAL EFFUSIONS

Symptoms:	Signs:
Dyspnea Cough Chest pain Chest heaviness Orthopnea Trepopnea	Dullness to percussion Decrease breath sounds Decreased fremitus Intercostal fullness Poor diaphragmatic excursion Tachypnea Decreased chest wall expansion

Table 8-4. SIGNS AND SYMPTOMS OF MALIGNANT PERICARDIAL EFFUSIONS

Symptoms:	Signs:
Dyspnea Cough Chest pain Orthopnea Palpitations Fatigue Dizziness Anxiety	Jugular venous distention Cardiomegaly Distant heart sounds Pericardial rub Pulsus paradoxus Hypotension Tachycardia

DIAGNOSIS
Radiology

Ascites

1. Abdominal flat plate: ground-glass appearance, obscured psoas shadow, floating loops of small bowel.
2. Ultrasound and computed tomographic (CT) scanning-sensitive tests to detect small amounts of ascites.

Pleural Effusion

1. Chest radiograph: blunting of the costophrenic angle, layering of fluid on lateral decubitus film, mediastinal shift.
2. CT scan and ultrasound-sensitive studies to demonstrate fluid.

Pericardial Effusion

1. Chest radiograph: enlargement of cardiac silhouette (water-bottle heart).
2. CT scan: demonstrates pericardial effusion earlier than chest radiograph.
3. Echocardiogram: most precise method of diagnosis.

Diagnostic Procedures

1. Ascites: Paracentesis.
2. Pleural effusion: thoracentesis; pleural biopsy—more sensitive than thoracentesis.
3. Pericardial effusion: electrocardiogram: low QRS amplitude, electrical alternans, tachycardia; pericardiocentesis.

Laboratory Findings

1. Ascites: bloody or serosanguinous fluid (>100 erythrocytes/μL) $>1,000$ leukocytes/μL in absence of infection, ascitic/serum protein ratio >0.4, ascitic/serum LDH >1.0, increased tumor markers (CEA, CA-125, CA 19-9, etc.), cytology is positive in $>50\%$ of cases.
2. Pleural effusion: effusion/serum protein ratio >0.5, ascitic/serum LDH >0.6, increased tumor marker-CEA, cytology is positive in 42 to 96% of cases.
3. Pericardial effusion: fluid frequently hemorrhagic, positive cytology in 80 to 90% of cases.

TREATMENT OPTIONS

Control of the tumor producing a malignant effusion is always the best treatment option. Unfortunately, when malignant effusions develop, curative therapy is rarely possible. Therefore, therapies for malignant effusions are palliative. Patient comfort and quality of life should be the primary concern in treating malignant effusions.

Ascites

The development of malignant ascites is often the first sign of recurrence of a number of cancers (ovarian, gastric, endometrial, and colorectal). Treatment is uncommonly associated with prolonged survival, but contributes substantially to quality of life.

1. **Diet and diuretics:** Sodium restriction and the use of diuretics are rarely effective in the treatment of malignant ascites.
2. **Paracentesis:** Repeat percutaneous paracentesis is an effective method for removing symptomatic or recurrent ascites. The patient is placed in a comfortable supine position and the amount of fluid determined through percussion. An area on an abdominal quadrant or in the midline is selected; distant from prior abdominal surgery and obvious skin infection. The skin is cleansed with a bactericidal soap and a sterile drape placed to shield the area. One percent lidocaine is infiltrated in the subcutaneous tissue to provide local anesthesia. A large-bore IV catheter is attached to a syringe and the skin is punctured. The catheter is carefully advanced until ascites is aspirated. The cath-

Table 8-5. ADVANTAGES AND DISADVANTAGES OF PARACENTESIS FOR MALIGNANT ASCITES

Advantages	Disadvantages
Simple Convenient Effective	Hypovolemia Electrolyte abnormalities Protein depletion Bleeding Infection Visceral injury

eter is advanced, the needle removed, and tubing attached to the catheter. The tubing is connected to a vacuum bottle and the fluid is drained. See Table 8-5 for potential side effects of this treatment.

3. **Peritoneovenous shunting:** This procedure takes advantage of the pressure difference between the abdominal cavity with ascites and the central venous pressure. The device consists of a length of tubing with multiple perforations that is placed in the abdominal cavity, a unidirectional valve, and tubing that is placed into the superior vena cava. The tubing is placed in a subcutaneous tunnel. See Table 8-6 for potential side effects of this treatment.

Table 8-6. ADVANTAGES AND DISADVANTAGES OF PERITONEOVENOUS SHUNTING FOR MALIGNANT ASCITES

Advantages	Disadvantages
Possible long-term relief of malignant ascites Single procedure Maintenance of intravascular volume	Surgical procedure required Occlusion Volume overload Disseminated intravascular coagulation (DIC) Infection

4. **Intraperitoneal therapy:** Intraperitoneal (IP) chemotherapy has a long history in the treatment of malignant ascites. Administration of IP chemotherapy produces a higher local concentration of chemotherapeutic agent(s). The use of indwelling peritoneal dialysis catheters and subcutaneously implanted reservoir catheter systems has allowed for safer and more reliable peritoneal access. An IP nuclear medicine scan is often performed after catheter placement to determine adequate distribution of injected material throughout the peritoneal cavity. From 10 to 20% of patients will have poor peritoneal distribution. Unfortunately, IP therapy's major drawback is the lack of effective chemotherapy agents to treat the cancers that commonly produce malignant ascites (Table 8-7). Epithelial ovarian cancer has

Table 8-7. ADVANTAGES AND DISADVANTAGES OF INTRAPERITONEAL CHEMOTHERAPY FOR MALIGNANT ASCITES

Advantages	Disadvantages
Tumor exposed to high local concentrations of chemotherapy agents Limited systemic absorption of chemotherapy Longer exposure of tumor to chemotherapy Potentially fewer systemic side effects from chemotherapy	Lack of effective chemotherapy agents for the majority of peritoneal malignancies Requires invasive procedure to administer therapy

been effectively treated with a variety of IP chemotherapeutic agents, most notably cisplatin. Gastrointestinal malignancies that commonly cause malignant ascites have been treated with 5-fluorouracil and bleomycin with limited success. In general, IP therapy responses are brief, with survival limited by the advanced state of the patient's malignancy. Response rates of percent are reported, with the best responses coming with low-volume ovarian cancer that is sensitive to cisplatin. See Table 8-8 for a list of intraperitoneal chemotherapy agents.

Table 8-8. INTRAPERITONEAL CHEMOTHERAPY AGENTS

Cisplatin	Phosphorus-32
Carboplatin	Mitomycin C
Fluorouracil	Paclitaxel

5. **Surgery:** Aggressive surgical resection of peritoneal tumor deposits has been performed with the goal of controlling or preventing tumor-related complications such as malignant ascites. This surgery is usually followed by IP chemotherapy. This procedure cannot be recommended outside centers with substantial

experience. See Table 8-9 for advantages and disadvantages of surgery.

Table 8-9. ADVANTAGES AND DISADVANTAGES OF SURGERY FOR MALIGNANT ASCITES

Advantages	Disadvantages
Treats tumor primarily May provide best palliation for low-grade intraperitoneal tumors	Major surgical procedure Noncurative

Malignant Pericardial Effusion

Involvement of the pericardium is an underrecognized complication of cancer care. Less than 30% of patients with malignant pericardial involvement will be diagnosed antemortem. Other causes of pericardial effusions in cancer patients are radiation-induced pericarditis and infection. The prognosis of malignant pericardial effusion depends on the patient's performance status, the effectiveness of systemic chemotherapy, and the responsiveness of the cancer to treatment.

1. **Pericardiocentesis and catheter drainage:** Pericardiocentesis is a method for removing fluid from the pericardial space to relieve the signs and symptoms of cardiac tamponade, or as a diagnostic aid to determine the etiology of a pericardial effusion. Echocardiography can determine the presence of hemodynamic compromise. Pericardiocentesis and catheter placement are most safely performed with echocardiographic guidance. Echocardiography allows more precise drainage and avoidance of likely complications: cardiac or coronary artery injury. The only significant contraindication is an uncontrolled bleeding diathesis. The patient is placed in a semirecumbent position. The left xiphocostal angle is identified, disinfected, and draped, and the skin is anesthetized with 1% lidocaine anesthesia. A syringe is attached to an 18- or 20-gauge spinal needle, inserted through the skin, and advanced toward the suprasternal notch under echocardiographic guidance. Continuous suction is maintained

until fluid is obtained. A sudden give may be noted when the pericardium is penetrated. Fluid is removed for diagnostic tests. A J-tip guidewire is advanced, the needle withdrawn, a dilator used to create an adequate opening, and a pigtail catheter placed for continuous drainage. See Table 8-10 for side effects of this treatment.

Table 8-10. ADVANTAGES AND DISADVANTAGES OF PERICARDIOCENTESIS FOR MALIGNANT PERICARDIAL EFFUSION

Advantages	Disadvantages
Prompt relief of symptoms Allows for diagnosis of etiology	Bleeding Infection Cardiac injury Dysrhythmias Pneumothorax Injury of adjacent structures Recurrence of pericardial fluid after catheter removed

2. **Instillational intrapericardial therapy:** Following catheter drainage, several sclerosing agents have been used to prevent reaccumulation of fluid (Table 8-11). There is no convincing data to support the use of one agent over another. Recurrence rates following pericardiocentesis without the use of a sclerosing agent are 20 to 50%. Following drainage of a pericardial effusion with a residual output <25 mL/24 hours and instillation of sclerosing agents, effusion recurrence rates of 18 to 25% have been reported. See Table 8-12 for side effects of this treatment.

Table 8-11. SCLEROSING AGENTS FOR MALIGNANT PERICARDIAL EFFUSION

Bleomycin Cisplatin Nitrogen mustard Phosporus-32

Table 8-12. ADVANTAGES AND DISADVANTAGES OF PERICARDIAL THERAPY FOR MALIGNANT PERICARDIAL EFFUSION

Advantages	Disadvantages
Prevention of effusion reaccumulation Well tolerated Simple procedure	Chest pain Fever Dysrhythmias

3. **Pericardial window:** This procedure involves the creation of a fenestration in the pericardial sac which allows fluid to drain into the peritoneal or left pleural cavities. This is commonly performed through a subxiphoid incision, and can be performed under general or local anesthesia. More recently, pericardiotomy has been accomplished with the use of a dilating balloon originally designed for cardiac valvuloplasty. This procedure can be performed at the same time as pericardiocentesis. A connection is created between the pericardial and left pleural spaces. A complete pericardiectomy, with complete removal of the pericardium, prevents significantly more effusion recurrences, but entails more extensive surgery. See Table 8-13 for side effects of this treatment.

Table 8-13. ADVANTAGES AND DISADVANTAGES OF PERICARDIAL WINDOW FOR MALIGNANT PERICARDIAL EFFUSION

Advantages	Disadvantages
Effective intervention Low recurrence rate Minimal morbidity	Bleeding Infection Pneumothorax Infection Invasive procedure required

4. **Pericardial Resection:** Involves removal of the entire pericardium through a thoracotomy incision. It is appropriate only for those patients with longer survivals and who can tolerate ag-

gressive surgery. This procedure is associated with the lowest recurrence rate. See Table 8-14 for advantages & disadavantages of this treatment.

Table 8-14. ADVANTAGES AND DISADVANTAGES OF PERICARDIAL RESECTION FOR MALIGNANT PERICARDIAL EFFUSION

Advantages	Disadvantages
Evaluate extent of thoracic disease Highest rate of diagnosis Lowest rate of recurrence	Requires general anesthesia and thoracotomy Significant morbidity and mortality

5. **Radiation therapy:** This therapy is most appropriate for exquisitely radiosensitive tumors such as lymphomas. It may be utilized for other cancers as well. Treatment is generally 20 to 30 Gy given daily for 2 to 3 weeks. See Table 8-15 for advantages & disadvantages of this treatment.

Table 8-15. ADVANTAGES AND DISADVANTAGES OF RADIATION THERAPY FOR MALIGNANT PERICARDIAL EFFUSION

Advantages	Disadvantages
Well tolerated Noninvasive	Limited efficacy for most common cancers Relatively poor efficacy

Malignant Pleural Effusion

The development of a new pleural effusion in a cancer patient requires an expeditious and thorough evaluation to determine the etiology of the effusion. Other causes for a pleural effusion should be sought in addition to malignancy, including heart and liver failure, infection, atelectasis, hemorrhage, and hypoalbuminemia. Malignant pleural effusions typically are exudative. However, malignant cells must be demonstrated in the pleural fluid or by pleural biopsy before the diagnosis of a malignant pleural effusion can be made with certainty.

1. **Supportive care:** may be an appropriate option for a patient with widely metastatic cancer and a brief life expectancy who is willing to accept hospice placement. Opiates and supplemental oxygen are the principal components of care. See Table 8-16 for advantages & disadvantages of supportive care.

Table 8-16. ADVANTAGES AND DISADVANTAGES OF SUPPORTIVE CARE FOR MALIGNANT PERICARDIAL EFFUSION

Advantages	Disadvantages
Readily applicable Easily implemented	May not utilize cancer-specific therapy May not provide optimal symptom control

2. **Thoracentesis:** can be performed simultaneously for diagnosis and relief of symptoms. Contraindications include an uncontrolled bleeding diathesis and patients unable to tolerate a pneumothorax. Patients receiving positive-pressure ventilation have a relative contraindication to thoracentesis. Anterior–posterior, lateral, and decubitus chest radiographs are performed prior to the procedure to document freely flowing pleural fluid. The patient is placed in an erect sitting position with the arms resting on a table in front of the patient. The superior margin of dullness is determined by percussion; ultrasonography or fluoroscopy may also be used. A spot approximately two rib interspaces lower is marked on the thorax. The skin is disinfected and draped. The skin is anesthetized with 1% lidocaine. A small-gauge needle is then attached to a syringe and advanced into the thorax along the superior margin of the rib; avoiding the neurovascular bundle located along the inferior margin of each rib. Continuous suction is applied. Entry into the pleural space is indicated by the aspiration of fluid. If no fluid is obtained, the patient is carefully leaned backwards or another site is chosen. The depth to which the needle penetrates is noted. A larger-gauge thoracentesis needle is attached to a syringe and advanced into the pleural space. Fluid is obtained for diagnostic studies. With some thoracentesis kits, a soft catheter is advanced

into the pleural space and further fluid removed for symptom relief. It is often recommended that no more than 1 L be removed at any one time, in order to prevent re-expansion pulmonary edema. See Table 8-17 for advantages and disadvantages of thoracocentesis.

Table 8-17. ADVANTAGES AND DISADVANTAGES OF THORACENTESIS FOR MALIGNANT PLEURAL EFFUSION

Advantages	Disadvantages
Simple, readily available procedure Diagnostic and therapeutic procedure Rapid relief of symptoms May be repeated as needed	Pneumothorax Hemothorax Empyema Vasovagal reaction Re-expansion pulmonary edema Hypoxemia Loculation

3. **Tube thoracostomy:** allows for complete drainage of a pleural effusion and introduction of a sclerosing agent to produce a symphysis of the visceral and parietal pleura. The patient is positioned with the pleural effusion located superiorly, and is provided with appropriate anxiolytic and analgesic premedications. A spot in the anterior axillary line in the sixth or seventh rib interspace is marked and sterilely prepared. The skin is anesthetized with 1% lidocaine. Intercostal nerve blocks may also be utilized by injecting several milliliters of local anesthetic agent with epinephrine at the inferior rib border at the angle of the rib. A small incision is made in the skin and carried through to the intercostal muscle. Curved scissors or a hemostat is used to dissect to the pleura and to puncture and spread the pleura. A finger is introduced to identify and break up adhesions. A size 28 or 32 French chest tube is then introduced until all the fenestrations are in the pleural space. The tube is secured with sutures and then bandaged. The chest tube is then connected to suction through an underwater seal system. Suction is main-

tained until fluid output from the chest tube is less than 150 mL/24 hours, and the lung has reinflated and remains so after the suction is discontinued and the chest tube placed under water-seal. If no further treatment is planned, the chest tube is then removed. Multiple chest tubes may be required to drain pleural-fluid loculations. The use of small-bore silastic chest tubes placed under ultrasound or fluoroscopy has gained favor recently. These tubes are more comfortable and seem to be as effective as larger chest tubes. See Table 8-18 for advantages & disadvantages of this treatment.

Table 8-18. ADVANTAGES AND DISADVANTAGES OF CHEST TUBE DRAINAGE FOR MALIGNANT PLEURAL EFFUSION

Advantages	Disadvantages
Rapid relief of symptoms Provides access for sclerotherapy	Lung injury Hemothorax Empyema Pain Re-expansion pulmonary edema Hypoxemia Requires hospitalization

4. **Thoracoscopy:** is a relatively old surgical procedure that has experienced a renaissance with the advent of better optics and instruments specifically used with a thoracoscope. Thoracoscopy is a valuable technique for diagnosing malignancy in patients with persistently negative cytology specimens from pleural fluid. Thoracoscopy is used to break up loculations of pleural fluid. Pleurectomy may also be performed through the thoracoscope. The thoracoscope allows drainage of pleural effusions and immediate sclerosis. See Table 8-19 for advantages & disadvantages of thoracoscopy.

Table 8-19. ADVANTAGES AND DISADVANTAGES OF THORACOSCOPY FOR MALIGNANT PLEURAL EFFUSION

Advantages	Disadvantages
Allows for diagnosis of cytologically negative effusions Avoids open thoracotomy Shorter hospital stay Fewer postoperative complications Sclerosis performed at same time as drainage	Requires general anesthesia May require conversion to open thoracotomy for complications Bleeding Infection Pneumothorax

5. **Thoracotomy:** is reserved for the rare patient with an undiagnosed pleural effusion or who requires surgery for relief of symptoms. These patients should have an excellent performance status and relatively long survival expectancy. See Table 8-20 for advantages & disadvantages of thoracotomy.

Table 8-20. ADVANTAGES AND DISADVANTAGES OF THORACOTOMY FOR MALIGNANT PLEURAL EFFUSION

Advantages	Disadvantages
Provides diagnosis great majority of cases Allows for pleurodesis even in cases which have failed chest tube sclerosis Full extent of intrathoracic tumor noted	Open thoracotomy Hospitalization Substantial morbidity

6. **Sclerosing agents** (Table 8-21): Few data from prospective randomized trials are available to guide a clinician in choosing sclerosing agent. The cost of the sclerosing agent (Table 8-22) should not be the major determinant in choosing an agent; an inexpensive agent may be ineffective and require multiple uses to achieve the success rates provided with a single application of a more expensive agent.

Table 8-21. SCLEROSING AGENTS FOR MALIGNANT PLEURAL EFFUSION

Sclerosing agent	Success rate	Dose	Comment
Talc	80–100%	2–10 g	No standard preparation
Bleomycin	13–87%	60 mg	Fever
Doxycycline	10–88%	500 mg	Multiple doses required
Minocycline	86%	300 mg	Vestibular symptoms
Mitoxantrone	80%	30 mg	Myelosuppression

Table 8-22. COST OF SCLEROSING AGENTS AT SFGH, 1995

Talc	$0.03/5 grams (sterilization costs not included)
Doxycycline	$21.07/100 mg
Bleomycin	$220/30 mg
Minocycline	$1.94/100 mg
Mitoxantrone	$550/30 mg

References

1. Buzaid AC, Garewal HS, Greenberg, BR, Managing Malignant Pericardial Effusion, West J Med 1989;150:174–179.
2. Chan, A, et al., Subxiphoid Partial Pericardiectomy With or Without Sclerosant Instillation in the Treatment of Symptomatic Pericardial Effusions in Patients with Malignancy, *Cancer* 1991;68:1021–1025.
3. Pass HI. Malignant pleural and pericardial effusions. In DeVita, VT, Jr., Hellman, S, Rosenberg, SA (eds.): Cancer: Principles and Practice of Oncology, 5th Ed. 1997 pg 2586–2598.
4. Walker-Renard, PB, Vaughan, LM, Sahn, SA, Chemical pleurodesis for malignant pleural effusions. Ann Intern Med 1994;120:56–64.
5. Weissberg, D and Ben-Zeev, I, Talc pleurodesis, Experience with 360 patients. J Cardiovasc Surg 1993;106:698–675.
6. Ziskind AA, et al, Percutaneous Balloon Pericardiotomy for the Treatment of Cardiac Tamponade and Large Pericardial Effusions: Description of Technique and Report of the first 50 cases. J Am Coll Cardiol 1993;21:1–5.

CHAPTER IX

Management of the Bone Marrow Transplant Patient

Betsy Althaus

MANAGEMENT OF FEBRILE NEUTROPENIA

The bone-marrow-transplant (BMT) patient experiences a period of profound neutropenia, which places the patient at high risk for infections. In order that all practitioners treat patients in a uniform, effective manner, institution-specific guidelines should be established for management of the febrile neutropenic patient. The guidelines should include decisions about empiric antimicrobial agents for gram-negative and gram-positive bacteria and fungal pathogens.

Early in neutropenia, the most common pathogens are bacterial. While infections with gram-positive organisms such as staphylococci and streptococci occur more frequently, gram-negative infections are more virulent. *Escherichia coli, Klebsiella* spp., and *Pseudomonas aeruginosa* are the most common gram-negative pathogens. Later in neutropenia, more resistant gram-negative organisms are cultured. The response to the first fever must include the initiation of antibiotics with broad-spectrum gram-negative activity. Established acceptable choices are an antipseudomonal beta-lactam drug with an aminoglycoside such as tobramycin or amikacin, or monotherapy with an antipseudomonal beta-lactam or monobactan. The initiation of vancomycin with the first fever is controversial. It may be appropriate if the patient shows clinical indications of a gram-positive infection, such as a reddened or tender central line site, or if gram-positive organisms are common and serious pathogens in an institution's BMT population.

Fungal infections occur in roughly 20% of BMT patients. The most common fungal organisms are *Candida* species and *Aspergillus*. Infections with *Candida* species may develop as early as in the first one to two weeks after BMT. Noncandidal fungal infections, such as with *Aspergillus* and *Fusarium*, tend to occur later.

425

Fungal infections are difficult to diagnose, with persistent fever while the patient is receiving antibiotics being the most common clinical indication of a fungal infection. Antifungal therapy should be started if the patient has a new or persistent fever while receiving broad-spectrum antibiotics. Once established, fungal infections, especially noncandidal infections, respond poorly to therapy. Because of the risk of *Aspergillus* infection, amphotericin is the antifungal agent of choice for initial empiric therapy.

INFECTION PROPHYLAXIS

BMT patients are at high risk for infection. Risk factors include prolonged and profound neutropenia, humoral and cellular immunodeficiency, and impairment of normal mucosal barriers secondary to mucositis and skin toxicity.

Allogeneic BMT recipients have the major added risk factor of therapy with immunosuppressive agents. The prophylactic use of antimicrobial agents in this high-risk population has generally produced a decreased frequency of infection and fewer days with fever, and has sometimes decreased mortality. Infection prophylaxis against bacteria, viruses, and fungus should be considered. The potential benefits of prophylaxis must be balanced against cost, patient acceptance, adverse reactions, drug interactions, and selection for resistant strains.

Bacterial Prophylaxis

The use of antibacterial prophylaxis in BMT patients is generally recommended, but the choice of drug, route of administration, and schedule vary widely among BMT programs. Several choices are available. The regimen should be active against aerobic gram-negative flora. Activity against gram-positive organisms may also be beneficial, depending on the infections usually acquired in a particular BMT program. Table 9-1 lists possible choices, with their advantages and disadvantages.

The time to begin antibacterial prophylaxis is unclear. It is generally started by day −2 (day 0 = day of hematopoietic graft infusion), and is sometimes started as early as day −7.

Patients with chronic graft-versus-host disease should receive daily oral antibacterial prophylaxis. Acceptable agents are penicillin 250 mg PO twice daily, an oral cephalosporin, or trimethoprim—sulfamethoxazole.

Table 9-1. **DRUG CHOICES FOR ANTIBACTERIAL PROPHYLAXIS**

Drug	Dose	Advantages	Disadvantages
Ciprofloxacin	500–750 mg PO twice daily or 500 mg every 8 hours	Reduced infections from gram-negative bacteria, generally well tolerated.	Possible increase in gram-positive infections.
Norfloxacin	400 mg PO twice daily		
Ofloxacin	200 mg PO twice daily		
Cotrimoxazole (trimethoprim-sulfamethoxazole)	160 mg/800 mg PO twice daily	Reduced infections from gram-negative and gram-positive bacteria, inexpensive.	Possible increase in duration of neutropenia, may increase *clostridium difficile* enterocolitis, may cause more allergic reactions
Oral nonabsorbable antibiotics (neomycin, gentamicin vancomycin, polymyxin B, colistin, bacitracin)	Various doses and combinations	Decreased bacterial infections.	Poor patient tolerance, expensive, gut decontamination only.
Vancomycin	15 mg/kg IV every 12 hours	Decreased gram-positive infections, decreased febrile days.	Possible increased risk of vancomycin-resistant enterococci. Expensive.

Herpes Simplex Prophylaxis

BMT patients are at a high risk for reactivation of Herpes simplex virus (HSV) infections for the first month after transplantation. The mucocutaneous lesions of such infections occur predominantly in the mouth, and may appear as severe mucositis. The lesions may extend extraorally, and may become superinfected with bacteria and fungi. Sites of HSV reactivation other than the mouth include the esophagus and the genital mucosa. Prophylaxis with IV acyclovir significantly reduces HSV reactivation in seropositive patients. Dosing schedules vary. One commonly used regimen is acyclovir 250 mg/m^2 or 5 mg/kg IV given every 12 hours, starting on day -2 of transplant, and continued until discharge or until the patient is no longer neutropenic and mucositis has resolved.

Herpes Zoster Prophylaxis

The risk of Herpes zoster virus (VZV) infections after BMT is 25 to 50%, with the majority of infections occurring between the second and tenth month. Some cases have developed as late as 10 years after BMT. The risk for VZV infection appears to be similar for autologous and allogeneic graft recipients. Between 60 and 70% of affected patients will have localized dermatomal disease, and the remainder will have disseminated, visceral, or CNS disease. More serious infections occur early after BMT. Disseminated VZV infection is rarely seen after the first 6 months. Prophylaxis with acyclovir delays but does not seem to prevent reactivation of the infection. The delay may provide the benefit of a decrease in more severe infections. The decision must be made to provide either prophylaxis or treatment. The patient may receive low-dose oral acyclovir prophylaxis for 6 to 12 months after transplantation, or may receive treatment doses of acyclovir IV initiated promptly upon onset of symptoms. (see Table 9-2)

Cytomegalovirus Prophylaxis

Cytomegalovirus (CMV) disease is a leading cause of morbidity and mortality in the allogeneic marrow-graft population. It is usually due to reactivation of latent virus in seropositive patients. The majority of cases occur between 30 and 90 days after BMT. The organs most commonly involved are the lungs and gastrointestinal tract. The most serious CMV disease is interstitial pneumonia. CMV in the gastrointestinal tract typically manifests as esophagitis or enteritis, with accompanying pain, nausea, or diarrhea. The CMV syndrome may produce

Table 9-2. ACYCLOVIR PROPHYLAXIS VERSUS TREATMENT FOR HERPES ZOSTER

Approach	Dose	Disadvantages	Advantages
Prophylaxis	200–400 mg PO thrice daily	Expensive May promote the development of resistant strains.*	Well tolerated. Effective for the duration of prophylaxis.
Treatment	500 mg/m² or 10 mg/kg IV every 8 hours for at least 7 days and for 2 days beyond the eruption of new lesions	Will usually require hospitalization. The patient may experience infection earlier in the post-transplant period than if prophylaxis had been used, which may result in a more serious infection. May promote the development of resistant strains.*	Effective. Avoids the need for long-term medication.

* It is unclear whether intermittent or continuous use of acyclovir is more likely to promote the development of resistance.

a variety of symptoms including arthritis, fever, hepatitis, leukopenia, and thrombocytopenia. CMV infection is common in autologous marrow recipients, but CMV disease is rare.

CMV disease can be significantly decreased by the early use of ganciclovir in high-risk allogeneic BMT patients. There are two main strategies for selecting high-risk patients for treatment with ganciclovir, (Table 9-3). One approach is to perform surveillance for CMV infection with either bronchoalveolar lavage (BAL) or CMV cultures, and to treat all patients with evidence of infection. This approach misses patients

Table 9-3. PATIENT SELECTION STRATEGIES FOR CMV PROPHYLAXIS

Approach	Advantages	Disadvantages
Treatment of all seropositive patients.	Reduces CMV disease. Includes patients with negative cultures who later develop disease.	Increases neutropenia. Treats patients who would not develop disease. Has not been shown to decrease mortality. Cost of additional drug.
Treatment of patients with CMV positive BAL or surveillance cultures.	Decreases CMV disease. Decreases mortality.	Cost of cultures or BAL. Fails to include patients who develop infection and disease before the next surveillance culture, or who become culture positive simultaneously with the onset of disease.

who develop infection and disease before the next surveillance culture, or who become culture positive simultaneously with the onset of disease. Approximately 12% to 22% of patients will fall into this category. A second approach is to treat all seropositive patients after marrow recovery. This strategy risks treating too many patients, including patients who would not develop CMV disease, and exposes them to the toxicity of ganciclovir. Neutropenia secondary to ganciclovir increases the risk of infection. The first strategy has been shown to reduce mortality, the second strategy has not.

Allogeneic BMT patients at high risk for developing CMV disease should receive early treatment or prophylaxis with ganciclovir (Table 9-4 and Table 9-5). The most effective approach for identifying high risk patients has not yet been determined.

Fungal Prophylaxis

Approximately 10% of BMT patients will acquire a *Candida* infection and 10% will acquire a noncandidal fungal infection. These infections are difficult to detect premortem, and carry a high mortality,

Table 9-4. TWO SCHEDULES OF GANCICLOVIR DOSES FOR CMV SEROPOSITIVE BMT PATIENTS

Time to Start	Dose	Schedule	Duration
a. One week before BMT b. When neutrophils are 1.0×10^{-9}	a. 2.5 mg/kg b. 6 mg/kg/day	a. Every 8 hours IV daily b. Monday through Friday	a. One week b. Until day 120 after BMT
a. When neutrophils are 0.75×10^{-9} or greater for 2 consecutive days b. After completion of course of treatment every 12 hours for 5 days	a. 5 mg/kg b. 5 mg/kg	a. Every 12 hours b. Daily	a. Five days b. Until day 100 after BMT

approaching 90 to 100% for invasive *Aspergillus* infections. As with other predictable infections in BMT patients, it is reasonable to attempt prophylaxis. A regimen that is both effective and nontoxic has yet to be established. There are two general approaches: use of fluconazole and use of low-dose amphotericin (Table 9-6). Prophylaxis with fluconazole decreased nonfungal mortality in one study. However, fluconazole is not active against *Aspergillus*, and some centers have reported an increase in infections with resistant candidal species, such as *Candida krusei*. Low-dose amphotericin has decreased mortality in some studies. Concern about the renal toxicity of amphotericin, especially when used in combination with cyclosporine, may limit its general acceptance.

Pneumocystis Carinii Prophylaxis

Allogeneic BMT recipients should receive prophylaxis against *Pneumocystis carinii* pneumonia (PCP) for 6 to 12 months after transplantation. Patients with chronic graft-versus-host disease (GVHD)

Table 9-5. GANCICLOVIR DOSES AND SCHEDULES FOR CMV POSITIVE BRONCHOALVEOLAR LAVAGE (BAL) or CULTURE POSITIVE PATIENTS

Time to Start	Dose	Schedule	Duration
a. If BAL is CMV positive at day 35 after BMT b. After completion of 2-week course of treatment every 12 hours	a. 5 mg/kg b. 5 mg/kg	a. Every 12 hours b. Daily	a. Two weeks b. Until day 100 after BMT
a. If surveillance culture is CMV positive after engraftment b. After completion of 1 week course of treatment every 12 hours	a. 5 mg/kg b. 5 mg/kg	a. Every 12 hours b. qDaily	a. One week b. Until day 100 after BMT

should continue to receive prophylaxis while they are receiving immunosuppressive agents. Trimethoprim–sulfamethoxazole double strength, given twice daily for 3 days of the week or two consecutive days (e.g., every Saturday and Sunday) is an effective, well-tolerated regimen. Some BMT programs prefer to wait until after engraftment to begin therapy with trimethoprim–sulfamethoxazole, through the concern that it may delay engraftment. Alternatives to trimethoprim–sulfamethoxazole are dapsone 50 mg PO given twice daily on Mondays, Wednesdays, and Fridays, or inhaled pentamidine 300 mg given once a month. PCP prophylaxis is generally not indicated for recipients of autologous marrow grafts.

Intravenous Immune Globulin

The use of IV immune globulin may be beneficial to the allogeneic marrow recipient. It may provide passive humoral immunity

Table 9-6. PROPHYLACTIC ANTIFUNGAL REGIMENS

Drug	Dose	Start	Duration
Fluconazole	400 mg PO or IV daily	First day of conditioning regimen.	Until neutrophils are $>1.0 \times 10^{-9}$ for 7 days, or amphotericin is started.
Amphotericin	0.1–0.25 mg/kg/day IV	First day of conditioning regimen, or day +1.	Until dose is increased in response to suspected fungal infection, or engraftment occurs.

against CMV and bacteria, and it may decrease GVHD. The most effective dose and schedule are not known. A variety of schedules and doses are employed. One regimen infuses a dose of 500 mg/kg weekly for the first 90 days, and then monthly for the first year. An alternative regimen is 500 mg/kg every 2 weeks for the first 90 days.

Graft Versus Host Disease (GVHD)

Prophylaxis

Recipients of non-T-cell-depleted allogeneic marrow grafts receive immunosuppressive therapy as prophylaxis against GVHD. Combination therapy with cyclosporine and methotrexate, cyclosporine and prednisone, or cyclosporine, methotrexate, and prednisone is used.

Cyclosporine

1. **Dose and Schedule:** Cyclosporine is usually started prior to marrow infusion (day −1). Beginning doses are 3 to 7.5 mg/kg/day IV, followed by a variety of dosing schedules. The doses for the first 2 to 4 weeks are usually given IV, either as a 24-hour continuous infusion or as two short, 1 to 4-hour infu-

sions. When the patient can tolerate oral agents, the dose is converted to oral cyclosporine. The total daily oral dose is usually three times the daily IV dose. The daily oral dose is divided into two equal doses given 12 hours apart. The dose should be decreased if the serum creatinine doubles from its baseline value, or is greater than 2 mg/dL (180 μmol/L).

2. **Monitoring Cyclosporine Levels:** It has not been clearly or consistently established how cyclosporine levels correlate with efficacy in preventing GVHD, or with toxicity. Interpretation of cyclosporine levels varies according to whether the level is measured in whole blood or plasma, with the temperature of the sample, and with the type of assay used. A general recommendation is to keep the cyclosporine level between 200 and 400 ng/mL by HPLC. See Table 9-7 for drug interactions that affect cyclosporine levels.

3. **Toxicity:** Therapy with cyclosporine can result in renal dysfunction, hypertension, gingival hyperplasia, neurologic toxicity

Table 9-7. DRUG INTERACTIONS WHICH AFFECT CYCLOSPORINE LEVELS

Drugs Which Increase Levels	Drugs Which Decrease Levels
Clarithromycin	Carbamazepine
Diltiazem	Phenobarbital
Erythromycin	Phenytoin
Fluconazole	Rifampin
Itraconazole	
Ketoconazole	
Nicardipine	
Verapamil	

including seizures and tremors, hirsutism, hypomagnesemia, and hemolytic uremic syndrome.

Tacrolimus

Tacrolimus (FK-506) is being used as an alternative immunosuppressant to cyclosporine. Its mechanism of action is similar. Efficacy in preventing or treating GVDH is at least equivalent to cyclosporine, and may be better. The usual dose is 0.03−0.04 mg/kg (lean body weight) IV continuous infusion over 24 hours. Although the desired level has not yet been established, the dose is usually adjusted to achieve a level in whole blood between 10–30 ng/ml. An upper level of 20 ng/ml is sometimes used. If the patient can tolerate oral drug, the daily dose is four times the IV dose, divided in two doses.

Toxicities seen with tacrolimus include renal dysfunction, hypertension, neurotoxicity, and hyperglycemia.

Methotrexate

1. **Dose and schedule:** The usual dose and schedule of methotrexate is 15 mg/m^2/day given IV on day $+1$, and then 10 mg/m^2 IV given on days 3, 6, and 11. The day 11 dose is not included in all regimens.
2. **Toxicity:** The usual toxicities of methotrexate are mucositis, myelosuppression, and hepatic toxicity. The dose may be reduced or held if the patients has severe mucositis, decreased renal function, or hepatic dysfunction.

   Methotrexate and trimethoprim–sulfamethoxazole should not be given on the same day, in order to avoid increased methotrexate levels.

Methylprednisolone, Prednisone Corticosteroids are sometimes added to methotrexate and cyclosporine for a three-drug prophylactic regimen. They may also form part of a two-drug regimen with cyclosporine or tacrolimus. There may be an increased risk of systemic fungal infections if corticosteroids are used without antifungal prophylaxis during the period of neutropenia at initial hospitalization. The dose and schedule for corticosteroids vary among institutions. IV methylprednisolone is usually started at about day $+7$ and continued until 6-months after BMT. A sample schedule appears in Table 9-8.

Treatment of Acute Graft-Versus-Host Disease (GVHD) Corticosteroids are the drugs of choice for primary therapy of acute GVHD. The usual

Table 9-8. AN EXAMPLE OF A THREE DRUG GVHD PROPHYLACTIC REGIMEN (cyclosporine and methotrexate, or cyclosporine and methylprednisolone may also be used as two drug regimens in the doses and schedules below)

Calendar	Cyclosporine	Methylprednisolone	Methotrexate
Day −2	5.0 mg/kg IV	0	0
Day 1	↓	0	15 mg/m² IV
Day 3	↓	0	10 mg/m² IV
Day 4	3 mg/kg IV	↓	0
Day 6	↓	↓	10 mg/m² IV
Day 7	↓	0.5 mg/kg/day IV (0.25 mg/kg every 12 hours)	
Day 15	3.75 mg/kg/day IV (may convert to oral dosing)	1 mg/kg/day IV (0.5 mg/kg every 12 hours)	
Day 29	↓	Prednisone 0.4 mg/kg PO twice daily	
Day 36	5 mg/kg PO twice daily	↓	
Day 43	↓	Prednisone 0.25 mg/kg PO twice daily	
Day 57	↓	Prednisone 0.1 mg/kg PO twice daily	
Day 84	4 mg/kg PO twice daily	↓	
Day 98	3 mg/kg PO twice daily	↓	
Day 120	2 mg/kg PO twice daily	Prednisone 0.05 mg/kg PO twice daily	
Day 180	0	0	

Table 9-9. AGENTS USED TO TREAT HIGH RISK OR REFRACTORY CHRONIC GVHD

Drug	Dose	Schedule
Cyclosporine	6 mg/kg PO every 12 hours	Every day, or every other day, alternating with prednisone.
Azathioprine	1.5 mg/kg/day, to the nearest 25 mg	With prednisone.
Tacrolimus	0.06–0.15 mg/kg q12 hours	Every day

dose is methylprednisolone 2 mg/kg/day given in divided doses from two to four times daily, followed by a slow taper in dose after 1 to 2 weeks.

Therapy for patients who fail to respond or have an inadequate response to steroids is usually unsuccessful. Antithymocyte globulin (ATG) given IV in doses of 10 to 15 mg/kg/day every other day for 1 to 2 weeks has sometimes been effective. Patients will have an increased infection risk, and prophylactic antibiotic, antiviral, and antifungal agents are appropriate.

Patients with refractory acute GVHD may benefit from investigational approaches.

Chronic Graft-Versus-Host Disease (GVHD) Chronic GVHD is treated with prednisone. A typical dose of prednisone is 1 mg/kg/day PO in divided doses for 1 month. The dose may be gradually shifted to 2 mg/kg every other day, then tapered slowly to 1 mg/kg every other day. Azathioprine has also been used as a single agent, in a dose of 1.5 mg/kg/day. Patients at high risk for GVHD or in whom primary therapy with steroids fails may be treated with a combination of prednisone and cyclosporine or prednisone and azathioprine. (Table 9-9)

Patients with refractory chronic GVHD may benefit from the use of investigational agents.

Selected References

Chao NJ, Schmidt GM, Niland JC, et al. Cyclosporine, methotrexate, and prednisone compared with cyclosporine and prednisone for prophylaxis of acute graft-versus-host disease. N Engl J Med 1993;329:1225–1230.

Ferrara JL, Deeg JH. Graft-versus-host-disease. N Engl J Med 1991;324:667.

Forman SJ, Blume KG, Thomas ED. Bone Marrow Transplantation. Blackwell Scientific Publications, Boston; 1994.

Goodrich JM, Boeckh M, Bowden R. Strategies for the prevention of cytomegalovirus disease after marrow transplantation. Clin Infect Dis 1994;19: 287.

Hughes WT, Armstrong D, Bodey GP, et al. Guidelines for the use of antimicrobial agents in neutropenic patients with unexplained fever. J Infect Dis 1990;161:381.

Momin F, Chandrasekar PH. Antimicrobial prophylaxis in bone marrow transplantation. Ann Intern Med 1995;123:205–215.

Pizzo PA, Meyers J, Freifeld AJ, Walsh, T. Infections in the cancer patient. *In*: DeVita VT, Hellman S, Rosenberg SA (eds.): Cancer: Principles and Practice of Oncology. Lippincott, Philadelphia, 1993.

Rowe JM, Ciobanu N, Ascensao J, et al. Recommended guidelines for the management of autologous and allogeneic bone marrow transplantation. A report from the Eastern cooperative Oncology Group (ECOG). Ann Intern Med 1994;120:143.

CHAPTER X

The Medical Management of Acute Disseminated Intravascular Coagulation (DIC) in Patients with Acute Leukemia

Lloyd E. Damon

GENERAL

There is no treatment algorithm for the acute disseminated intravascular coagulation (DIC) of acute leukemia that can be considered standard. The goal of treatment is to minimize the risk of fatal intracranial hemorrhage. No prospective, randomized trial has been performed that establishes that the treatment of acute DIC has achieved this goal. However, clinical experience indicates that modern treatments have reduced the incidence of fatal intracranial hemorrhage (historically, 20 to 30% of patients undergoing induction chemotherapy during acute DIC). The type of treatment applied for this problem is variable and depends on the oncologist involved. At the very least, transfusion therapy is utilized (platelets, fresh-frozen plasma, and/or cryoprecipitate). Some oncologists will also utilize heparin, antifibrinolytic agents, both, or neither. The following algorithm is utilized at the University of California, San Francisco Adult Leukemia and Bone Marrow Transplantation unit.

PATHOPHYSIOLOGY

DIC is a syndrome, not a disease, and its clinical expression and severity are a spectrum. This spectrum represents a relative balance of pathologic thrombosis and bleeding. In the acute DIC of leukemia, bleeding predominates the clinical picture. In acute leukemia, procoagulant substances released from malignant cells (during active cellular proliferation and/or death) drive pathologic soluble coagulation-factor consumption (via excess thrombin generation and excess plasmin formation), overstimulation of the fibrinolytic system, and platelet activation and consumption. The acute DIC of leukemia can result in severe and life-threatening hemorrhage due to hypofibrinogenemia, proximal coagulation-factor exhaustion, circulating fibrin/fibrinogen degradation products (which exhibit *in vivo* anticoagulant effects), and thrombocytopenia. The relative contribution of each of these factors to a patient's bleeding or bleeding risk is variable and patient-specific. For instance, in some patients, overactivity of fibrinolysis outweighs thrombin generation as the source of fibrinogen consumption. Such patients will benefit more from antifibrinolytic agents than from heparin.

All subtypes of acute myelogenous leukemia (AML) can cause acute DIC. Acute promyelocytic leukemia (M3) is universally associated with DIC. Many oncologists begin prophylactic heparin in patients with the M3 subtype of AML even if there is no laboratory evidence of DIC at diagnosis (DIC uniformly occurs as induction chemotherapy is started). Acute myeloblastic leukemias (subtypes M1 and M2) often cause DIC but run a distant second to M3 in terms of its incidence. DIC can also occur in acute lymphoblastic leukemia (ALL). The DIC of ALL is notable for a relative sparing of platelet consumption compared to AML.

DIAGNOSIS OF ACUTE DIC

Test	Result	Etiology	Comment
Prothrombin time (PT)	Prolonged	Fibrinogen/Fibrin degradation products (FDP)	Severe prolongation due to factor VII consumption
Activated partial thrombo-plastin (aPTT)	Normal	APTT insensitive to FDP	As proximal factors are consumed, PTT begins to prolong

continued

Test	Result	Etiology	Comment
Thrombin time (TT)	Prolonged	FDP Hypofibri- nogenemia	
Fibrinogen	Low (or falling)	Thrombin formation (via extrinsic and intrinsic coagulation pathways) Plasmin formation	
Plasmin Activity	Increased	Direct activation by leukemic substances Physiologic response to fibrin formation Endothelial release of tissue- and urokinase-plaminogen activators (t-PA, u-PA)	
Platelets	Low (or falling)	Activation due to thrombin formation Decreased bone marrow production	
Red Blood Cell morphology	Schistocytes	Fibrin formation in microcirculation	Number of schistocytes does not correlate with the clinical severity of DIC.
α_2-plasmin Inhibitor (α_2-PI)	Normal or Decreased	Response to pathologic fibrinolysis	Low α_2-PI implies excess fibrinolysis; antifibrinolytic therapy indicated

continued

Test	Result	Etiology	Comment
Fibrinogen D-Dimers	Increased	Fibrin formation and crosslinking followed by fibrinolysis	
FDP	Increased	Excess plasmin formation	

TREATMENT

Some acute DIC of acute leukemia is mild enough that specific treatment is not warranted. There are no firm guidelines for this decision, and it must be individualized on a case-by-case basis. The following are treatment recommendations for average-sized adults.

Transfusion Therapy

1. Platelet Transfusions
   a. Six random units or a single apheresis collection.
   b. Keep platelet count >30,000/μL.
   c. Check platelet count every 8 to 12 hours.
2. Cryoprecipitate
   a. Keep fibrinogen >100 mg/dL.
   b. Ten units given per transfusion.
   c. Check fibrinogen every 8 to 12 hours.
3. Fresh frozen plasma
   a. Give 4 to 6 units (10 to 12 ml/kg) per transfusion. Administered when aPTT is prolonged and not felt to be due to excess heparin (see below) or antithrombin III is found to be very low.

Heparin Therapy

1. Begin heparin if the fibrinogen is low (<175 mg/dL) or falling, or if the patient has M3 and a normal fibrinogen level.
2. Goals of heparin is to keep fibrinogen stable or rising and the aPTT normal.
3. Dosing
   a. 1,500-unit IV bolus.
   b. 500 units/hour drip initially; titrate dose to achieve above goals.
   c. May need up to 1,200 to 1,500 units/hour in severe DIC.

Anti-fibrinolytic Therapy

1. Begin antifibrinolytic therapy if fibrinogen consumption cannot be controlled by aggressive heparin/cryoprecipitate administration or clinical bleeding is ongoing despite optimal transfusion/heparin therapy.
2. Dosing
   a. Aminocaproic acid 4 G IV bolus, then 1 G/hr IV drip.
   b. Tranexamic acid 10 mg/kg IV every 8 hours (alternative to aminocaproic acid).
   Recommend use of antifibrinolytic agents always in conjunction with heparin to minimize the risk of pathologic thrombosis.

All-*Trans* Retinoic Acid

1. All-*trans* retinoic acid (ATRA) has been shown to induce complete remissions in patients with acute promyelocytic leukemia (M3) without bone marrow aplasia and with little or no acute DIC. It interacts with the retinoic acid receptor-alpha (RARα) to cause terminal differentiation of leukemic promyeloblasts. RARα is the product of a mutated gene created by the classic acute promyelocytic leukemia chromosomal rearrangement (t(15,17)).
2. Dosing
   45 mg/m²/day orally (in morning with fatty meal)
3. Side effects
   a. Cutaneous: dry skin, cheilitis, photosensitivity, rash.
   b. Ocular: dry eyes, night blindness.
   c. Musculoskeletal: myalgias, arthralgias, weakness.
   d. Neurologic: headache, pseudotumor cerebri.
   e. Hepatic: elevated liver blood tests.
   f. Lipid: hypertriglyceridemia, hypercholesterolemia, pancreatitis.
   g. Fetal: craniofacial malformations, CNS abnormalities, thymic aplasia, cardiac abnormalities.
   h. All-*trans* retinoic acid syndrome: leukocytosis, dyspnea, hypoxemia, fever, hypotension, extremity edema (potentially fatal; if present, stop ATRA and treat with corticosteroids).

References
1. Tallman MS, Kwaan HC. Reassessing the hemostatic disorder associated with acute promyelocytic leukemia. Blood 1992;79: 543–552.

2. Rodeghiero F, Avvisati G, Castaman G, et al. Early deaths and anti-hemorrhagic treatments in acute promyelocytic leukemia. A GIMEMA retrospective study in 268 consecutive patients. Blood 1990;75:2112–2117.
3. Bick RL, Baker WF Jr. Disseminated intravascular coagulation syndromes. Hematol Pathol 1992;6: 1–24.
4. Warrell RP Jr., de The H, Wang Z-Y, Degos L. Acute promyelocytic leukemia. N Engl J Med 1993;329: 177–189.

Subject Index

445